SYSTEMS BIOLOGY AND ITS APPLICATION IN TCM FORMULAS RESEARCH

T0311952

SYSTEMS BIOLOGY AND ITS APPLICATION IN TCM FORMULAS RESEARCH

Edited by

WEI-DONG ZHANG

Second Military Medical University, Shanghai, PR China

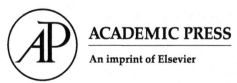

ACADEMIC PRESS

An imprint of Elsevier

Academic Press is an imprint of Elsevier
125 London Wall, London EC2Y 5AS, United Kingdom
525 B Street, Suite 1800, San Diego, CA 92101-4495, United States
50 Hampshire Street, 5th Floor, Cambridge, MA 02139, United States
The Boulevard, Langford Lane, Kidlington, Oxford OX5 1GB, United Kingdom

Notices
Knowledge and best practice in this field are constantly changing. As new research and experience
broaden our understanding, changes in research methods, professional practices, or medical treatment
may become necessary.

Practitioners and researchers must always rely on their own experience and knowledge in evaluating
and using any information, methods, compounds, or experiments described herein. In using such
information or methods they should be mindful of their own safety and the safety of others, including
parties for whom they have a professional responsibility.

To the fullest extent of the law, neither the Publisher nor the authors, contributors, or editors, assume
any liability for any injury and/or damage to persons or property as a matter of products liability,
negligence or otherwise, or from any use or operation of any methods, products, instructions, or ideas
contained in the material herein.

Library of Congress Cataloging-in-Publication Data
A catalog record for this book is available from the Library of Congress

British Library Cataloguing-in-Publication Data
A catalogue record for this book is available from the British Library

ISBN: 978-0-12-812744-5

For information on all Academic Press publications
visit our website at https://www.elsevier.com/books-and-journals

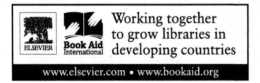

Working together
to grow libraries in
developing countries

www.elsevier.com • www.bookaid.org

Publisher: Mica Haley
Acquisition Editor: Rafael Teixeira
Editorial Project Manager: Tracy I. Tufaga
Production Project Manager: Poulouse Joseph
Cover Designer: Christian J. Bilbow

Typeset by SPi Global, India

CONTENTS

CONTRIBUTORS

Peng Jiang
Shanghai Hutchison Pharmaceutical Limited Company, Shanghai, PR China

Runui Liu
Second Military Medical University, Shanghai, PR China

Chao Lv
Second Military Medical University, Shanghai, PR China

Dale G. Nagle
University of Mississippi, University, MS, United States

Shikai Yan
Shanghai Jiao Tong University, Shanghai, PR China

Changsen Zhan
Shanghai Hutchison Pharmaceutical Limited Company, Shanghai, PR China

Weidong Zhang
Second Military Medical University, Shanghai, PR China

Jing Zhao
Shanghai University of Traditional Chinese Medicine, Shanghai, PR China

Junjie Zhou
Shanghai Hutchison Pharmaceutical Limited Company, Shanghai, PR China

YuDong Zhou
University of Mississippi, University, MS, United States

Xianpeng Zu
Second Military Medical University, Shanghai, PR China

Introduction

In the clinical practice of Traditional Chinese Medicine (TCM), formulae refers to a major type of medication with features and advantages typical of traditional medicine in China. Using high technology to clarify the science underlying formulae is critical for the modernization of TCM. In the first section of this book, we introduce strategies and technologies established by our research group during the long-term study of TCM formulae. The first chapter describes the establishment of the modern research system for investigating formulae, and it provides the readers with an overview of this field; the second chapter summarizes the theories, strategies, and methods for studying the material, therapeutic basis for formulae, and progress in this field. From the third to sixth chapters, we present various new technologies for the study of formulae. In the second section of the book, we focus on the Shexiang Baoxin Pill (SBP), a well-known formula with significant therapeutic effect in clinical use, and we use it as an example to highlight the latest formulae-based achievements under the established, modern systems of TCM.

This is a reference book for researchers, postgraduates, and undergraduates who are involved in research and development, pharmaceutical production, and quality control of TCM. It is also suitable for interested readers in medical schools, institutes, and pharmaceutical companies.

Ideas and Methods for the Modern Research of TCM Formulas

CHAPTER 1

Strategy for Modern Research of Traditional Chinese Medicine Formulae

Shikai Yan*, Jing Zhao†, Dale G. Nagle‡, YuDong Zhou‡, Weidong Zhang§
*Shanghai Jiao Tong University, Shanghai, PR China
†Shanghai University of Traditional Chinese Medicine, Shanghai, PR China
‡University of Mississippi, University, MS, United States
§Second Military Medical University, Shanghai, PR China

Abstract

One of the key tasks in the strategy to modernize traditional Chinese medicine (TCM) is efficient methodology development. Based on systems biology and network biology, we proposed a methodology for the study of TCM compound prescriptions that combines the theory of TCM with modern biological techniques. The methodology involves both theories of reductionism and holism at both the macroscopic and microscopic levels, for in vivo and in vitro analyses. The proposed methodology is composed of four research platforms: chemical, pharmacology, systems biology and network biology. The proposed methodology provides a powerful tool to modernize the study of TCM compound prescriptions, which may be important to fully reveal the essential principals of TCM, and to promote new drug discovery based on TCM formulae as well as the dissemination and further development of TCM theory.

Keywords: Traditional Chinese medicine compound prescription, Modernization of TCM, Systems biology, Network biology, Holism, Reductionism, TCM formulas.

Historically, traditional Chinese medicine (TCM) formulae are major prescription forms for the clinical application of TCM, which represent the characteristics and advantages of TCM. Their complicated chemical composition, profound compatibility rules, and functional diversity have long hindered the progress of TCM research. As a result, it is very difficult to describe the essential features of TCM using modern scientific language. This gap in TCM's scientific translation tends to hinder its worldwide acceptance and widespread application. Thus, it is urgently important to establish a modern strategy for TCM formulae research.

Based on TCM theory and modern chemical, biological, and informatics technologies, we propose an innovative research system for TCM formulae that combines holistic principles and reductionist methods with macro- and microsystem studies, in vivo and in vitro research. This TCM formulae research system includes basic chemical substance research, modern pharmacology, and systems and network biology. It uses modern technologies to provide systematic research ideas to explore traditional theory and examine TCM formulae. Thus, it facilitates the application of TCM formulae for new drug R&D while concurrently revealing the scientific foundation of TCM to enhance and develop its precious legacy.

1.1. CURRENT RESEARCH ON TCM FORMULAE

For some time, TCM research has relied on many of the same approaches applied to western medicine such as active ingredient(s) screening and constituent isolation, which enables the discovery of bioactive components and, to some extent, the TCM mechanism of action studies. However, due to multicomponent and multitarget characteristics of TCM formulae, it is often difficult to interpret the scientific implications of TCM. Therefore, there is an urgent need to develop a modern research system appropriate for TCM research.

In this century, a policy of TCM modernization has been gradually carried out in China, and TCM formulae research has seen remarkable development. A series of ideas has been put forward for TCM research such as the "1-2-3-4" strategy established by Professor Guoan Luo,[1] pharmaceutical chemistry recommended by Professor Xijun Wang,[2] and multicomponent combinatorial TCM proposed by Professor Boli Zhang.[3] The "1-2-3-4" strategy means one combination (combination of chemistry and pharmacology), two clarifying general levels (to clarify the material basis and its efficacy), three stages (stages of Chinese materia medica, effective section, and active components), and four levels (animal, tissues, cells, and subcellular, molecular). Pharmaceutical chemistry focuses on the exogenous substances and TCM-active chemicals absorbed into the bloodstream. Multicomponent combinatorial TCM suggests developing new modern drugs by recombination of multiple effective TCM components.

During the late 20th century and early 21st century, biological research has experienced many innovations at both the micro- to macrolevels, and a more comprehensive description of life phenomena related to various functional molecules has become a reality.[4,5] By bioinformatics and computer modeling approaches,[6] omics technologies are expected to provide more insights and clues to the mechanisms of biological processes and functions. Therefore, this may build up a theoretical framework for modern life science, including that for TCM research.[7,8] As an example, Professors Zhu Chen and Saijuan Chen revealed the synergistic action mechanism of the *Realgar-Indigo naturalis formula (RIF)* for the treatment of acute promyelocytic leukemia using a systems biology approach.[9] In addition, Professor Guoan Luo further expanded the concept of "system" that the action of TCM on a patient composed of a systematic interaction process between two complicated systems, and thus put forward a new concept of "chemomics" for TCM research.[10]

There is already consensus regarding the application of an integrative or holistic method to TCM study, as systems biology, bioinformatics, and network biology[11] have gradually become key technologies of TCM research. However, available systems biology and bioinformatics approaches are often confined to the global description of a biological system, often ignoring the specific characterizations of the detailed dynamic biological processes. Therefore, we should not only study the global effects of TCM but must also endeavor to reveal TCM mechanisms at the more detailed molecular and network levels as well as to explore reasonable solutions to the problem of modernizing TCM.

1.2. PRINCIPLES FOR THE STUDY OF TCM FORMULAE

Most TCM formulae can be considered as a combination of natural chemical constituents derived from diverse medicinal materials in accordance with compatibility principles, which generally agree with the characteristics of multicomponent, multipathway, multitarget, and global synergistic action. Due to the complexity of their composition and pharmacological mechanisms, TCM formulae require a set of unique and effective research methods. Such a system should follow certain principles, for example, the combination of holism and reductionism, the combination of micro- and macro-based research, and the combination of in vivo and in vitro studies.

1.2.1 Holism and Reductionism

Reductionism accesses a bottom-up research mode that dissects and disassembles the whole research object into detailed parts to study, envisioning the whole as the sum of each part. In contrast, holism is a top-down study mode that does not simply consider the whole system as the sum of each part. From the perspective of a logical view, reductionism emphasizes analysis and deduction, focusing on the understanding of the local parts at a micro level. The holistic approach is composed of synthesis and induction, focusing on the macro level and an overall understanding.[12]

In the field of medicine and life science, reductionism has played a great role in the formation of classical physiology, pathology, and anatomy. It has also greatly promoted the development of biochemistry, cell biology, and molecular biology. However, along with the expansion of medical research, reductionism gradually shows its limitations. The reductionist approach often disassembles a system into subtle parts. As a result, it may lead to unexpected deviations in interpretation. People have come to recognize that using only the reductionist method is not enough to accurately characterize the complexities of life science. Accordingly, along with the rapid development of systems biology and bioinformatics in the 1990s, holistic approaches have gradually become popular and are at the forefront of technological methods in life science. Holistic methods also have certain limitations, sometimes revealing the overall nature of biological phenomena, but they may lack detailed information in regard to key mechanistic elements. Therefore, application of either a holistic or reductionist approach alone is not above reproach. It is necessary to use a combination of both to fully understand the essence of an object, especially if the object is as complex and functionally integrated as TCM.

Early TCM studies were largely based on a philosophy of holism, focusing on a global curative effect being observed. Along with the widespread application of western science and modern technology at the beginning of the 20th century, the philosophy of reductionism was gradually accepted and bioactive compound isolation and discovery from TCM became the mainstream research model at that time. This reductionist-based research approach played an important role for TCM development and application. One of the most prominent examples was the discovery of artemisinin. However, researchers have come to recognize the limitation of reductionism. For example, about 300 compounds can be easily isolated from a single plant preparation; a TCM formula consisting of four or five medical herbs can include anywhere from 1000 to 2000 chemical compounds. However, although the chemical structures and pharmacological activities for a particular compound may have become increasingly clear, we still cannot fully understand many of the mechanisms involved in the overall effects of TCM formulae. Since the beginning of the 21st century, systems biology and bioinformatics have been widely applied in the study of TCM and have made remarkable progress at resolving some of its complexities. Alternatively, we can now sometimes understand the overall pharmacological characteristics of TCM formulae, but we still often cannot completely resolve the origin and nature of their effects, especially the synergistic mechanisms among active ingredients in more complex medicinal products.

Therefore, in order to fully understand TCM formulae, we should combine the philosophies of holism and reductionism. Modern separation and analysis technologies should be applied to discover active ingredients from TCM. On the other hand, we should use holistic-based systems biology and bioinformatics for the characterization of the effects of TCM formulae and the discovery of effective components from top-down models.

1.2.2 Macro- and Microstudies

It is a crucially important task for the modernization of TCM to explore the action mechanism(s) of TCM formulae. In spite of thousands of years of TCM application, modern pharmacological TCM research has a history of less than 100 years, beginning with the study of Ephedra in the 1920s by Professor Kehui Chen.[13] Since that time, modern TCM research has gradually matured.

To a large extent, previous pharmacological TCM studies used western medicine-based approaches, including research at various whole animal, tissue, subcellular, and molecular biological levels. These studies mostly describe the overall characterization of TCM formulae, but often lack more detailed biological function information at the gene, protein, and small-molecule metabolite levels.

Most TCM formulae are a combination of many compounds with different structures and functions. The action of TCM formulae on patients is actually the process of multiple active components comprehensively modulating biomolecular networks, including adjusting complex gene, protein, and metabolite systems. Using only a macrolevel approach to TCM research is not sufficient; it is necessary to investigate the interactions between active TCM components and their molecular targets. Because of the limitations of methods and techniques, it is especially challenging to study TCM formulae at the molecular level. The rapid development of systems biology and network analysis makes it possible to construct models of TCM formulae-based molecular interaction networks. Systems biology describes the pathological and physiological states of an organism through the integration of genomics, proteomics, metabolomics, and other multiple parameter information, and then constructs disease-related networks and drug-intervening networks. Further comparative analysis on disease-related networks and drug-intervening networks before and after TCM administration will help us understand the pharmacological mechanisms of TCM formula and identify the key active components thereof.[14]

Therefore, the use of only a macrolevel approach to TCM formulae research is not enough; modern technologies available to study systems biology and network biology at the micro level are also required. The combination of macro and micro research allows the understanding of inherent characteristics and the molecular network-based mechanisms of TCM formulae so as to realize the modernization and international acceptance of TCM.

1.2.3 In Vitro and in vivo Studies

Pharmacological TCM studies have primarily relied on in vitro assays for the discovery of bioactive constituents and for their pharmacological evaluation due to the suitability of in vitro methods for high-throughput screening and for their relative efficacy and simplicity. Insufficient attention has often been paid to the need for in vivo studies, which are, however, also necessary because the majority of drugs must first be absorbed into the bloodstream before exerting their pharmacological actions (except for those that directly act on the gastrointestinal tract and intestinal flora). Professor Xijun Wang put forward the concept of "TCM serum pharmaceutical chemistry," which suggests that TCM research should not only focus on the ingredients of the TCM itself but must also consider the availability of TCM components in the serum of model animals following TCM administration. The premise behind this concept is that the actual composition of ingredients absorbed into the bloodstream is most likely to play a significant role in TCM efficacy, and our research should focus on those physiologically available components.

In recent years, the concept of "TCM serum pharmacology" has also been rapidly developing, suggesting that we should consider the drug-containing serum as a new "preparation" for pharmacological TCM research. The serum pharmacology approach combines in vivo and in vitro assays, a suitable concept for the study of TCM formulae. This is especially true because of the extreme complexity of TCM constituents and multiple interference factors; in vitro pharmacological experiments often produce only false-negative or false-positive results and unreliable scientific conclusions. Serum pharmacology methods more closely model actual processes involved in drugs acting on organisms in vivo, and overcome some of the limitations of simple in vitro cell assays.

Both in vivo and in vitro assays should be applied in TCM formulae research. in vitro studies take advantage of convenient, fast, high-throughput screening, while in vivo analysis better models drug-induced biological processes and more accurately represents pharmacological TCM activities. The combination of both study types should be considered for a more accurate interpretation of the biochemical and biomedical implications of TCM formulae.

1.3. MODERN TCM FORMULAE RESEARCH

In accordance with the inherent characteristics of TCM formulae and the principals of combining holism and reductionism, macro and micro research, macro and micro analysis, and in vitro and in vivo assays, we put forward a proposed strategy to develop a modern system of TCM formulae research (Fig. 1.1). This system includes four research fields: therapeutic material basis, modern pharmacology, systems biology, and network biology.

1.3.1 Research on Therapeutic Materials Basis

The study of therapeutic materials basis is the premise and foundation of TCM research. Thus, it plays an important role in the modern research system of TCM formulae. There are two approaches for the research of therapeutic materials basis. The first, with the aim of lead compound discovery, is to isolate constituents from TCM formulae or its individual medicinal components and to find single active ingredients, mainly using various modern technologies of bioassay-guided chromatographic separation and spectroscopy-based structure identification. The other approach, with the guidance of TCM theory, is to perform active ingredient mixed constituent screening and multicomponent combinatorial optimization.

As a typical research method derived from western medicine, the first approach primarily focuses on the purification and activity testing for single active ingredients and then generalizes to the therapeutic material basis of TCM formulae. This bottom-up idea completely ignores the potential correlation and interactions of a large number of TCM constituents, and cannot accurately reflect the inherent combinatorial characteristics of TCM. The second research method focuses on the whole TCM formulae under the guidance of TCM theory, follows the principals of whole to part with a top-down approach, and progressively determines the active ingredients of TCM. Its most common study strategy is as follows: medicinal materials of TCM formulae—chemomics (constituents of whole TCM formulae)—chemical composition in vitro (serum pharmaceutical

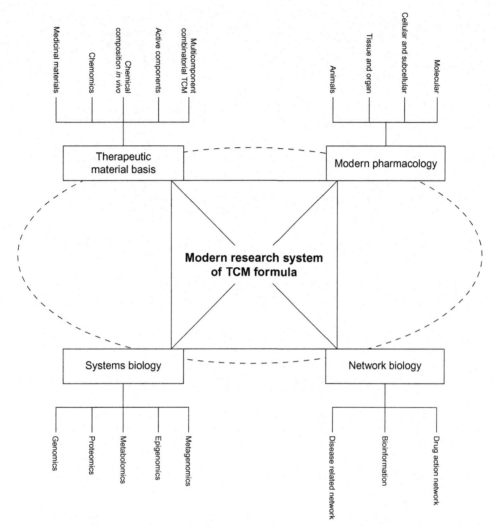

Fig. 1.1 Strategy outline of a modern research system for TCM formulae research.

chemistry)—active components—multicomponent interactions. This research strategy has become accepted by an ever-growing number of scientists.

The proposed strategy of therapeutic material basis research combines both ideas of top-down and bottom-up, as shown in Fig. 1.2. On one hand, chemical separation and screening is performed top-down on TCM formulae and medicinal materials under the guidance of TCM theory, then serum pharmacochemistry studies determine active components in vitro. On the other hand, based on a comprehensive understanding of structural and pharmacological studies on active ingredients, multicomponents interaction and compatibility are studied to develop new drugs of multicomponent combinatorial TCM in a bottom-up fashion.

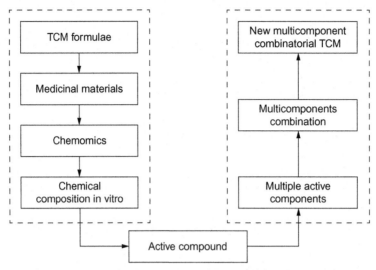

Fig. 1.2 Strategy of therapeutic material basis research that combines both top-down and bottom-up approaches.

The combined idea, following the roadmap of TCM formulae—medicinal materials—chemomics—chemical composition in vitro—active compound—multiple active components—multiple components combination—new multicomponent combinatorial TCM—is a promising new tool for TCM formulae research and drug development.

1.3.2 Modern Pharmacology

Pharmacological TCM formulae research should be guided by TCM theory and carried out at both the macro and micro scales with a combination of top-down and bottom-up strategies.

1.3.2.1 Top-Down: Holistic Pharmacology and Active Components Screening

Under the guidance of TCM theory, the holistic pharmacological properties of TCM formulae and medicinal materials are studied first. Then we investigate the pharmacological activities of specific components, which is the most common strategy used to screen bioactive TCM components. In this top-down approach, the main focus is macrolevel research, including pharmacological studies on whole animals, tissues, organs, and at the cellular, subcellular, and molecular levels.

1.3.2.2 Bottom-Up: Pharmacological Evaluation of Key Active Components and Multicomponent Compatibility

The discovery of bioactive components permits further pharmacological investigation on key active components and multicomponent compatibility. The study should be performed with a bottom-up approach, using microlevel pharmacological methods such as systems biology, bioinformatics, structural biology, and molecular network technology. The evaluation of multicomponent synergy and compatibility is expected to develop new multicomponent combinatorial TCM.

1.3.3 Systems Biology

The concept of systems biology was first proposed nearly 20 years ago by Professor Leory Hood.[4,5] Systems biology involves the computational and mathematical modeling of complex biological systems. It is a biology-based interdisciplinary study that focuses on complex interactions within biological systems and on how these interactions give rise to the function and behavior of that system (e.g., the enzymes and metabolites in a metabolic pathway or a heart rhythm), using a holistic approach (rather than traditional reductionism) to biological research. Systems biology includes a series of "omics" techniques, such as genomics, transcriptomics, proteomics, and metabolomics.

Systems biology is characterized by integral and systematic concepts, and is consistent with the nature of TCM theory. Therefore, soon after its emergence, systems biology rapidly gained the attention of TCM researchers. At present, systems biology is widely applied in many aspects of TCM research, and its application shows excellent prospects for resolving many of the complex interactions that are characteristic of TCM.

1.3.3.1 Genomics

Genomics is the study of genes, their functions, and related techniques, such as applications of recombinant DNA, DNA sequencing methods, and bioinformatics to sequence, assemble, and analyze the function and structure of genomes. Advances in genomics have triggered a revolution in discovery-based research to understand even the most complex biological systems.

According to its theory, TCM does not emphasize a selective direct fight against pathogenic factors, but rather enhances the body's resistance to disease and adjusts the body's functional status. Generally, drugs work directly or indirectly by modifying the expression or functions of specific molecular targets or genes while the treatment effects of TCM are more likely to play an important role in regulating or modifying the expression of disease-related genes and gene products. Genomics can be used for identifying TCM targets by monitoring genomic responses to TCM treatment. Thus, it is possible to explore the mechanism of TCM formulae at the gene expression level, further clarifying the scientific basis of TCM.[15]

Genomics can be used for the high-throughput screening of active components in TCM formulae. In specific pathological models, the screening of active TCM components can be realized by comparative analysis of the differentially expressed genes in tissues or organs before and after TCM administration. In the pharmacological evaluation of TCM formulae, chemical genomics-based studies on the yeast *Saccharomyces cerevisiae* can produce important results, which can be systematically interpreted to the more integrative and systemic effects of active TCM ingredients on basic cell physiology. Genomics-based models can be constructed by comprehensive analysis of data and other results from existing pharmacology, TCM constituent studies, and established yeast cell genomics. It is expected to grow as an important tool for the discovery of bioactive TCM components and for the understanding of TCM mechanisms.

1.3.3.2 Proteomics

Proteomics is the large-scale study of protein expression. Proteins are vital parts of living organisms with many functions. The proteome is the entire set of proteins, produced or modified by an organism or system.[16] Administration of TCM formulae in the human body will inevitably lead to structural and functional changes at every level, from individual molecules to that of the whole organism, and produce specific changes in the proteome. Proteomics can be used for TCM target discovery and for the description of the pharmacological process.

In addition, proteomics can be used to investigate the potential synergistic compatibility of TCM formulae by comparatively studying proteomic changes within model systems with single component and multiple-component combination intervention strategies. It is helpful to understand multitarget and multipathway action mechanisms and to further reveal the scientific basis of TCM formulae.

1.3.3.3 Metabolomics

Specifically, metabolomics is the systematic study of the unique chemical fingerprints that specific cellular processes leave behind and the study of their small-molecule metabolite profiles.[17] The metabolome represents the collection of all metabolites in a cell, tissue, organ, or organism, which are the biochemical products of cellular processes. Each type of cell and tissue has a unique metabolome that can be used to elucidate organ or tissue-specific information while the study of biofluids can give more generalized though less specialized information. Commonly examined biofluids include urine and plasma, as they can be obtained by relatively noninvasive means.

Metabolomics can be used for the efficacious evaluation of TCM. According to metabolimic principles, in the "pathological" state the metabolome would inevitably show abnormal changes while a successful drug intervention can correct the metabolic profile back to a "normal" state. Metabolomics is often based on the overall analysis of urine, blood, saliva, and cell or tissue extracts of a series of samples, and pattern recognition is used to highlight variations in metabolomic changes before and subsequent to TCM treatment. Therefore, metabolomics can be employed to objectively evaluate the therapeutic effects of TCM as well as explore its mechanism by reverse backtracking related metabolic pathways or metabolic networks and their dynamic changes. In addition, metabolomics can also be used to evaluate the safety and toxicology profiles of TCM formulae.

1.3.3.4 Epigenomics

Epigenetic modifications play an important role in gene expression and regulation, and are involved in numerous cellular processes such as differentiation, development, and tumorigenesis. Epigenomics is the study of the complete set of epigenetic modifications on the genetic material of a cell. Epigenetic modifications are reversible modifications on a cell's DNA or histones that affect gene expression without altering the DNA sequence. Epigenomic maintenance is a continuous process that plays an important role in the stability of eukaryotic genomes by taking part in crucial biological mechanisms such as DNA repair. Two of the most characterized epigenetic modifications are DNA methylation and histone modification.

The destruction of epigenetic equilibrium is understood as an important index to study the mechanistic pathogenic basis of various diseases, and may play a crucial role in disease prevention and treatment. This is especially true in the study of stem cell differentiation and development, and in the study of hypertension, coronary heart disease, type II diabetes, osteoporosis, tumors, autoimmune disease, and metabolic diseases.[18]

Since 2003, the human epigenome project (HEP)[19] and the alliance of human epigenome in development and disease (AHEAD)[20] have been implemented to study DNA methylation patterns in human tissues, primarily focusing on stem, breast cancer, CD34 + hematopoietic stem, liver, and liver parenchyma cells.

1.3.3.5 Metagenomics

The human gastrointestinal tract has the extremely complex and huge microbial colonies with 10^{13}–10^{14} microbes residing in the human colon,[21] almost 10 times the number of cells in the human body itself; this large bacterial community is generally regarded as "super human organs".[22,23] Therefore, Joshua Lederberg proposed the concept of the human body as a super organism that is composed of both eukaryotic cells and symbiotic microbial communities.[24]

Metagenomics is the study of genetic material recovered directly from environmental samples. While traditional microbiology and microbial genome sequencing and genomics rely upon cultivated clonal cultures, early environmental gene sequencing cloned specific genes (often the 16S rRNA gene) that can be used to produce a profile of diversity in a natural sample. Because of its ability to reveal the previously hidden diversity of microscopic life, metagenomics offers a powerful lens for viewing the microbial world that has the potential to revolutionize our understanding of the entire living world. As the price of DNA sequencing continues to fall, metagenomics currently allows microbial ecology to be investigated at a much greater scale and with increasing detail than ever before. The NIH officially launched the Human Microbiome Project (HMP)[25] in 2007, and in 2010 the EU funded another human gut metagenome plan to study human gut microbial communities and to understand the relationships between human health and the distribution of bacterial species in the gut.[26]

Metagenomics is critically important for TCM formulae research. The vast majority of TCM is administrated orally, and the active ingredients interact with intestinal microflora to produce complex interactions within the gastrointestinal tract. To some extent, the intestinal flora can be regarded as a novel target of TCM.

1.4. NETWORK BIOLOGY AND TCM NETWORK PHARMACOLOGY

Large numbers of complex real world systems can be described by networks. Individuals within systems and their interactions are represented by vertices and edges in networks, respectively. In 2004, Barabasi and coworkers proposed the concept of "network biology".[27] They built network models to express interactions within complex cellular biological systems and tried to get better understanding of these systems through topologies and features of networks. Network biology studies various molecular networks at different biological levels. It is known that in cells, genes and their products typically interact or communicate with each other so as to perform particular cellular tasks. Such interactions can be expressed with molecular networks with different meanings at distinct levels. Specifically, at the genomic level, gene regulatory networks are collections of interactions between transcription factors and their target genes in the processes of regulating mRNA and protein gene expression levels.[28,29] At the proteomic level, protein–protein interaction (PPI) networks represent the physical interactions between proteins.[30] At the metabolomic level, the relationships between metabolites and catalytic enzymes can be represented by metabolic networks.[31]

Over the last decade, important progress has been made in network biology research. For example, it has been revealed that many molecular networks are scale-free,[32] small-world networks[33] that exhibit hierarchical organization features.[34] Meanwhile, these features are closely related to the functions and evolution of corresponding biological systems.

In cells, different levels of biological processes are closely related to the occurrence and development of diseases. On one hand, multiple genes associated with the same disease often interact with each other and form a complex disease network[35]; on the other hand, the interactions between genes of different diseases usually lead to comorbidity.[36] Drugs play their therapeutic effects by binding to drug target proteins. Considering the existence of disease-associated protein network interactions, multiple protein regulation may be expected to produce better disease-associated therapeutic effects. Therefore, in recent years, network modeling for complex diseases and drug discovery has become a hot topic.[37–39] Important scientific problems that attract the attention of the global medical and scientific community include how to correctly understand the molecular mechanisms and network regulation mechanisms of complex diseases, how to correctly identify the key nodes in disease network regulation systems, and how to effectively intervene within specific pathogenic disease network structures.

TCM has unique efficacy in the treatment of complex chronic diseases. However, due to its complex composition and unclear theory, it is still a difficult task to fully clarify TCM action mechanisms in the context of modern biological science and biomedical technologies. Typical TCM formulae usually consist of combinations of several plant or animal products, each of which contains a variety of chemical compounds. The low molecular weight biochemicals from natural product components exhibit a high degree of structural diversity.[40,41] Specific chemical compounds achieve their effect of inhibiting the disease by targeting and regulating distinct proteins while also exerting potential side effects and toxicity.[42] Through the analysis of the chemical compounds found in TCM formulae, many of these products have been found to functionally overlap with established western medicines. From the molecular point of view, multicomponent and multitargeted TCM formulae, like multicomponent western medicine, act by multi-dimensional mechanisms. It can be deduced that the therapeutic effect of TCM formulae is the cumulative sum of the effects generated by each multicomponent molecular combination on the complex biological molecular networks within the human organism. Therefore, an emerging trend is to apply the ideas and methods of network biology to TCM pharmacology to decipher the action modes of TCM formulae in the context of molecular networks. Thus, "TCM network pharmacology" has appeared as a new field of research.

One of the key problems of TCM network pharmacology is to evaluate potential synergistic effects of multiple TCM targets on disease-associated networks. According to the complex component features of TCM, their unclear targets, and their potential to treat diseases by regulating complex disease-associated networks, we proposed a workflow for network-based TCM pharmacology.[37] This workflow includes four steps: (1) to identify biologically active TCM compounds; (2) to identify the biochemical and physiological targets of active TCM compounds; (3) to identify disease-associated genes and construct disease-specific networks; and (4) to identify signaling pathways and networks regulated by TCM formula and to evaluate the effects of TCM formula on complex disease-associated networks. These four steps are further illustrated in Chapter 4.

The spectrum of human diseases has changed considerably over the past century. Because TCM is believed to function through comprehensive regulatory phenomena that result from its multiple-component, multiple-target, and multiple-dimensional effects, it has certain advantages over single-target western medicine in the treatment of complex chronic diseases. Additionally, the important outcome of multiple drug anti-HIV "cocktail" therapy has further stimulated considerable interest in developing multicomponent, multitargeted medicines. The global medical and scientific communities have begun to pay increasing attention to TCM formulae. With this consideration, there is great benefit to intensifying the study and development of TCM formulae. However, the pharmacodynamic material basis of TCM formulae and its sophisticated modes of pharmacological action make their characterization a rather complex task. The lack of accepted systematic and scientific methodologies to guide their evaluation hinders the study of TCM formulae and produces a bottleneck in the TCM modernization process.

With the recent development of systems biology, systems-based methods and top-down study approaches have been widely applied in TCM research. However, it is worth noting that we cannot just emphasize the global system alone nor can we merely focus on its individual parts. In fact, both purely holistic (top-down) approaches and reductionist (down-top) approaches are singularly one-sided methodologies. Only through their efficient combination can it be possible to uncover the underlying regulatory mechanisms responsible for the physiological effects of TCM formulae. The research system we propose applies modern chemistry, biology, and information technology in the study of TCM pharmacology, which integrates systems and reductionism perspectives, macro- and microtargeted studies, and both in vivo and in vitro experimentation. Using systems and network biology for primary technical support, this research system studies TCM formula from the perspective of basic chemical material groups, modern pharmacology, and both systems and network biology. This research system provides a strategy that integrates modern science and technology in the research of TCM theory. Further, it provides methodological approach to evaluate TCM formulae and further sheds light on the functional material base and functional principles of TCM. Such methods may also help to scientifically clarify the basis of TCM formulae and stimulate TCM formulae-based drug development so as to further enhance the global acceptance and understanding of TCM theory.

REFERENCES

1. Luo GA, Wang YM. Chemical research system of traditional Chinese medicine compound prescription. *World Sci Technol/Mod Tradit Chin Med* 1999;**1**(1):16–9.
2. Wang XJ. Studies on serum pharmacochemistry of traditional Chinese medicine. *World Sci Technol/Mod Tradit Chin Med* 2002;**4**(2):1–4.
3. Zhang BL, Wang YY. Fundamental research on the key scientific problems of TCM prescriptions: the development of modern Chinese medicine. *Chin J Nat Med* 2005;**3**(5):258–61.
4. Hood L. Systems biology: new opportunities arising from genomics, proteomics and beyond. *Exp Hematol* 1998;**26**:681.
5. Ideker T, Galitski T, Hood L. A new approach to decoding life: systems biology. *Annu Rev Genomics Hum Genet* 2001;**2**:343–72.
6. Li S. Frame work and practice of network based studies for Chinese herbal formula. *Chin J Integr Med* 2007;**5**:489–93.
7. Wang M, Lamers RJ, Korthout HA, et al. Metabolomics in the context of systems biology: bridging traditional Chinese medicine and molecular pharmacology. *Phytother Res* 2005;**19**(3):173–82.
8. Verpoorte R, Crommelin D, Danhof M, et al. Commentary: "A systems view on the future of medicine: inspiration from Chinese medicine?" *J Ethnopharmacol* 2009;**121**(3):479–81.

9. Wang L, Zhou GB, Liu P, et al. Dissection of mechanisms of Chinese medicinal formula Realgar-Indigo naturalis as an effective treatment for promyelocytic leukemia. *Proc Natl Acad Sci U S A* 2008;**105**:4826–31.

10. Luo GA, Liang QL, Liu QF, et al. Chemomics-integrated global systems biology: a holistic methodology of study on compatibility and mechanism of formulas in traditional Chinese medicine. *World Sci Technol/Mod Tradit Chin Med* 2007;**9**(1):10–6.

11. Barabaosi AL, Oltvai ZN. Network biology: understanding the cell's functional organization. *Nat Rev Genet* 2004;**5**:101–13.

12. Li S, Wang YY. Relationship between systems theory and reductionism in medical research. *J Beijing Univ Tradit Chin Med* 2005;**28**(1):1–5.

13. Meng XF, Luan HB, Wang PJ. Pharmacology research under the guidance of traditional Chinese medicine theory. *Chin J Inf Tradit Chin Med* 2006;**13**(12):7–51.

14. Herrgård MJ, Swainston N, Dobson P, et al. A consensus yeast metabolic network reconstruction obtained from a community approach to systems biology. *Nat Biotechnol* 2008;**26**:1155–60.

15. Auffray C, Chen Z, Hood L. Systems medicine: the future of medical genomics and healthcare. *Genome Med* 2009;**1**(1):2.

16. Dove A. Proteomics: translating genomics into products. *Nat Biotechnol* 1999;**17**(3):233–6.

17. Nicholson JK, Wilson ID. Understanding "global" systems biology: metabonomics and the continuum of metabolism. *Nat Rev Drug Discov* 2003;**2**(8):668–76.

18. Martin H, Marco AM. Epigenetics and human disease. *Int J Biochem Cell Biol* 2009;**41**(1):136–46.

19. Bradbury J. Human epigenome project—up and running. *PLoS Biol* 2003;**1**(3). e82.

20. Jones PA, Archer TK, Baylin SB, et al. Moving AHEAD with an international human epigenome project. *Nature* 2008;**454**:711–5.

21. Guarner F, Malagelada JR. Gut flora in health and disease. *Lancet* 2003;**361**(9356):512–9.

22. O'Hara AM, Shanahan F. The gut flora as a forgotten organ. *EMBO Rep* 2006;**7**(7):688–93.

23. Cho I, Blaser MJ. The human microbiome: at the interface of health and disease. *Nat Rev Genet* 2012;**13**(4):260–70.

24. Lederberg J. Infectious history. *Science* 2000;**288**(5464):287–93.

25. Peterson J, Garges S, Giovanni M, et al. The NIH Human Microbiome Project. *Genome Res* 2009;**19**(12):2317–23.

26. Qin J, Li R, Raes J, et al. A human gut microbial gene catalogue established by metagenomic sequencing. *Nature* 2010;**464**(7285):59–65.

27. Barabasi AL, Oltvai ZN. Network biology: understanding the cell's functional organization. *Nat Rev Genet* 2004;**5**(2):101–13.

28. Werhli AV, Grzegorczyk M, Husmeier D. Comparative evaluation of reverse engineering gene regulatory networks with relevance networks, graphical gaussian models and bayesian networks. *Bioinformatics* 2006;**22**(20):2523–31.

29. Wang RS, Zhang XS, Chen L. Inferring transcriptional interactions and regulator activities from experimental data. *Mol Cell* 2007;**24**(3):307–15.

30. Rual JF, Venkatesan K, Hao T, et al. Towards a proteome-scale map of the human protein–protein interaction network. *Nature* 2005;**437**(7062):1173–8.

31. Zhao J, Yu H, Luo JH, et al. Complex networks theory for analyzing metabolic networks. *Chin Sci Bull* 2006;**51**(13):1529–37.

32. Barabasi AL, Albert R. Emergence of scaling in random networks. *Science* 1999;**286**:509–12.

33. Watts DJ, Strogatz SH. Collective dynamics of 'small-world' networks. *Nature* 1998;**393**:440–2.

34. Ravasz E, Somera AL, Mongru DA, et al. Hierarchical organization of modularity in metabolic networks. *Science* 2002;**297**:1551–5.

35. Goh KI, Cusick ME, Valle D, et al. The human disease network. *Proc Natl Acad Sci U S A* 2007;**104**(21):8685–90.

36. Lee DS, Park J, Kay KA, et al. The implications of human metabolic network topology for disease comorbidity. *Proc Natl Acad Sci U S A* 2008;**105**(29):9880–5.

37. Zhao J, Jiang P, Zhang W. Molecular networks for the study of TCM pharmacology. *Brief Bioinform* 2010;**11**(4):417–30.

38. Ideker T, Sharan R. Protein networks in disease. *Genome Res* 2008;**18**(4):644–52.
39. Liu ZP, Wang Y, Zhang XS, et al. Network-based analysis of complex diseases. *IET Syst Biol* 2012;**6**(1):22–33.
40. Zhao J, Zhang WD. Systems biological based study of multi-target and multi-component drugs. *Chin Pharm J* 2010;**45**(15):1121–6.
41. Jiang P, Dou SS, Liu RH, et al. Research idea and methods on pharmacodynamic material basis of traditional Chinese medicine. *World Sci Technol/Mod Tradit Chin Med Meteria Med* 2008;**10**(1):11–6.
42. Yang HQ, Li XJ. Chemical proteomics and discovery of drug targets. *Acta Pharm Sin* 2011;**46**(8):877–82.

CHAPTER 2

Theories and Methods for the Evaluation of the Pharmacodynamic Material Basis of Traditional Chinese Medicine

Peng Jiang*, Dale G. Nagle†, YuDong Zhou†, Weidong Zhang‡
*Shanghai Hutchison Pharmaceutical Limited Company, Shanghai, PR China
†University of Mississippi, University, MS, United States
‡Second Military Medical University, Shanghai, PR China

Abstract

With growing worldwide attention to traditional Chinese medicine (TCM) research, TCM formulae have found increased demand. Subsequently, new scientific hypotheses and modern technologies have emerged to study the pharmacodynamic material basis of TCM formulae. This chapter reviews the concepts and research methods that have been developed over the past 10 years to examine the pharmacodynamics material basis of TCM formulae. The advantages and potential deficiencies of each new approach are analyzed and critiqued to provide perspective and enlighten readers regarding the scientific principles that build the foundation of the pharmacodynamic material basis concept of TCM formulae.

Keywords: Traditional Chinese medical formulae, Pharmacodynamic material basis, Effective components, Serum pharmacology, Serum pharmacochemistry, Molecular biological chromatography.

The pharmacodynamic material basis of traditional Chinese medical formulae is the concept that the efficacy of a traditional Chinese medicine (TCM) preparation toward any particular symptom or disorder results from the sum of all its effective components. The source of these chemical constituents is complex and not only includes the original composition of raw medicinal herbs in the medicine, but also products formed during the preparation process (e.g., processing methods, decocting preparation, etc.). The pharmacodynamic material basis of traditional Chinese medical formulae does not simply consider the additive effects of all the components but treats the TCM preparation as a potentially synergistic combination of its various active substances.

Recent advances in cell and molecular biology, computer science, chromatographic methods, genetic recombination technologies, genetically modified animal-based disease model systems, cellular genetic probes, engineered genetic technologies, TCM chemical fingerprinting, high-throughput screening (HTS), and combinatorial chemistry methods are now becoming widely used in the study of the pharmacodynamic material basis of

Systems Biology and Its Application in TCM Formulas Research
https://doi.org/10.1016/B978-0-12-812744-5.00002-3

TCM. The application of advanced science and technologies greatly enhances the ability to clarify the scientific foundation and functional mechanisms of TCM while also serving to promote TCM modernization and internationalization.

2.1. THE DEVELOPMENT OF RESEARCH ON THE PHARMACODYNAMIC MATERIAL BASIS OF TCM

Since the 1990s, the study of the pharmacodynamic material basis of TCM entered into a new period with many theories provided from several researchers, and some theories and ideas are still in use today. Therefore, it is important to understand the history and development of research on the pharmacodynamic material basis of TCM.

As early as 1991, Huang[1] put forward the hypothesis of "syndrome and treatment pharmacokinetics," which suggested that the state of a disease or syndrome could significantly change the pharmacokinetic parameters of prescriptions. In 1997, he further enhanced the theory of "prescription active component dynamics," which emphasized that prescription component interactions and compatibility have a great influence on the dynamic parameters of the active ingredients in vivo.

Xu and Lei[2] proposed the "formulae shotgun theory" in 1996, which considered that TCM formulae are composed of a variety of effective components and that, through their interactions in the human body, produce new active substances that play a combined specific drug effect. This theory has enriched our understanding of the formulae, emphasized the integrity of the formulae, and provided an important theoretical basis for subsequent research. In 1998, at the meeting of the "global Chinese modernization of traditional Chinese medicine academic research seminar," Zhou[3] put forward the "quantitative composition activity relationship" concept to study integrated TCM systems, paving the way to examine structure-activity relationships of multicomponent formulae and form multivariate pharmacodynamic indexes. This method is consistent with the dialectical thinking mode in Chinese medicine theory, which has a positive significance in explaining the drug action mechanisms of a prescription, screening for the effective components as single drugs and so forth.

In 2000, Cao[4] proposed the theory of coordination chemistry in the study of the effective chemical composition in TCM prescriptions. This approach considers that the effective substance is the combination of organic matter and trace metal elements and compounds that serve to coordinate the activity; this combination can reflect the material basis of TCM more than any one set of specific pure organic compounds. This theory has opened up a new way to study TCM prescriptions, and recent experimental results have come to validate this theory.[5–9]

In 2001, Wang and Zhou[10] put forward a different view for the study of TCM prescriptions. Their proposed system suggests that the material basis for the analysis of prescriptions should distinguish between major and minor components, and proposed a theory that "major active ingredient and minor active ingredients combined effect."

In 2003, Liu[11,12] believed that the material basis of TCM prescriptions should be considered to be based on their clinical efficacy, and established animal, organ, and cell models to study TCM prescription activity in order to clarify the pharmacodynamic material basis of TCM.

In 2007, Luo et al.[13] put forward a theoretical research system for the study of the pharmacodynamic material basis of TCM prescriptions, "a combination, two basic clarifying, three chemical levels, four pharmacological level," and combined this with modern scientific methods and advanced analytical tools to better clarify the pharmacodynamic material basis of TCM.

Recently, using the mathematical model to identify the active components was also popular. For example, Liu et al.[14] synchronized the results of multiple component pharmacokinetics (PK) and multiple indicator pharmacodynamics (PD) to determine the relevant active components of TCM prescriptions, and then interpreted the pharmacodynamic material basis of TCM prescriptions.

2.2. NEW METHODS FOR THE STUDY OF THE PHARMACODYNAMIC MATERIAL BASIS OF TCM

Along with the emergence of various theories for the pharmacodynamic material basis of TCM prescriptions, new theory-based research methods are also rapidly developing. From the earliest single-herb, system-separation method of research that examines disassembled prescriptions to whole prescription-based research, plant chemistry provides a powerful tool. After many years of research, these methods have made an outstanding contribution to the interpretation of the material basis of prescriptions.[15–18] Due to the rapid development of analytical technologies and the integration of interdisciplinary science, the research methods and techniques used to examine TCM prescriptions are rapidly advancing. The following is a general introduction to the application of various new technologies and methods.

2.2.1 Combined Chemical Technologies for the Study of TCM

In 1998, Yang et al.[19] suggested a combinatorial chemistry-based traditional Chinese medical research method, which is based on the concept that TCM prescriptions are like natural combinatorial chemical libraries (NCCL), and that under the guidance of TCM theory, indicated that these preparations cure pathological physiology and impact pharmacological evaluation indexes through the combination of many single components acting at many sites or targets in a potently synergistic manner. As an example of a combinatorial Chinese medical chemistry research methodology, Yang et al.[19] used a dual-index library screening method for rhizoma ligustici wallichii and *Gastrodia elata* extract formulae. After analysis and comparison, they observed that two groups of active components, namely the Rhizoma Chuanxiong alcohol extract and the *G elata* alcohol extract, exhibited the strongest antiplatelet activity in the combination formulae that released 5-HT and functionally blocked vascular endothelial cell calcium channel function.

Luo et al.[20] applied the combinatorial chemistry research concept to carry out the study of the mechanism of the effect of TCM prescription drug action mechanisms, and in 2006 developed the metabolomics-like method of "chemomics." A chemical "fingerprint" of a Qingkailing injection was established by a chemomics-based model. Cellular models were evaluated with a total of 51 pharmacological indexes to eventually determine that the potential of Qingkailing to treat cerebral ischemia injury appears to be based on four kinds of effective components: bile acids, baicalin, cyclohexene iridoids, and a mother of pearl preparation. Together, the four kinds of substances form the active material group of a Qingkailing injection, thus revealing the material basis for its efficacy.

This combinatorial chemistry-based approach to TCM formulae can be used to simplify the molecular diversity of prescriptions and develop simplified formulae of "useful molecules." This approach not only fit the entire concept of TCM theory, but also accord with the theory of dialectical analysis of TCM. These combinatorial chemistry methods provide important avenues for the further exploration of Chinese medicine prescriptions.

2.2.2 Serum Pharmacology and Serum Pharmacochemistry Method

The Japanese scholar Tashiro Shin-ichi presented the theory of "Serum Pharmacology" and "Serum Chemistry" in the 1980s. While in China, Wang Xijun proposed the theory of "Serum Pharmacochemistry of Chinese Traditional Medicine" and how this concept could be implemented by combining methods to determine serum pharmacological activity in vitro and to isolate and identify effective components from the serum. Using this method, the in vitro activity of prescription compounds absorbed into the bloodstream is assayed and the effective components of the prescription and its physiological metabolites are identified. Homma et al.[21] studied Chaipo decoctions using the serum pharmacology and serum chemistry methods. Analysis from high-performance liquid chromatography with diode-array detection (HPLC-DAD) indicated that, after administration, three new peaks were observed in serum samples. These substances were subsequently shown to be magnolol, 8,9-dihydroxymagnolol, and glycyrrhizin. Therefore, it was concluded that these three components were most likely to contribute to the pharmacological activity of the decoction.

The application of the serum chemistry approach was eventually picked up in China, but quickly grew. For example, Wang et al.[22] used a rat serum pharmacochemistry-based method to establish that the efficacy of the Liuwei Dihuang Pill was related to five serum components and that the pharmacodynamic action of these components intensified the physiological stability of its active ingredients. Wang and coworkers studied the serum components associated with oral ingestion of the Danggui Buxue Decoction by rats using HPLC-DAD/MS and found 46 unique compounds, 10 prototype components, and

21 probable physiological metabolites.[23] Using HPLC/EI-MS, Jiang analyzed the in vivo serum chemistry of rats given the Shexiang Baoxin Pill.[24] Seventeen prototype constituents and four metabolites were identified and their structures were confirmed. Using the same method, Hu studied the serum components following ingestion of the Huang Lian Jie Du decoction; a total of 22 prototype components and eight physiological metabolites were identified. From that study, a preliminary efficacy and material basis of the decoction of rhizoma was postulated.[25]

Serum pharmacology and serum pharmacochemistry theories were used to establish new drug efficacy evaluation systems, which have proven valuable for the evaluation of the functional basis of TCM while also providing new methods for the development of second generation "enhanced" TCM prescriptions. At their current level, however, serum pharmacology-based approaches still some have significant shortcomings,[26] such as the inability to determine the potential physiological impact generated by the different composition of intestinal flora between humans and animal-based model systems. Animal-based serum methods may also produce experimental artifacts caused by different absorption characteristics and drug metabolism enzymes that exist between humans and animals. Therefore, human clinical serum samples are more likely to produce more reliable results. However, precise disease diagnoses, clinically observable therapeutic effects, and serum samples of sufficient size are required for patient-based serum pharmacology-based TCM studies.

2.2.3 Analysis of Spectrum-Effect Relationships

The spectrum–effect relationship concept is based on TCM chemical fingerprint research. Useful chemical information is derived from the application of chromatography, spectroscopy, and associated technologies. It combines TCM formulae chemical fingerprint compositions with TCM efficacy results. The purpose of the profile-effect study is to make standard chemical controls that can truly reflect the inherent quality of the TCM products. Ning et al.[27] has studied the material basis for the efficacy of the TCM product known as the Wuzhuyu decoction. Results indicated that the material basis of the Wuzhuyu decoction was found to be produced chiefly by the chemical constituents contained in chromatographic peaks or fractions called X_4, X_9 (rutaecarpine), X_{10} and X_{12}. Similarly, Lu et al.[28] found a corresponding relationship between the fingerprint of *Houttuynia condata* injections and their therapeutic effects. GC-MS results indicated that chromatographic peaks from 17 to 21 min primarily associated with the bioactivity of *Houttuynia condata* injections. These peaks were found to be produced by methyl *n*-nonyl ketone, decanoylacetaldehyde, lauryl aldehyde, caprylaldehyde, β-pinene, β-linalool, *l*-nonanol, 4-terpineol, α-terpineol, bornyl acetate, *n*-decanoic acid, acetic acid, and geranyl acetate. Three of the compounds were consistent with results from previous studies. Recently, Jin et al.[29] applied the spectrum-effect relationship method to study the therapeutic material basis of the Carapax Trionycis decoction on hepatic fibrosis. In this study, the pattern and strategy for the dose-dependent effect and fingerprinting-effect relationships were based on the concept of target constituent "knock-out and knock-in." Mao et al.[30] established a mathematical expression for evaluating the potential anticancer efficacy of *Zanthoxylum nitidium* samples to human tumor cells based on their infrared spectroscopy-based fingerprints. This model indicated that alkaloids in *Z. nitidium* were responsible for the major effects of this product on tumor cells. Fingerprint analysis studies by Huang et al.[31] correlated with the pharmacodynamic constituents in Herba Erigerontis injections against neurotoxicity induced by beta-amyloid peptide. Constituents referred to as "B" and "C" showed clear activity and observed peaks numbered 4 and 7–12 positively correlated the fingerprints with the pharmacology studies. This study suggests the possible validity of this approach to deduce active TCM constituents. Kang et al.[32] used the chromatography-activity relationship method to examine the effect of Curcumae Rhizoma (stir baked with vinegar) on the stagnation of vital energy and blood stasis syndrome influencing hemorheology. The results showed that among 16 common chromatographic peaks in the HPLC fingerprint, peaks referred to as numbers 6, 7, and 9–13 strongly correlated with the activity. It is clear that the fingerprint-based technique and pharmacodynamic evaluation systems need to be closely integrated, and the validity of the efficacy evaluation model is of primary importance. Otherwise, the spectrum-effect relationship method cannot accurately reflect the therapeutic material basis of TCM preparations.

2.2.4 HTS of Multiple Targets

The curative effects of TCM products are believed to be produced by a combination of effective components that act synergistically to target multiple biological targets. High-throughput multiple target-based screening technologies are being applied to TCM research. Such approaches facilitate the ability to adapt complex TCM prescription compositions to modern ligand-receptor drug theory by using multiple-target analysis to determine effective TCM components.[33]

Complex TCM components can be simultaneously evaluated against multiple potential biochemical targets in a high-throughput manner with recently developed new biochip, gene, receptor, and enzyme-based methods.[34] Sun et al.[35] used extracellular patch clamp methods with in vitro cultured cortex neurons to examine and identify TCM products for the *N*-methyl-D-aspartic acid receptor antagonism. These experiments showed that the aqueous extract of Radix Scutellariae, Radix Stephania Tetrandra, herb *Salvia japonica*, and others blocks the *N*-methyl-D-aspartic acid pathway. Similarly, el-Mekkawy et al.[36] found that *Ganoderma lucidum* fruiting bodies contain the compounds ganoderiol F and ganodermanontriol that have anti-HIV-1 receptor activity. Li et al.[37] established a high-throughput anti-HIV screening method that targets the 90-positive transcriptional elongation factor b (p-TEFb) and successfully applied this method to evaluate TCM preparations to yield two positive medicines, Cibotii Rhizoma and Radix Scutellariae.

New ultrahigh-throughput screening (UHTS) technologies that can screen tens of thousands of samples daily at reduced costs are replacing the HTS methods. Application of UHTS shows promise to speed up the modernization TCM research. However, one potential drawback of even the best UHTS systems is that many protein, enzyme, and simple cell-based in vitro UHTS techniques are limited because they do not fully reflect in vivo pharmacology and cannot model the complexity of human physiology.

2.2.5 Molecular Biological Chromatography Technique

Due to the development of modern molecular biology techniques and their combination with medicinal chemistry, new molecular biological chromatography technologies have been developed. These techniques are based on the use of biological macromolecules to separate and determine the structures and potential functions of active compounds, including medicinal ingredients in TCM preparations.[38] These techniques include fixed-serum protein biochromatography, fixed-biofilm chromatography, and HPLC-microdialysis. Biochromatography studies by Wang et al.[39] examined the binding status of the *Artemisia* methanol extract on columns prepared with human serum albumin (HSA), and found five peaks with the capacity to bind serum albumin. Two of the compounds were identified as the biologically active compounds scoparone and capillarisin. Mao et al.[40] screened the effective components of *Angelica sinensis* by using immobilized liposome column chromatography (ILC) and found 10 peaks from the ILC chromatogram, including two identified as ferulic acid and ligustilide, both of which have been reported to be the most important ingredients in *Angelica*. Huang et al.[41] used a microdialysis HPLC technique to screen bioactive substances from Rhizome Chuanxiong, analyzed Rhizoma Chuanxiong and Chuanxiong plasma conjugates, and identified ferulic acid and 3-butyl phthalate lactone from the peaks in the HPLC chromatograms. The 3-butyl phthalate lactone exhibited strong adhesion, indicating its potentially strong activity. Molecular biology-based chromatography techniques can not only be used to study the material basis of prescription efficacy, but may also help to explain the distribution, excretion, metabolism, activity, toxicity, and in vivo biological transformation of drugs. It is likely that these methods will have a great impact in the future study of the medicinal material basis of TCM.

2.2.6 Metabolism Method

After taking Chinese medicine, only a portion of the ingredients are absorbed into the body; these ingredients are those most likely to a play a role in forming physiologically active metabolites. A growing number of studies have shown that the chemical composition of many TCM formulae has biological activity after biological transformation and formation of metabolites. Therefore, it is logical to clarify the material basis TCM prescriptions, the potentially synergistic principles, and the mechanism responsible for their action by combining metabolic product dynamics studies with research on the naturally occurring prototypical components of the original preparations.[42] Several methods are often used to study TCM metabolism and these are usually used in various combinations.

The first is the use of an in vivo method to separate and analyze metabolites in animal blood, urine, bile, gastric juice, intestinal fluid, and feces following TCM administration, so as to identify substances that may play an active mechanistic role in the material basis of the TCM product.[38]

Following oral administration of licorice Aconite decoction, cinnamic acid and *6E, 12E*–tetradece 8,10-diene-1,3-diol diacetylene were analyzed by Kano.[43] Tan et al.[44] compared the change of active ingredients of the Mahuang decoction in artificial gastric conditions, intestinal juice, and serum following intragastric administration in rats. These experiments assessed different time period exposures of gastric, intestinal juice, and in blood, and further confirmed ephedrine and glycyrrhizic acid, respectively, as rapidly absorbed potentially active ingredients.

Another method is through analysis of the absorble components and their metabolic conversion characteristics of the prescriptions in artificial gastric juice, intestinal juice, and intestinal flora, combined with the pharmacodynamic results from the isolated active ingredients in the prescription. Metabolism and other processes can effectively eliminate the interference of a large number of ineffective components so as to more quickly find the role(s) of the physiologically effective components.[44] Yang et al.[45,46] has found considerable success with the use of these in vitro metabolic study methods, working with antitumor Buckeye saponins. The intestinal bacteria metabolites studies with escin-Ia found that deacetylated Buckeye saponin I metabolites also have antitumor activity.

Metabolic studies on TCM prescriptions provide new opportunities to discover missing answers, the embarrassing dilemma that has long-plagued Chinese medicine—"to know that it works, but not to know why." They are also laying a solid foundation for the construction of ADME/Tox new drug screening platforms in line with the principles of Chinese medicine.

2.2.7 System Biology Method

Systems biology is the study of the composition of all the integrated components that compose a biological system (genes, mRNA, proteins, metabolites, etc.), as well as the dynamic relationships that exist between these components under specific conditions.[47] Systems biology combines genomic, proteomic, and metabolomic science to study the differences of intermolecular effects all around. From extrapolation to environmental chemistry in species interactions, mathematical models are established to evaluate the differences or changes in mRNA, protein and metabolite levels that lead to phenotypically unique biological and biomedical outcomes.

Chinese medicine theory is characterized by an integrated philosophy of mind and body. While the prescription may be the primary application of TCM treatment, its efficacy assumes a multitargeted synergistic in vivo effect to produce a comprehensive set of results. In this respect, the approach and scope of systems biology is largely consistent with the overall theory of Chinese medicine, which can provide a powerful tool to unravel the mechanistic black box-like mystery sometimes attributed to TCM.

Fu[48] clarified the serum components and variable composition of Qisheng Yiqi Pills by a chemomics-based method to validate the material basis of TCM systems biology research. Based on these results, a rat myocardial infarction model system was established and used to examine the integrated physiological effect of Qisheng Yiqi Pills. The results were combined with computer simulation filtering and biochip technologies to establish network pharmacology-related pathways and targets that predict an overall model of systemic function. Ultimately, these studies indicated that the substances primarily responsible for the efficacy of Qisheng Yiqi Pills were a set of saponins, flavonoids, and phenolic acids that function at a specific set of integrated targets and related pathways to improve the symptoms and pathology of myocardial infarction. Similarly, Ran et al.[49] used a systems biology approach to validate the in vivo physiological basis of acupuncture in the treatment of asthma.

A hot new area of systems biology couples metabolomic-based methods with biological system studies. Wang et al.[50] used metabolomics to characterize Yinchenhao Decoctions, and unambiguously characterized the five endogenous biomarkers of rat liver injury. The callback function on makers of Yinchenhao decoction has shown significant preventive effect on hepatitis, and given a new explanation for the prevention and treatment of liver injury from the drug metabolism. Metabolomics studies by Yu et al.[51] resolved the active antimicrobial substances found in *Aquilegia vulgaris* and helped establish that magnoflorine was the primary anti-*Staphylococcus aureus* constituent. This group further suggested that the activity was due to its effect on similar mechanistic ribosomal protein translation targets attributed to *Columbine* and antibiotics such as clindamycin, chloramphenicol, streptomycin, and tetracycline. Jiang et al.[52,53] used metabolomics to examine serum and urine metabolism to correlate specific metabolites and the therapeutic effects observed with the Shexiang Baoxin Pill for the treatment of myocardial infarction in a rat-based model. Results from these studies indicate that the Shexian Baoxin Pill can greatly regress the symptoms of myocardial infarction; it may also reduce myocardial infarction risk by regulating cellular energy metabolism and inhibiting inflammatory processes.

Because the use of systems biology-based TCM research is only in its infancy, it will take time before it can reach its exciting full promise for use as a tool for clinically based TCM research. With the development of new systems biology techniques and improvement in data analysis methods, it will likely provide valuable insights to help mechanistically explain important material basis aspects of Chinese medicine formulae.

REFERENCES

1. Huang X. *The scientific basis and prospect of the combination of traditional Chinese medicine and Western medicine in twenty-first century with the hypothesis of "syndrome and treatment pharmacokinetics"*. Beijing: China Medical Science and Technology Press; 1991. p. 207–16.

2. Xu Y, Lei QJ. *The "shotgun" theory of traditional Chinese medicine: the modern research of traditional Chinese medicine*. Beijing: China Environmental Science Press; 1996. p. 102–3.

3. Zhou LD. In: *Recommendations for the establishment of "quantitative structure-activity relationship" in research of traditional Chinese medicine. Global academic seminar on Chinese herbal medicine modernization.* **2**; 1999. p. 33–4.

4. Cao ZQ. New thinking about study of pharmacodynamic material basis and functional mechanism in Chinese materia medica—study on the relation between morphology and biological activity of chemical species in Chinese materia medica. *J Shanghai Univ Tradit Chin Med* 2000;**14**(1):36–40.

5. Wang J, Jia RY, Li XM. Study on the modern efficacy and inorganic elements of traditional Chinese medicine. *J Trace Elem Electrolytes Health Dis* 1996;**13**(4):29–31.

6. Li SF, Liang SR, Geng HH. The pharmacodynamics of baicalin-metal ion chelation. *Chin Arch* 1999;**10**(2):152–3.

7. Zhou JM. Synergistic effect of trace elements and organic components in plant. *Inf Chin Tradit Med* 1993;**10**(5):23–4.

8. Wang XP. The study of statn on the heavy metal in the Liu Shen Wan and interact with organic constitnets. *Stud Trace Elem Health* 2003;**20**(4):27–8.

9. Ou Yang JM. Citrate inhibits the chemical basis of urinary calculi formation. *Chinese J Inorg Chem* 2004;**20**(12):1377–82.

10. Wang BX, Zhou QL. Cognition of active ingredients of traditional Chinese medicine and its research methods. *Chin J Chin Mater Med* 2001;**26**(1):10–3.

11. Liu JX, Ren JG. Discussion on substance basis of traditional Chinese medicine compound. *Res Inf Tradit Med* 2004;**6**(12):8–11.

12. Fu JH, Fu Y, Liu JX. On the hypothesis of "component pharmacy" *Chin J Inf TCM* 2006;**13**(1):52–4.

13. Luo GA, Liang QL, Liu QF, et al. Chemomics-integrated global systems biology: a holistic methodology of study on compatibility and mechanism of formulas in traditional Chinese medicine. *World Sci Technol/Mod Tradit Chin Med Materia Med* 2007;**9**(1):10–6.

14. Liu JX, Lin L, Zhang Y, et al. Further study of indicated pharmacokinetics of traditional Chinese medicine. *World Sci Technol/Mod Tradit Chin Med Materia Med* 2012;**14**(13):1562–6.

15. Kou JP, Liu Y, Zhu DN, et al. Preliminary study on material basis of different laxative potency of Xiao Chengqi-Tang and other two prescriptions. *Lishizhen Med Mater Med Res* 1999;**10**(6):401–3.

16. Xiao HB, Xia XH, Piao ZD, et al. Pharmacodynamic and separating prescription studies of Xiaofengsan. *Chin J Exp Tradit Med Formul* 1999;**5**(4):21–3.

17. Zhu DN, Li ZM, Yan YQ, et al. Study on the relationship between chemical dynamic changes and pharmacodynamics of Shengmai San compound—study on compound chemistry of Shengmai powder (II). *Chin J Chin Materia Med* 1998;**23**(5):291–3.

18. Zhu DN, Yan YQ, Li ZM. Study on the relationship between chemical dynamic changes and pharmacodynamics of Shengmai San compound—study on compound chemistry of Shengmai powder (III). *Chin J Chin Materia Med* 1998;**23**(8):483–5.

19. Yang K, Guo L, Zhou MM, et al. A preliminary study on chemical combination of traditional Chinese medicine. *Pharmacol Clin Chin Materia Med* 1998;**14**(3):42–4.

20. Luo GA, Ql L, Zhang RL, et al. Study on chemical substances and traditional Chinese medicine prescriptions—also on the material basis of Qingkailing's compound. *World Sci Technol/Mod Tradit Chin Med Materia Med* 2006;**8**(1):6–15.

21. Homma M, Oka K, Taniguchi C, et al. Systematic analysis of post-administrative Saiboku-To urine by liquid chromatography to determine pharmacokinetics of traditional Chinese medicine. *Biomed Chromatogr* 1997;**11**:125–31.

22. Wang XJ, Zhang N, Sun H, et al. Preliminary study on serum pharmacochemistry of Liu Wei Di Huang Wan. *Chin J Nat Med* 2004;**2**(4):219–22.

23. Wang P, Liang Y, Zhou N, et al. Screening and analysis of the multiple absorbed bioactive components and metabolites of Danggui Buxue decoction by the metabolic fingerprinting technique and liquid

chromatography by/diode-array detection mass spectrometry. *Rapid Commun Mass Spectrom* 2007;**21**:99–106.

24. Jiang P, Liu R, Dou S, et al. Analysis of the constituents in rat plasma after oral administration of Shexiang Baoxin pill by HPLC-ESI-MS/MS. *Biomed Chromatogr* 2009;**23**(12):1333–43.

25. Hu Y, Jiang P, Wang S, et al. Plasma pharmacochemistry based approach to screening potential bioactive components in Huang-Lian-Jie-Du-Tang using high performance liquid chromatography coupled with mass spectrometric detection. *J Ethnopharmacol* 2012;**141**(2):728–35.

26. He YZ. A survey of studies on "serum pharmacology" and "serum medicinal chemistry" in Japanese. *Foreign Med Sci Chin Med Vol* 1998;**20**(5):3–7.

27. Ning LL, Bi KS, Wang R, et al. Methodological study on the material basis for the efficacy of the traditional Chinese medicine Wuzhuyu decoction. *Acta Pharm Sin* 2000;**35**(2):131–4.

28. Hongmei L, Yizeng L, Pin Q. Profile effect on quality control of *Houttuynia cordata* injection. *Acta Pharmacol Sin* 2005;**40**(12):1147–50.

29. Jin SX, Li XY, SS F, et al. Carapax trionycis pharmacodynamic material basis and quality control research. *Globa Tradit Chin Med* 2012;**5**(6):433–5.

30. Mao XL, Tan Y, Juan C, et al. Infrared fingerprint of *Zathoxylum nitidum* and its effect on inhibition of tumor cell. *J Infrared Millimeter Waves* 2013;**32**(1):91–6.

31. Huang Y, Qi XL, Guan ZZ, et al. Study on fingerprints correlated with pharmacodynamic of constituents in Herba Erigerontis against neurotoxicity induced by beta-amyloid peptide. *Chin J Chin Materia Med* 2010;**35**(8):1038–41.

32. Kang W, Zhang JM, Fu S, et al. Chromatography-activity relation of stagnation of vital energy and blood stasis syndrome influencing hemorheology by stir-baked *Curcumae rhizoma* with vinegar. *Chin Tradit Patent Med* 2013;**35**(2):330–4.

33. Guo LM, Wang CY, QQ G, et al. Research methods and development trend of Chinese herbal compound effect substance. *Chin Tradit Patent Med* 2007;**29**(1):118–21.

34. Gui GH. Application of high-throughput screening in drug development. *Basic Med Sci Clin* 2001;**21**(4):289–93.

35. Sun X, Chan LN, Gong X, et al. *N*-Methyl-D-aspartate receptor antagonist activity in traditional Chinese stroke medicines. *Neurosignals* 2003;**12**:31–8.

36. el-Mekkawy S, Meselhy MR, Nakamura N, et al. Anti-HIV-1 and anti-HIV-1-protease substances from *Ganoderma lucidum*. *Phytochemistry* 1998;**49**:1651–7.

37. Li F, Li YH, XL W, et al. Establishment of high-throughput screening model for anti-HIV drugs with p-TEFb as target and its application in screening Chinese meteria medica. *Chin Tradit Herb Drug* 2014;**45**(5):679–85.

38. He XJ, Qiu F, Yao XS. Present situation and thinking of Chinese traditional compound medicine research. *Prog Chem* 2001;**13**(6):481–4.

39. Wang H, Zou H, Ni J, Kong L, Gao S, Guo B. Fractionation and analysis of *Artemisia capillaris* Thunb. By affinity chromatography with human albumin as stationary phase. *J Chromatogr A* 2000;**870**(1–2):501–10.

40. Mao X, Kong L, Luo Q, et al. Screening and analysis of permeable compounds in Radix *Angelica Sinensis* with immobilized liposome chromatography. *J Chromatogr B* 2002;**779**:331–9.

41. Huang X, Kong L, Li X, et al. Strategy for analysis and screening of bioactive compounds in traditional Chinese medicines. *J Chromatogr B* 2004;**812**:71–84.

42. Feng NP, Di B, Liu WY. Drug metabolism and modernization of traditional Chinese medicine. *World Sci Technol/Mod Tradit Chin Med* 2003;**5**(2):5–7.

43. Kano XII Y. Pharmacological properties of plant medicament drug ingredients of traditional Chinese medicine oral administration of Gancaofuzi Decoction in rats in the portal vein blood. *Foreign Med Chin Med Sci* 1990;**12**(4):236–8.

44. Tan Y, Li G, Dong XP. A comparative study of Mahuangtang body metabolism. *Pharmacol Clin Chin Materia Med* 2002;**18**(2):1–4.

45. Yang XW, Zhao J, Cui JR. Studies on the biotransformation of escin Ia by human intestinal bacteria and the anti-tumor activities of desacylescinI. *J Peking Univ Health Sci* 2004;**36**(1):31–5.

46. Yang XW, Xing ZT, Cui JR, et al. Studies on the metabolism of cinobufagin and cinobufotalin by human intestinal bacteria. *J Peking Univ Health Sci* 2001;**33**(3):199–204.

47. Liu CX. Modern research on systems biology and traditional Chinese medicine (I). *J Tianjin Univ Tradit Chin Med* 2006;**25**(3):115–8.
48. Fu JZ. *Study on the effective substance basis and system biology of Shenqi Yiqi dripping pills* [Master's thesis]. Tianjin: Nankai University; 2012.
49. Ran J, Yin LS, Wnag Y, et al. Bioinformatic analysis of differentially expressed proteins in anti-asthma acupuncture. *Shanghai J Acupunct Moxib* 2014;**3**(9):875–8.
50. Wang XJ, Sun WJ, Sun H, et al. Metabonomics of CCL4-induced rat liver injury and interfering effects of the Yin Chen Hao Tang extract. *World Sci Technol/Mod Tradit Chin Med* 2006;**8**(6):101–6.
51. Yu Y, Yi ZB, Liang YZ. Validate antibacterial mode and find main bioactive components of traditional Chinese medicine *Aquilegia oxysepala*. *Bioorg Med Chem Lett* 2007;**17**:1855–9.
52. Jiang P, Dai W, Yan S, et al. Potential biomarkers in the urine of myocardial infarction rats: a metabolomic method and its application. *Mol BioSyst* 2011;**7**:824–31.
53. Jiang P, Dai W, Yan S, et al. Biomarkers in the early period of acute myocardial infarction in rat serum and protective effects of Shexiang Baoxin pill using a metabolomic method. *J Ethnopharmacol* 2011;**138**:530–6.

CHAPTER 3

Application of Systems Biology in the Research of TCM Formulae

Shikai Yan*, Dale G. Nagle[†], YuDong Zhou[†], Weidong Zhang[‡]
*Shanghai Jiao Tong University, Shanghai, PR China
[†]University of Mississippi, University, MS, United States
[‡]Second Military Medical University, Shanghai, PR China

Abstract

In the postgenomic era, biological studies are characterized by the rapid development and wide application of systems biology, which is often based on global analyses of biological samples using high-throughput analytical approaches and bioinformatics and may provide new insights into biological phenomena. In this chapter, the development and advances of systems biology made over the past decades are reviewed, especially genomics, transcriptomics, proteomics, and metabolomics. The applications of systems biology are then summarized in regard to their use in studying the action mechanisms of TCM formulae, TCM syndrome, TCM formulae component interactions and compatibility, and TCM formulae pharmacokinetics as well as in TCM-based drug discovery and development.

Keywords: Omics, Genomics, Transcriptomics, Proteomics, Metabolomics, TCM formulae, TCM syndrome, Component interactions, compound compatibility, Pharmacokinetics, TCM-based new drugs.

During the late 20th and early 21st century, biological research has experienced considerable development, from microlevel advances to macrolevel innovations. This progress has led to a more comprehensive description of life phenomena and a better-illustrated picture of biochemical and physiological processes. One example is the sequencing of the human genome in 2003 by the International Human Genome Sequencing Consortium that stands as a crucial milestone in the history of genetic research. This has paved the way for genome studies and "genomics" research and initiated the so-called "postgenomic era" in biomedical research.[1] In the postgenomic era, determining the primary sequences of informational macromolecules is no longer a limiting factor in trying to understand the biological functions of cells and organisms.[2] Consequently, the research focus has moved beyond the genome to the role of specific genes, which is a much more challenging task. This includes the need to understand transcriptional gene regulation, the biochemical functions of gene products and gene product interactions, and the mechanisms that influence how gene products control cellular physiology, biochemistry and metabolism.

Systems Biology and Its Application in TCM Formulas Research
https://doi.org/10.1016/B978-0-12-812744-5.00003-5

3.1. OMICS IN SYSTEMS BIOLOGY

Inspired by the term "genomics," a number of terms have been coined with the suffix "-ome" and "-omics" over the last two decades, such as transcriptomics, proteomics, metabolomics, glycomics, and lipidomics. Traditional biochemical methods are relatively inefficient and time-consuming while omics technologies are based on global high-throughput analytical methods such as microarrays, two-dimensional gels, and two-dimensional LC/MS techniques that produce large-scale data sets. By means of bioinformatics and computer-based modeling methods, omics technologies show great promise in providing important new insights and valuable clues to help understand the mechanisms responsible for biological processes and functions, and thus may build a comprehensive theoretical framework for modern life science.

The postgenomic era spurred both the development of omics technologies and their application to biomedical and pharmaceutical research. Compared with traditional research methods, omics-based methods allow for the efficient exploration of the genome, transcriptome, and proteome in an increasingly broad manner with greater sensitivity and resolution. Omics technologies provide new methods to identify and validate novel therapeutic targets, to assess potential drug toxicity and safety issues, to explore pharmacology, to establish a molecular-based patient diagnosis and prognosis, and to personalize healthcare. Meanwhile, these omics technologies produce vast data sets that pose a specific challenge: how to deal with such complicated data? As an indispensable tool for omics, bioinformatics derives knowledge from the computer-based analysis of omics data by retrieval and analysis of genetic code information, experimental results from various sources, patient statistics, and the scientific literature. The field of bioinformatics has developed a number of novel methodologies for processing, analyzing, and efficiently interpreting omics data over the past 20 years, and the combination of omics and bioinformatics enables integral analysis of multiple forms of omics data. It is now generally accepted that an efficient investigation of any biological process should be conducted from multiple viewpoints; for example, just one strategy in systems biology is to look from the viewpoint that connects the cell-chromosome-DNA-RNA-protein-metabolite.

Instead of analyzing individual components or aspects of the organism through routine biochemical methods such as individual gene function, protein or biochemical reaction, omics technologies can simultaneously focus on many components and their interactions within a localized cellular system or biochemical process. Omics reflects the evolution of collective thoughts and data, and is often considered the most essential part of systems biology. Diverse high-throughput approaches have become routine for accumulating a wealth of omics-scale data, providing a unique and distinctive view of the cell-chromosome-DNA-RNA-protein-metabolite continuum (Fig. 3.1).

Omics data generally describe the "wholeness" of biological systems and may not always provide useful, highly specific information directly or in detail. However, through bioinformatic analysis, further useful information can be discovered, such as the

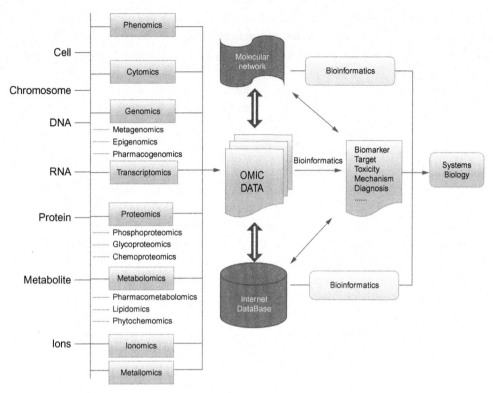

Fig. 3.1 Various omics techniques and their roles in systems biology.

identification of diagnostic biomarker(s), potential therapeutic target(s), and key disease-specific pathway(s), to name just a few. Network biology is another important tool for omics data processing, especially for the analysis of multiomics data. Molecular networks can visualize multiomics data and reveal the relationships between various functional biochemical and other molecules, which are essential for a comprehensive understanding of a biological process from multiple perspectives. Public databases available on the Internet now play an increasingly important role in biological research, and bioinformatics applies and connects them to interpret experimental omics data. Therefore, based on omics data, public databases, and molecular networks, it is possible to view biological processes with regard to pathway maps, protein interactions, functional ontologies, gene-disease associations, mechanisms of drug action, and personalized medicine, which is also an aim of systems biology. Various omics, bioinformatics, systems biology, and other research methodologies are closely associated with each other, as shown in Fig. 3.1.

Over the past two decades, omics-based methods have emerged as efficient tools for the global study of the interactions between drugs and functionally important biomolecules. Results from single drug-gene or drug-protein interactions are not sufficient to explain complex phenotypes: it is necessary to understand drug responses at an entire system level. Omics often denotes the study of an entire set of entities in a class, which may be known as "pharmacogenomics,"[3] "pharmacotranscriptomics," "pharmacometabolomics," and "pharmacoproteomics".[4] Herein advances in omics technologies are reviewed, alongside a brief historical and futuristic perspective of omics applications in pharmaceutical research, especially in the fields of drug target discovery, toxicity evaluation, personalized medicine, and traditional Chinese medicine (TCM).

3.1.1 Genomics

Genomics is a genome-scale technology and can be applied to all areas of biological investigation. In general, genomics research includes both structural genomics and functional genomics. Structural genomics seeks to describe the three-dimensional structures of proteins encoded by a given genome, and allows for a high-throughput method of structure determination through a combination of experimental and modeling approaches. Even today, one major branch is still concerned with sequencing the genomes of various organisms, especially with patterns of gene expression under various conditions. Functional genomics attempts to describe gene and protein functions and their interactions. Microarrays and bioinformatics are the most important tools for genomics research, such as in the serial analysis of gene expression (SAGE), cDNA microarrays, DNA chips, and sequence-tagged fragments display. Genomics is a broad concept that can be used in different research fields, but of particular importance is pharmacogenomics, metagenomics, and epigenomics.

3.1.1.1 Pharmacogenomics

Every person has a unique pattern of genomic variation, which leads to individual differential responses to drugs. Pharmacogenomics examines how genes affect a person's response to drugs so as to develop effective and safe medications and to determine appropriate patient-specific doses. It embraces the discovery of new disease-associated genes and investigates the effects of genetic factors on medications with the aim of predicting the individual's clinical response. Adverse drug reactions are reported as a significant cause for hospitalizations and deaths in many countries.[5] Pharmacogenomics enables researchers to better understand how inherited differences in genes affect the body's response to medications, which can be applied to predict whether the drug is effective or ineffective and whether it may cause specific side effects for a particular patient. For instance, McDermott and Benes[6] applied pharmacogenomics to the discovery of new biomarkers for the sensitivity and resistance to cancer therapeutics and identified a marked sensitivity of Ewing's sarcoma cells harboring the EWS-FLI1 gene translocation to poly (ADP-ribose) polymerase (PARP) inhibitors. Hayden[7] reported the pharmacogenomic prediction of anthracycline-induced cardiotoxicity (ACT) in children, with multiple genetic variants in SLC28A3 and other genes (i.e., ABCB1, ABCB4, and

ABCC1) being identified as associated with ACT. This information can be used to identify potentially high-risk patients before initiation of anthracycline-based chemotherapy.

3.1.1.2 Metagenomics

The term "metagenomics" was first used by Handelsman and colleagues in 1998.[8] It studies the collection of gene sequences from the environment in a way analogous to the study of a single genome. A large number of microorganisms exist in the gastrointestinal (GI) tract of humans and animals. It is reported that the gut bacterial population in humans has about 3 million genes, almost 150 times of the number of human genes,[8] and that these genes are closely associated with the physiological functions of the host. The first metagenomics study was conducted on a woolly mammoth (*Mammuthus primigenius*) sample using emulsion polymerase chain reaction and the pyrosequencing technique.[9]

Microbial communities play a key role in preserving human health. Metagenomics has been widely applied in the research of obesity, providing evidence for the important role of intestinal microbiota for obesity. Ley and coworkers demonstrated that, in obese rats, the proportion of Acteroidetes and Firmicutes bacteria in the cecum varies significantly.[10] Turnbaugh observed analogous differences in the distal gut microbiota of obese versus lean individuals, and the relative abundance of Bacteroidetes increases as obese individuals lose weight.[11] A recent study of the gut microbiota of 123 nonobese and 169 obese patients has suggested that a high bacterial richness, particularly in eight species, may protect against obesity.[12] Metagenomics studies have also demonstrated an imbalanced microbiota composition in various diseases, such as Crohn's disease,[13] necrotizing enterocolitis,[14] polyposis or colorectal cancer,[15] and type 2 diabetes.[16]

3.1.1.3 Epigenomics

Epigenetics refers to the heritable changes in gene expression without any alteration in the DNA sequence. Epigenomics deals with the global analysis of epigenetic changes across the entire genome in order to reveal the genetic information in addition to the DNA sequence, which may affect gene function. Epigenetic regulation can be complemented by five different mechanisms: DNA methylation,[17] histone posttranslational modification,[18] histone variants,[19] RNA interference,[20] and nuclear organization.[21] Methylation is the most common flexible genomic parameter that can change genome function under exogenous influence and usually occurs in CpG islands, a CG rich region, or in the DNA (e.g., promoter regions, regulatory domains, and also in intergenic regions).[22] The Human Epigenome Project (HEP) was initiated in October 2003 by the Human Epigenome Consortium, with the aim of identifying, cataloging, and interpreting genome-wide DNA methylation patterns of all human genes in all major tissues.[23] The HEP is widely supported by cancer research scientists from all over the world. Studies have described DNA hypomethylation in several tumor types, such as colorectal and gastric cancers and melanomas.[24] Another important epigenetic alteration is histone modification in cancer cells that can affect gene transcription through local relaxation of nucleosomal structure and through recruitment of nonhistone proteins,[25] which can be chemically modified by distinct enzymes at their external N- and C-terminal tails as well as at internal histone-fold domains.

3.1.2 Transcriptomics

The transcriptome is the set of all RNA molecules, including mRNA, rRNA, tRNA, and other noncoding RNAs produced in the cell, which, unlike the genome, is able to vary under the influence of external environmental conditions. Transcriptomics investigates the way the entire transcriptome changes under a variety of biological conditions. The sequence of RNA mirrors the sequence of the DNA from which it was transcribed, and the RNA transcription process is the first step in gene expression. However, although the same genome exists in almost every cell in humans or other organisms, different cell types express distinctly different sets of genes. Retrieval of a transcriptome database can help researchers determine when and under what conditions each gene is turned on or off, thus providing valuable clues to its possible function. Through the collection and comparison of transcriptome patterns from the cells of healthy or diseased organisms, researchers can interpret the functional elements of the genome and gain a better understanding of the biological functions of specific cell types and their role(s) in disease pathogenesis. Currently, approaches for transcriptome data acquisition and analysis are primarily based on chip technology, including cDNA microarray and oligonucleotide chips[26]; SAGE[27]; and massively parallel signature sequencing (MPSS).[28] Modern RNA-Seq is a recently developed approach to transcriptome profiling that uses deep-sequencing technology to reveal a snapshot of the presence and quantity of RNA from a genome at a given moment in time.[29–31]

Transcriptomics can facilitate the identification of disease-related gene expression patterns and thus is a valuable tool for clinical diagnosis. For example, patients with Alzheimer's disease (AD) can display altered neuronal gene expression profiles that are associated with neurofibrillary tangles, and those corresponding transcriptome patterns have emerged as a potential resource for the discovery of new AD-associated biomarkers.[32,33] Transcriptomics is also a meaningful method for the diagnosis of diseases that lack an easily identifiable "gold standard" symptomatic diagnostic pathology, such as autism.[34] Currently, the diagnosis of autism relies on a subjective assessment from more than 10h of clinical evaluation in order to make a judgment while by comparing the transcriptomic differences between the normal population and patients, disease-related specific expression can be discovered for an autism diagnosis. Transcriptomics has also exhibited great potential for use in personalized medicine,[35] drug-induced toxicity studies,[36] tumor profiling,[37,38] and in stem cell research.[39]

3.1.3 Proteomics

The proteome is the entire set of proteins[40] produced or modified by an organism or system, which varies in accordance with genetic and environmental factors. Proteomics is the large-scale, high-throughput, and systematic-level study of the structures and functions of the proteome of a specific type of cell, tissue, or bodily fluid.[41,42] Proteomics is a complement to genome translation and modification studies and is an efficient tool that can be used to form a comprehensive picture of overall gene expression.

With advances in related high-throughput analytical technologies and mass spectrometry (MS), proteomics has been rapidly developed in various research fields. Two-dimensional gel electrophoresis (2-DE) is a traditional approach to study proteomes that is still widely used. With improved capacity, sensitivity, resolution, and detection accuracy, two-dimensional fluorescence difference, two-dimensional gel electrophoresis (2-D DIGE) has emerged as a more efficient proteomics method which uses narrow pH-gradient gel separation combined with high-sensitivity protein staining techniques.[43,44] Currently, two-dimensional chromatography with mass spectrometric detection (2DLC-MS),[45] two-dimensional gel electrophoresis-liquid chromatography with mass spectrometric detection (2DE-LC-MS),[46] capillary electrophoresis with mass spectrometric detection (CE-MS),[47] and other chromatographic techniques are increasingly being applied to proteomic studies. For example, 2D LC-MS, with the first dimensional separation based on the molecular protein size and the second dimensional separation by reversed-phase chromatography or strong cation exchange chromatography, are superior to methods relative to the use of two-dimensional gels due to their greater separation capacity, higher resolution, and increased speed. In recent years, new 2D-LC and related technologies have rapidly developed and are fast becoming the major methods for proteomic research.

MS is an essential tool in proteome analysis. Traditionally, proteins were identified by sequence analysis. Due to the rapid development of modern MS techniques, target protein identification can now be quickly and efficiently realized with only a minute amount of sample (typically a few nanograms or micrograms are sufficient). In addition, MS can also differentiate proteins with posttranslational modifications. Based on different ion sources, proteomic MS methods include matrix-assisted laser desorption time-of-flight mass (MALDI-TOF-MS), and electrospray ionization time-of-flight mass (ESI-TOF-MS). In addition to TOF-MS, other useful mass spectrometer systems include quadrupole and ion trap mass spectrometers. Traditional 2DE-based analysis is inherently limited by its low resolution, poor reproducibility, and potentially serious factors that can introduce biased results. To overcome these shortcomings, quantitative proteomic methods were developed. There are two primary strategies for proteome quantification: label-free methods[48] and stable isotope labeling methods. The most important techniques for quantitative proteomics are ICAT (isotope-coded affinity tag),[49] iTRAQ (isobaric tag for relative and absolute quantitation),[50] and SILAC (stable isotope labeling with amino acids in cell culture).[51]

Proteomics has provided a new understanding of medical and life science research and has produced remarkable achievements over the past two decades. In early clinical cancer diagnosis, a series of cancer-related biomarker proteins has been discovered, such as cathepsin B,[52] heat shock protein 27,[53] mRNA junction protein P62,[54] oral squamous cell carcinoma-related protein of HPA/sAa/K-10/GA-HAS,[55] and Pfetin.[56] Drug development is among the most promising areas for the applications of proteomics. Proteomics is already an invaluable tool with even greater potential in the discovery and validation of drug targets, elucidation of drug action mechanisms, toxicology assessment, and in drug metabolism studies.

3.1.3.1 Phosphoproteomics

Phosphorylation is one of the most important posttranslational modifications of proteins in the cell. Phosphoproteomics is a branch of proteomics that studies those proteins that contain posttranslational phosphate substituents. Protein phosphorylation regulates nearly every aspect of cell life from gene expression, signaling, and metabolism to the processes involved in cell growth, division, differentiation, and development. Moreover, the dysregulation of protein phosphorylation can result in numerous pathogenic conditions, most notably cancer, diabetes, heart disease, and AD.

In recent years, the development and application of proteomics has provided technological support for the qualitative, quantitative, and functional studies of phosphorylated proteins, and made possible the large-scale systematic study of protein phosphorylation. The identification and detection of phosphorylated proteins are key technologies in phosphoproteomics research. Technologies applied in phosphoproteomics include diphase phosphate polypeptide spectra (2D-PP), two-dimensional gel electrophoresis (2DE), two-dimensional high-performance liquid chromatography (2D-HPLC), and immobilized metal affinity chromatography (IMAC). Phosphorylated proteins are isolated and enriched and then structurally identified or directly analyzed by LC/MS.

Phosphoproteomics plays an important role in the study of disease pathogenesis and pharmaceutical research, where it can be applied to the discovery of targets, especially phosphorylated targets.[57,58] In addition, phosphoproteomics can be used to screen for potential diagnostic or prognostic markers by comparing the abundance of protein phosphorylation between patients and healthy subjects. Protein phosphorylation is a highly dynamic process that is very sensitive to the use of pharmaceutical agents. Thus, phosphoproteomics can also be used as a powerful tool in personalized medicine. Currently, phosphoproteomics research has made great progress in the study of kidney disease, largely promoting the study of changes in various hormones and cytokines in kidney function and pathology. An example is in the study on the effects of vasopressin on renal collecting duct cells.[59,60] Similarly, it has been used to assess renal tubular epithelial cell function and epithelial-mesenchymal transition induced by angiotensin II and transforming growth factor-β (TGF-β).[61,62] In addition, Gonzales[63] found that the serine-811 phosphorylation sites in the thiazide-sensitive Na–Cl cotransporter, NCC, are potential biological targets for renal disease and that another phosphorylation site of serine-256 in the water channel aquaporin-2 (AQP2) can be used to assess the activity of vasopressin and then monitoring the process of the disease.[64]

3.1.3.2 Glycoproteomics

Glycoproteomics is a branch of proteomics that identifies, catalogs, and characterizes those proteins that contain carbohydrates as posttranslational modifications.[65] Glycosylation, which exists in over 50% of proteins, is recognized as an important posttranslational modification.[66] Protein glycosylation is involved in cellular immunity, cell adhesion, regulation of protein translation, protein degradation, and a variety of other biological processes. Glycoproteomics research includes the identification of glycoproteins, elucidation of glycosylation sites, and the analysis of glycosylation in the structure and function of proteins. Currently, common glycoproteomics methods include the separation and enrichment of glycoproteins and glycopeptides,[67,68] mass spectrometric analysis of protein glycosylation sites,[69] real-time and high-throughput analysis of carbohydrate chains,[70] and structural and functional analysis of glycoproteins.

Protein glycosylation patterns can change during the process of tumor development and the identification of these events may facilitate early cancer diagnosis and enhance the ability to monitor neoplastic disease progression. Further, the identification of altered protein glycosylation patterns during tumor development may reveal tumor cell regulatory mechanisms at the molecular level. Glycoproteomics is now widely used for the discovery and characterization of biomarkers for the diagnosis of cancers of the breast,[71] lung,[72] stomach,[73] and ovaries[74] as well as for other disorders such as liver fibrosis[75] and AD.[76]

3.1.3.3 Chemoproteomics

Chemoproteomics uses a chemistry-based approach to characterize protein structure and function. In general, functionally active small molecules are used to interfere with certain aspects of the proteome, and target proteins may be detected and isolated due to alteration in observed chemical-protein interactions. Unlike qualitative or quantitative proteomics, chemoproteomics focuses on chemical-protein interactions and provides a possible new technology for drug target discovery,[77] which is considered as a promising new potential for function-based proteomics.[78]

The most common chemoproteomics research process is as follows: first, protein extracts are incubated with a chemical probe or small-molecule chemicals. Then, the proteins are separated using affinity chromatography and identified by high-resolution MS. Finally, further bioinformatics analysis is conducted to characterize the protein structure and function.[79] The process usually involves several approaches, including activity-based protein profiling (ABPP),[80] compound-centric chemical proteomics (CCCP),[81,82] protein chip or protein microarray,[83] and network analysis.[84]

Chemoproteomics is a form of function-based proteomics that has been increasingly applied to drug target discovery and validation. In drug target discovery, for example, it has been successfully used to identify targets to block the invasion of malarial *Plasmodium* species into red blood cells. Cysteine proteases are necessary enzymes for *Plasmodium falciparum* survival. Greenbaum[85] prepared chemical probes targeted to cysteine protease, and found falcipain 1 to be cysteine proteolysis active, which led to the screening of a compound as a falcipain 1 inhibitor. Similarly, Chen developed chemoproteomics-based approaches to elucidate the mechanisms involved in the response of acute promyelocytic leukemia (APL) to treatment with arsenic trioxide and concluded that oncoprotein PML-RAR (promyelocytic leukemia—retinoic acid receptor alpha) may function as a direct drug target for APL.[86]

3.1.4 Metabolomics

The term "metabolome" refers to the complete set of small-molecule metabolites to be found within a biological sample, such as from a single organism. Metabolomics is defined as "the quantitative measurement of the dynamic multiparametric metabolic response of living systems to pathophysiological stimuli or genetic modification".[87] The approach was pioneered by Jeremy Nicholson at Imperial College London. Nuclear magnetic resonance (NMR), LC/MS, and GC/MS are the most common technologies in metabolomics research. The data generated in metabolomics usually consist of measurements performed on subjects under various conditions; these measurements may be digitized spectra, or a list of metabolite levels. Several pattern recognition methods and statistical programs are currently available for the analysis of both NMR and MS data, such as principal components analysis (PCA) and partial least squares (PLS).[88] Freely available comprehensive software XCMS developed at the Scripps Research Institute can be used to analyze global MS-based metabolomics datasets.[89,90] Other popular metabolomics programs for mass spectral analysis are known by such acronyms as MZmine,[91] MetAlign,[92] and MathDAMP.[93]

Any disturbance to living systems, regardless of whether physiological, pathological, or from other factors, causes changes in cellular and organismal metabolite profiles. Therefore, the metabolome represents the physiological or pathological status of organisms. Therefore, metabolomics can be used in the toxicology assessment,[94] disease diagnosis,[95,96] molecular pathology,[97] and for a number of other important applications.

3.1.4.1 Pharmacometabolomics

The concept of "pharmacometabolomics" was first proposed by Clayton in 2006.[98] From the changes in the metabolome for an individual patient caused by drug administration, pharmacometabolomics can provide a detailed mapping of drug effects on certain metabolic mechanistic pathways implicated in a patient's individual treatment response. Such metabolic profiles represent a complete overview of individual metabolite or pathway alterations, providing a more detailed biochemical depiction of disease phenotypes. This approach can be applied to the prediction of response to pharmaceuticals by patients with a particular metabolic profile.

Personalized medicine is a very important application of pharmacometabolomics. Prior to drug administration, the metabolic phenotype of an individual patient is studied and employed in a predictive manner to determine the potential responses of therapeutic agents. In 2006, Clayton[98] applied ^{1}H NMR-based metabolomics to study an acetaminophen-induced liver toxicity model. For the first time, it was demonstrated that an individual's response to a drug can be predicted by their metabolome, and that there is an association between the predose urinary composition and the extent of liver damage sustained after paracetamol administration. In our group, a metabolomic approach was proposed to assess the feasibility of chemosensitivity prediction in a mouse xenograft model of human gastric cancer. Based on the data of metabolic profiles and the k-nearest neighbor algorithm, a prediction model for chemosensitivity was developed. An average accuracy of 90.4% was achieved, suggesting that pharmacometabolomics can be used for chemosensitivity prediction in the treatment of cancer.[99] In addition to personalized medicine, pharmacometabolomics is also a powerful tool for drug toxicity assessment,[100,101] pharmaceutical efficacy evaluation,[102] and to examine mechanisms of drug action.[103]

3.1.4.2 Lipidomics

Lipids are the structural components of cell membranes, serving as energy storage sources and also participating in many important cellular functions. Clinical studies have established that many critical diseases are associated with disorders in lipid metabolism, such as AD, diabetes, and even some infectious diseases. Studies have shown that mammalian cells contain 1000–2000 kinds of lipids. In 2003, Han and coworkers proposed the concept of lipidomics.[104] The lipidome is the complete lipid profile within a cell, tissue, or organism, and is a subset of the metabolome. Lipidomics is the large-scale study of pathways and networks of cellular lipids in biological systems.[104–106] Although it is often considered as a branch of the more general "metabolomics," lipidomics itself is a distinct discipline due to the uniqueness and functional specificity of lipids relative to other metabolites.

Lipidomics analysis is based on multidimensional LC/MS, and mainly includes the following steps: lipid extraction, separation, detection, identification, quantification, and data processing. Lipids are often extracted by acid, alkali, or a neutral solvent with traditional procedures established by Bligh/Dyer and Floch.[107] The simplest method of lipid separation is the use of thin-layer chromatography (TLC), although TLC has limited resolution capacity; thus solid-phase extraction (SPE) and LC are extensively used. Lipid detection is often conducted by using electrospray ionization or matrix-assisted laser desorption/ionization (MALDI) mass spectrometry. Mass spectrometric identification of lipids is primarily achieved through qualitative analysis and comparative MS^n analysis to authentic reference samples. Further development of the quantitative analysis of lipids is based on isotope labeling. Finally, bioinformatics is used to process the qualitative and quantitative results.

Lipidomics can determine key lipids and enzymes that may suggest potential abnormal pathways or pathogenic mechanisms, and is an effective manner for diagnosis and treatment plan development. In recent years, lipidomics has been increasingly studied, especially in regard to the discovery of diagnostic lipid disease biomarkers,[108] lipid metabolism-related drug targets,[109] and to deduce lipid-associated pharmacological mechanisms.[110]

3.1.5 Other "Omics" Technologies

3.1.5.1 Phenomics

Phenomics is the study concerned with the measurement of the phenome as changes occur in response to genetic mutation and environmental influences. In 1996, the concept was first proposed at the University of Waterloo in a speech. The term phenotype refers to the entire physical and biochemical traits of an organism, including skin color, eye color, weight, and specific individual characteristics. Specific phenotypes result from the combined effects of genetic and environmental factors, and phenotypic variation between individuals may be due to environmental or genetic variation, such as single nucleotide polymorphism-based resistance (SNPs). Phenomics has come to be used to bridge the genotype and phenotype of the organism.

The research on phenomics is mainly performed on a phenotype-microarray platform that enables one to monitor simultaneously the phenotypic reaction of cells to environmental challenges observed on microtiter plates. In 2006, Niculescu and his colleagues proposed PhenoChipping as a quantitative method for phenomics analysis. Phenomics has been mainly used to study genotype-phenotype relationships,[111] the genetic basis of complex traits,[112] and in agriculture for crop improvement.[113]

3.1.5.2 Immunomics

Immunomics studies the response and regulation process of the immune system on pathogens, which deals with all immune-related molecules, together with their targets and functions. Immunomics includes the techniques of genomics, proteomics, and bioinformatics. On the basis of genomics and proteomics research, immunomics makes full use of bioinformatics, biochip technologies, structural biology, high-throughput screening, and systems biology methods to study the immune system and immune responses so as to discover susceptibility-related genes and immune-related molecules.

The immune system shows great diversity compared with other body systems. For such a highly complex system, traditional research methods are largely limited. While immunomics may become a powerful new approach, immunomics is currently applied primarily in vaccine development,[114,115] target identification,[116] and disease diagnosis.[117]

3.1.5.3 Metallomics

Metal elements play an important role in biology despite their relatively low abundance in physiological systems. It is estimated that one third of proteins requires metal ions (usually a transition metal ion, such as copper, iron, zinc, and molybdenum) as a cofactor to perform their biological functions; these are often called "metal proteins." In 2002, Haraguchi proposed the term "metallomics" for the systematic study of metals or metalloid elements in cells, organs, or biological tissues.[118] Metallomics can be defined as the "comprehensive analysis of the entirety of metal and metalloid species within a cell or tissue type"[119] that can be considered as a branch of metabolomics, although metals are not typically considered as metabolites. Metal elements in metallomics include the biological metals combined with biological macromolecules, such as metal proteins, metal enzymes, metal nucleic acid fragments, metal-containing ligands (organic acids, amino acids, etc.), metal polysaccharides, and also free alkali and alkaline earth metal ions. Metallomics aims to reveal the physiological functions and biological effects of the metallome. The key problem is associated with the structure elucidation of a biologically active metallome.

As the most commonly used approaches, inductively coupled plasma mass spectrometry (ICP-MS) and neutron activation analysis (NAA) enable the simultaneous quantitative analysis of multiple elements.[120] Synchrotron radiation X-ray microfluorescence analysis (SR-μXRF), and synchrotron radiation microfluorescence beam-based CT, EDX, PIXE, SIMS, and LA-ICP-MS, are also used to study the distribution of the metallome.[121] Metallomics is also applied to the field of environmental research[122] and in drug discovery.[123,124]

3.1.5.4 Cytomics

Cytomics involves research on the structure and function of cellular systems, subsystems, and their functional components at the single-cell level. Cytomics research is often based on genome databases, and also uses genomics or proteomics technologies. Sensitive, noninvasive and fluorescence-based methods are most widely employed in cytomics to conduct the integrated analysis of a single cell. The comprehensive analysis of cell morphology can be performed according to cell fluorescence quantitative data and cell imaging. Currently, the cytomics technologies include flow cytometry, laser capture microdissection (LCM), confocal laser scanning microscopy (CLSM), laser scanning cytometry (LSC), high-content screening (HCS), and bioimaging.

Cytomics provides new strategies and effective approaches to pharmaceutical research, such as in target validation,[125] drug development[126] and pharmacological and toxicological evaluation[127] as well as establishing the potential clinical efficacy of predictive and personalized medicine.[128]

3.1.5.5 Ionomics

It is generally known that ions play a crucial role in all biological functions within an organism, especially in energy metabolism, enzyme activity, intracellular signaling, and biochemical transportation. In 2003, Salt and colleagues proposed the concept of ionomics.[129] Ionomics studies the measurement and biological processes of elementals of an organism to address biological problems. Various techniques can be used to measure the elemental composition in ionomics. The most important methods are inductively coupled plasma-mass spectrometry (ICP-MS), X-ray fluorescence (XRF), inductively coupled plasma optical emission spectroscopy (ICP-OES), synchrotron-based microXRF, and NAA.[130] Ionomics is currently applied to the fields of functional genomics,[131] modern plant nutrition studies,[132] and in other research areas.

3.1.5.6 Interactomics

The interactome is the whole set of molecular interactions that occur within a particular cell. The term interactome was originally coined in 1999 by a group of French scientists headed by Bernard Jacq,[133] and is often described in terms of biological networks. Interactomics is a discipline at the intersection of bioinformatics and biology that deals with studying both the interactions and the consequences of those interactions between and among proteins and other molecules within a cell.[133] Molecular interactions can occur between molecules belonging to different biochemical families or within a given family, such as proteins, nucleic acids, lipids, and carbohydrates. Interactomes may be described as biological networks, and most commonly, interactome refers to protein–protein interaction (PPI) network and protein-DNA interaction networks (also called gene regulatory networks), or subsets thereof. Therefore, a typical interactome includes transcription factors, chromatin regulatory proteins, and their target genes. Interactomics aims to compare such networks of interactions between and within species in order to discover patterns of network preservation and/or variation. Interactomic methods are currently being used to predict the function of proteins with no known function, especially in the field of drug discovery.[134]

3.2. APPLICATION OF SYSTEMS BIOLOGY IN THE RESEARCH OF TCM FORMULAE

Systems biology has gained worldwide attention. Currently, the production of large "omics" data sets has become routine, and pharmaceutical research has entered into this burgeoning omics era. Pharmaceutical research increasingly relies on genomics, transcriptomics, proteomics, and metabolomics, and even the combination of multiple omics technologies. In almost every aspect of pharmaceutical research and drug development, including drug target discovery, efficacy evaluation, safety assessment, drug mechanism research, and personalized medicine, omics techniques can be used as efficient and powerful tools.

Omics research is the most essential part of systems and network biology, and omics methods make it possible to more fully understand the pathological disease processes as well as to reveal the important pathways and possible mechanisms involved in pharmaceutical action and therapy. Moreover, omics studies may highlight potential new therapeutic targets for drug development and allow for efficient safety assessments targeted to increasingly personal medicine. Omics techniques have been extensively applied to TCM and other ethnomedical practices. Because of its overall global approach to analysis, omics-based methods fulfill many of the requirements needed to study even the most complicated areas of research, such as TCM. Therefore, omics technologies have come to be recognized as powerful methods in modern pharmaceutical research, and are especially suited for the study of TCM formulae.

3.2.1 Action Mechanisms of TCM Formulae

The rapid development of systems biology provides new ideas for TCM formulae research, and exciting progress has been made in this regard. Chen and Chen[135] applied proteomics to investigate the therapeutic mechanisms of the TCM product Realgar-Indigo naturalis formula (RIF) on murine and cell-based models of APL. These studies suggested that RIF tablets produced multitargeted synergistic effects to achieve enhanced activity for the treatment of APL.

Bai and coworkers[136] applied a network pharmacology-based approach to clarify the antiinflammatory and antitussive (cough suppressing) mechanisms of the Chinese medicinal preparation Chuanbei Pipa Dropping Pills (CBPP). The chemical constituents of CBPP were identified by UPLC/Q-TOF-MS, and potential antiinflammatory ingredients were selected and analyzed using bioinformatics to predict the target proteins and target-related pathways, respectively. Following RNA-sequencing (RNA-Seq) analysis to investigate differential gene expression patterns in the lung tissue of rats with chronic bronchitis, it was found that six primary constituents affected 19 different pathways. The expression of 34 genes involved in different therapeutic functions was significantly decreased following CBPP treatment: immunosuppression, antiinflammation action, collagen formation, and muscle contraction. The active components acted on the mitogen-activated protein kinase (MAPK) and TGF-β pathways, altered focal adhesion, and tightened junctions and the cytoskeletal action to exert antiinflammatory effects, resolve phlegm, and relieve cough. This novel global chemomics-integrated systems biology approach represents an effective and increasingly accurate strategy for the study of TCM that often involves the interplay between multiple components with multiple target mechanisms (Fig. 3.2).

Sheng-ma-bie-jia-tang (SMBJT) is a TCM formula that is widely used in China for the treatment of systemic lupus erythematosus (SLE). However, no molecular mechanisms have been identified for SMBJT. Huang[137] systematically analyzed targets of the ingredients in SMBJT to evaluate its potential molecular mechanism. First, 1267 potential targets were collected from the Traditional Chinese Medicine Integrated Database (TCMID). They performed gene ontology and pathway enrichment analyses for these targets and determined that they were enriched in metabolism (amino acids, fatty acids, etc.) and signaling pathways (chemokines, Toll-like receptors, adipocytokines, etc.). Ninety-six targets, which are known SLE disease proteins, were identified as essential targets and the remaining 1171 targets were defined as common targets of this formula. The essential targets directly interacted with SLE disease proteins. In addition, some common targets also exhibited essential connections to both key targets and SLE disease proteins in enriched signaling pathways, such as the toll-like receptor-signaling pathway. The study found distinct functions of essential and common targets in immune system processes. This multilevel approach to decipher the underlying mechanisms responsible for the efficacy of SMBJT in the treatment of SLE illustrates the enormous potential of such methods to help increase our understanding of TCM formulae.

Jia[138–140] conducted GC/MS- and LC/MS-based metabolomic analysis of kidney and liver tissues from animal models to investigate disease pathology, potential TCM efficacy, and toxicity, and suggested that metabolomic studies can play an important role in TCM research. Genomics primarily relies on microarray techniques, which can be used to study TCM formulae that are typically characterized by multicomponent and multi-targeted mechanistic processes.[141] Luo[142] used a gene chip-based system to study the Shuanglong prescription, identifying a gene network regulated by the major active components in the Shuanglong prescription that was associated with its efficacy in the treatment of myocardial infarction.

Luo[143] postulated that, in the human body, the process through which TCM formulae exert their pharmacological effects can be regarded as biological interactions between two complicated systems—an intervention system (TCM) and a response system (human body)—and that systems biology methods should be applied in combination with bioinformatics and network biology so as to clarify TCM mechanisms that synergistically integrate multiple components, pathways, and targets. Based on patterns of treatment similarity, chemical structure similarity, and PPI networks, Li[144] developed the drugCIPHER tool for drug target identification. Xu[145] studied the interactions between active TCM components and targets in the treatment of chronic kidney disease, and found that molecular docking and network pharmacology methods can be used to rapidly screen for

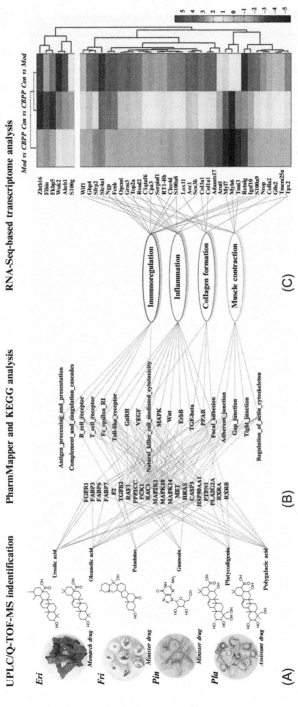

Fig. 3.2 Pathway prediction and RNA-Seq analysis of CBPP. (A) Structures of five representative active compounds that were identified by UPLC/Q-TOF-MS; (B) Main targets and pathways as analyzed by PharmMapper and KEGG, respectively (network analysis); (C) RNA-Seq-based transcriptome analysis by clustering and the functional classification of 34 up-regulated genes.[136]

bioactive TCM compounds and in target discovery, which can provide an important means for both basic TCM research and new drug development.

The emergence and continuous advancement of many forms of biological information databases provide a wealth of resources for the construction of biological networks. Large institutions have established gene, protein, and metabolite databases (see Table 3.1). For example, the OMIM database collects known human genetic diseases and disease-related genes; the DrugBank database contains detailed drug and drug target information; the HPRD database collects human protein interaction information; and the KEGG database is a relatively complete collection of biochemical metabolic reaction data. These databases are valuable resources for the study of TCM formulae mechanisms through the application of systems and network biology.

3.2.2 The Concept of a Syndrome in TCM

The formal concept of "syndrome," in relation to TCM, was first proposed in the second National Conference on TCM syndromes in 1986.[146] In Chinese medicine, as in western medicine, the term "syndrome" is used to specifically describe a relatively fuzzy concept or condition that lacks uniform, objective, qualitative, or quantitative indicators. Scientific methods to define and characterize such phenomena described in TCM as syndromes have met with little success. However, compared with traditional research approaches, metabolomic-based methods hold great promise as more efficient tools to help understand such conditions.

Shen[147] used an aging rat model to study physiological kidney deficiency syndrome and its treatment with TCM, and found gene expression variations in the hypothalamus-pituitary-adrenal-thymus (HPAT) axis associated with the aging process and with drug intervention, and numerous sites of molecular network regulation within the HPAT axis. Li et al.[148] used metabolomics to examine the syndrome known as blood stasis due to the Qi Deficit syndrome (QDBS). Urine samples from QDBS rats and control rats were comparatively analyzed with ^1H NMR. It was found that the metabolic profile of QDBS rats was significantly different from that of the control rats. This analysis included a series of related biomarkers, especially formate, creatinine, and citrate, which showed significant changes in levels, indicating that the syndrome may be associated with basic biochemical metabolic pathways. Using a nontargeted metabolomics method, Wang and colleagues[149] discovered potential biomarkers associated with jaundice syndrome (JS) which are also used in its diagnosis. Multivariate data analysis was used to identify potential biomarkers. Forty-four JS-associated marker metabolites were shown to be distinctly different in JS, relative to healthy controls. Metabolic pathways involving the metabolism and synthesis of alanine, aspartate, and glutamate, and pathways related to ketone degradation were found to be dysregulated in JS patients. Such studies demonstrate the

Table 3.1 Examples of important human gene, protein, and metabolism databases

Category	Database	URL	Remarks
Gene	Ensembl	http://www.ensemble.org/	Ensembl annotate genes, computes multiple alignments, predicts regulatory function, and collects disease data
	HGNC	http://www.genenames.org.org/	HGNC is responsible for approving unique symbols and names for human loci, including protein coding genes, RNA genes, and pseudogenes, to allow unambiguous scientific communication
	Entrez Gene	http://www.ncbi.nlm.nih.gov/ sites/entrez?db=gene	Entrez Gene is NCBI's repository for gene-specific information, including DDBJ, EMBL, GenBank, OMIM, etc.
	HGMD	http://archive.uwcm.ac.uk/uwcm/ mg/hgmd/search.htL	The Human Gene Mutation Database (HGMD) represents an attempt to collate known (published) gene lesions responsible for human inherited disease
Protein	Uniprot	http://www.uniprot.org/	UniProt provide the scientific community with a large, comprehensive, high quality, and freely accessible resource for protein sequence and functional information
	SWISS-PROT	http://us.expasy.org/sprot/	The Swiss-Prot is the best-annotated protein database and as such is an absolute requirement in the toolbox of any protein chemist. The database is maintained by SIB and EBI
	PIR	http://pir.georgetown.edu/	The world's first database of classified and functionally annotated protein sequences
	HPRD	http://www.hprd.org	Human Protein Reference Database, a database of curated proteomic information pertaining to human proteins

Continued

Table 3.1 Examples of important human gene, protein, and metabolism databases—cont'd

Category	Database	URL	Remarks
Metabolites	Metlin	http://metlin.scripps.edu/	METLIN includes an annotated list of known metabolite structural information that is easily cross-correlated with its catalogue of high-resolution Fourier transform mass spectrometry spectra, tandem mass spectrometry spectra, and LC/MS data
	HMDB (human metabolome database)	http://www.hmdb.ca/	The Human Metabolome Database is a freely available electronic database containing detailed information about small-molecule metabolites found in the human body
	GMD (the Golm Metabolome Database)	http://gmd.mpimp-golm.mpg.de/	The Golm Metabolome Database facilitates the search for and dissemination of reference mass spectra from biologically active metabolites quantified using GC/MS
	BiGG Models	http://bigg.ucsd.edu/	BiGG Models: a platform for integrating, standardizing, and sharing genome-scale models
Pathway	KEGG	http://www.genome.ad.jp/kegg/	Kyoto Encyclopedia of Genes and Genomes, a database resource for understanding high-level functions and utilities of the biological system
	BioCyc	http://biocyc.org/	The BioCyc database collection is an assortment of organism specific pathway/genome databases, and provides reference to genome and metabolic pathway information for thousands of organisms
	HumanCyc	http://www.humancyc.org/	Encyclopedia of Human Genes and Metabolism provides an encyclopedic reference on human metabolic pathways
	Reactome	http://www.reactome.org	A free online database of biological pathways. There are several Reactomes that concentrate on specific organisms. The largest of these is focused on human biology, the following description concentrates on the human Reactome
Drug	DrugBank	http://redpoll.pharmacy.ualberta.ca/drugbank/index.htL	A unique bioinformatics and cheminformatics resource that combines detailed drug information. It contains 8261 drug entries, including 2021 FDA-approved small-molecule drugs, 233 FDA-approved biotech drugs, 94 nutraceuticals, and more than 6000 experimental drugs

potential of metabolomics as a diagnostic tool for diseases and to provide new mechanistic insights into previously undefined pathophysiological processes.

To identify potential plasma biomarker molecules for unstable angina (UA) patients with Qi Deficiency and Blood Stasis syndrome (QDBS), Zhao et al.[150] performed LC-MS analysis on UA patients with QDBS and with no QDBS symptoms, and in healthy control patients. Six possible plasma biomarker proteins were isolated by polyclonal antibody affinity column. Actin were found only expressed, and FN, ApoH and ANXA6 were found highly expressed in plasma of patients with UN-QDBS, suggesting they might be the special molecules for the disease. Moreover, as compared with health persons, SAA, CP, MYH11, and C6 showed high expression, and the six proteins, for example, A1 BG, ApoA4, GSN, HBB, HBD and TF, showed low expression in the plasma of UA-QDBS patients. It concluded that UA-QDBS might belong to a kind of inflammatory reaction. There are simultaneous existence of myocardial injury, blood coagulation factor abnormality, lipid metabolic disorder and oxygen transport obstacle in patients of UA-QDBS. They interact mutually and influence each other. The newly discovered differentially expressed proteins provide clues for the discovery and investigation of potential new therapeutic targets for antiangina drugs. Label-free quantitative proteomics has become an efficient new method for disease and syndrome biomarker research.

Table 3.2 shows examples of the application of systems biology to TCM syndromes.

3.2.3 Active Component Compatibility (or Synergy) in TCM Formulae

In western medicine, the concept of drug compatibility refers to the ability of drugs to not interact with each other in a negative fashion when combined. For example, one agent may promote the chemical degradation or metabolism of the other, one drug may interfere with the pharmacological activity of the other, or one drug may increase the toxicity of the other. In TCM, "compatibility" refers to the concept of multiple agents acting synergistically to enhance the therapeutic benefits of the combination. Nearly all TCM formulae contain two or more materials to produce synergistic effects, reduce side effects, or to otherwise improve therapeutic outcomes. Aconiti Lateralis Radix Praeparata (Fuzi in Chinese) is commonly used clinically as a cardiotonic, antiinflammatory, and analgesic to relieve antimyocardial ischemia through an antihypoxic effect. However, its alkaloidal components may cause toxic reactions such as cardiotoxicity. Thus, it is combined with other Chinese herbs to reduce its toxicity. It is now generally accepted that combining Fuzi and Rhei Radix Et Rhizoma (Dahuang in Chinese) reduce their overall toxicity while synergistically enhancing their effects. However, if TCM compatibility is improper or unbalanced, it will produce toxic effects and even cause damage to the human body. This phenomenon is known a "incompatibility."

Most TCM formulae compatibility research has been based on pharmacology, chemical composition, and pharmacokinetic (PK) studies on the whole formulae and various

Table 3.2 Systems biology research on common TCM syndromes

Corr. author	TCM syndrome	TCM formula	Disease	Sample	Method	Biomarkers	Main conclusion	Ref.
Zhou Wenxia	Kidney Yin deficiency		Diabetes	Patient	Metabolomics proteomics	Creatinine, citrate, TMAO, phenylalanine, tyrosine, alanine, glycine, and taurine	KYDS is associated with alterations in amino acid metabolism, energy metabolism, and gut microflora	151
Chen Jianxin	Qi deficiency Qi Stagnation			Literature	Bioinformatics Network biology	Qi deficiency: CD4, CHAT, EPO, GCG, INS, PTH, PRL, REN, SHBG, and MAOA Qi Stagnation: EGF, EGFR, INS, PRL, SHBG, SNAP25, BDNF, COMT, DRD4, CD4, and IL6	CHD of Qi deficiency pattern emphasizes the imbalance of the immune system, while that of Qi stagnation patients focuses on the imbalance of the nervous system	152
Jia Wei	Kidney Yang deficiency	*Cistanche deserticola*		Rat	Metabolomics		It demonstrated the protective effect of total ginsenosides (TGs) on stressed rats	139
Su Shibing	Damp heat and blood stasis Liver stagnation and spleen deficiency		Posthepatitic cirrhosis	Patient	Microarray	PNP, AQP7, PSMD2	DHAS is most likely related to the system process while the functions overrepresented by LDSDS are most related to the response to stimulus	153

Author	Syndrome	Formula	Disease	Sample	Methods	Biomarkers	Conclusion	Ref
Duan Jinao	Cold coagulation and blood stasis	Shaofu Zhuyu decoction	Coronary heart disease	Rat	Metabolomics Network biology	Urine: 5α-tetrahydrocortisol, 5-dehydro-4-eoxyglucose, 2-phenylethanoid glycoside, hippuric acid, normeperidinic acid glucuronide Plasmar: PC (0:0/18:0), 17-phenyl trinor PGF2α methyl ester, LysoPC (22:6), LysoPC (17:0)	SFZYD did regulate the TCM CCBS by multiple targets, and biomarkers and SFZYD should be used for the clinical treatment of CCBS syndrome	154
Yu Gui	Blood stasis		Angina pectoris	Patient	Microarray	miR-146b-5p, miR-199a-5p, CALR, TP53		155
Wang Xijun	Liver stagnation and spleen deficiency			Patient	Metabolomics	Prolylhydroxyproline, L-cystine succinyladenosine, methionine sulfoxide, kynurenic acid, 2-octenoylcarnitine, adrenaline, α-N-phenylacetyl-L-glutamine	Biomarker-based diagnosis model, over 93% accuracy	156
Wang Xijun	Heart-Qi deficiency	Wenxin capsule		Patient	Metabolomics	Glyceric acid 1,3-biphosphate, 1,3-bisphosphoglycerate, 9(S)-HODE, 9-HODE, 13-HODE, etc.	Glycolysis or gluconeogenesis metabolism, biosynthesis of unsaturated fatty acids metabolism, fatty acid biosynthesis, and purine metabolism networks were acutely perturbed by HQD	157

Continued

Table 3.2 Systems biology research on common TCM syndromes—cont'd

Corr. author	TCM syndrome	TCM formula	Disease	Sample	Method	Biomarkers	Main conclusion	Ref.
Xie Shiping	Lung Qi deficiency		HIV/AIDS	Patient	Metabolomics	Glycyl-L-leucine, L-valine, α-aminobutyric acid, methyl succinic acid, glycine propionyl, etc.	Part of the potential existing markers contributed to the clinical diagnosis of TCM syndrome differentiation of AIDS	158
Liang Heng	Kidney Yang deficiency		Aging	Patient	2-DE proteomics	33 Proteins	33 Proteins potentially related to human kidney Yang deficiency syndromes, and will be helpful to understand mechanism of human kidney Yang deficiency syndromes	159
Song Jiannan	Phlegm stasis		Atherosclerosis	Patient	2-DE proteomics		Variation of functional protein constitution may be the marker proteins for making diagnosis and prognosis of PSS in H&A	160
Jin Guangliang	Phlegm stasis	Xiaoyaosan		Rat	Bioinformatics	GSK3b, St3gal5	GSK3β and St3gal5 related to Phlegm stasis symptom	161

deconstructed formulae.[162] More than 60 commonly used TCM formulae have been examined through a deconstructed or reverse-engineered component strategy,[163] including Guizhi Decoction, Buzhongyiqi Decoction, Buyanghuanwu Decoction, and Rehmanniae Decoction of Six Ingredients.

Systems biology has the potential to reveal the compatibility principles of multiple-component TCM formulae at the molecular level. Thus, it has attracted much attention by TCM researchers. Studies of TCM compatibility require not only investigation of the synergistic effects between various medicinal materials, but must also take into consideration the chemical and physiological stability and reactivity of the potentially active constituents.

The combination of *Salvia miltiorrhiza* and *Panax notoginseng* is a commonly used medicinal pair in TCM practice.[164] It is called a medicinal pair because additional synergistic effects appear when the two herbs are used together. Chen et al.[165] used systems biology approaches to predict the functional networks for the synergistic mechanisms of the *S. miltiorrhiza* and *P. notoginseng* combination. TCMGeneDIT was used for text mining to retrieve association information regarding various genes affected by *S. miltiorrhiza* and *P. notoginseng*. PPI between these genes were obtained from databases and literature searches and visualized using Cytoscape. Differences between networks were identified by the Merge program. Highly connected regions were detected by the IPCA algorithm to infer the significant complexes or pathways in this network. The most relevant functions and pathways were extracted from subnetworks by the BiNGO tool. Twenty-one and 41 genes were found to be associated with *S. miltiorrhiza* and *P. notoginseng*, respectively, including nine common genes associated with both drugs, indicating that 53 genes are only associated with the action of one or the other in combination. Human genomic scale PPI networks consist of thousands of proteins. The subnetworks made up of overlapping proteins between *S. miltiorrhiza* and *P. notoginseng* networks were more than the subnetworks reconstituted by PPI information concerning the nine overlapping genes. A new subnetwork emerged by the network about drug combination removed the *S. miltiorrhiza* and *P. notoginseng* networks. The most relevant functions and pathways extracted from four highly connected regions in the subnetworks were related to apoptosis, cell proliferation, and small G-protein signaling pathways. Taken together, protocols such as the one developed for this study may lead to a deeper understanding of a "whole" system perspective of drug combination mechanisms. In this case, the *S. miltiorrhiza* and *P. notoginseng* combination may act synergistically against coronary heart disease by altering programmed cell death, cell proliferation, and small G-protein signaling pathways.

Trying to address the possible beneficial effects of TCM formulae, Chen[135] used Realgar-Indigo naturalis formula (RIF, also named as Compound *Huangdai* tablets), which has been shown to be very effective in treating human APL as a model. The main components of RIF are Realgar, *Indigo naturalis*, and *S. miltiorrhiza*, with tetra'arsenic tetra-sulfide (A), indirubin (I), and tanshinone IIA (T) as major active ingredients, respectively. The study reports that the ATI combination acts synergistically in the treatment of an in vivo murine APL model and in the induction of APL cell differentiation in vitro. The ATI combination causes intensified ubiquitination-mediated proteasomal degradation of promyelocytic leukemia (PML)-retinoic acid receptor alpha (RAR-α) oncoprotein, strongly reprograms myeloid differentiation regulators, and enhances G(1)/G(0) arrest in APL cells through multiple target perturbation, relative to the effects of the individual agents. Furthermore, ATI intensifies the expression of the aquaglyceroporin, aquaporin 9, and facilitates the transportation of A (tetra-arsenic tetra-sulfide) into APL cells, which in turn enhances A-mediated PML-RAR-α degradation and increases the therapeutic efficacy. The data also indicate that A is the principal component of the formulae, whereas T (tanshinone IIA) and I (indirubin) serve as adjuvants. This study suggests that dissecting the mode of action of clinically effective formulae at the molecular, cellular, and organism levels may be a good strategy to explore the value of TCM (Fig. 3.3).

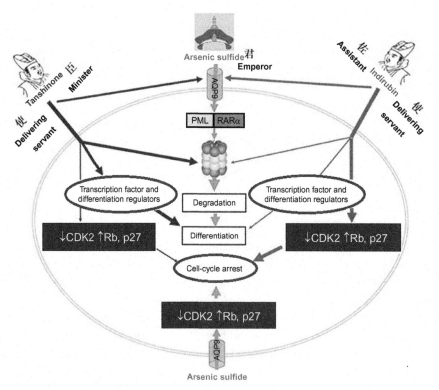

Fig. 3.3 Synergistic effects of RIF TCM formulae. *From http://news.sjtu.edu.cn/info/1002/89738.htm.*

3.2.4 Pharmacokinetic Studies of TCM Formulae

PK and pharmacodynamic (PD) TCM studies draw on pharmaceutical kinetic theory and analytical methods to describe quantifiable interactions and transformations of TCM components, and play an important role in the course of TCM modernization.[166] As suggested by the previously discussed Realgar-Indigo naturalis formula results, it makes sense to clarify the foundation of effective TCM components and pharmacological mechanisms. Use of PK methods could provide great value in the design and optimization of dosage regimens and help facilitate TCM-based new drug development.

Increasing attention is being paid to the scientific evaluation of TCM. As many TCMs are capable of biotransformation in the GI tract, awareness of the capacity of the GI tract-based biotransformation of TCM formulae may lead to the discovery of its active components and their corresponding mechanisms of action. Host metabolic enzymes and intestinal bacteria may be responsible for significant metabolism of TCM components. Increased understanding of the in vivo processes that act upon TCM formulae in the GI tract should help guide the development of metabolic TCM studies that use human-derived in vitro model systems. Such systems will improve our understanding of TCM as safe and effective therapeutic agents.[167]

PK TCM studies began with rhubarb (*Rheum rhabarbarum*) by Qionghua Chen in 1963.[168] Since the beginning of the 1990s, TCM PK has been prosperous, and its results have generated important new theories and methods.[169,170] However, due to the extreme complexity of TCM and the previous lack of interdisciplinary studies on its chemistry, PK, and pharmacology, there remained only vague impressions of the mechanistic material basis of TCM herbal formulae. Currently, most TCM PK studies have only examined the PK profiles of single TCM components, rather than examine the potential interplay between the ingredients as a whole. As a result, validated PK methods used to evaluate single-component known drug entities may not produce accurate results when used to examine materials with unknown components, especially the often complex mixtures used in TCM formulae. However, modern methods need to be adapted to determine the PK and PD profiles of Chinese herbal formulae to clarify the mechanistic basis of TCM and provide science-based direction for the application of these clinically important medications.

Due to the complex mixtures of ingredients in TCM formulae, their mechanisms of action often remain unclear and scientific data to their efficacy and dose-response relationships can lead to a bottleneck in the process of TCM modernization and internationalization. To overcome such limitations will require the integration of Chinese medicine theory, modern data analysis, and data mining technologies to build novel research models to adequately characterize TCM prescriptions. In this light, Zhang et al.[171] provided an overview of TCM serum pharmacochemistry, PK (pharmacodynamics), and systems biology theory and its practice in order to establish an integrated three-dimensional "serum pharmacochemistry-pharmacokinetics (pharmacodynamics)-systems biology" approach for scientific TCM prescription research that will help reveal the pharmamaterial basis, mechanisms of action, and potential synergistic "compatibility" relations with these medicines.

3.2.5 Discovery and Development of TCM-Based New Drugs

In the period between 1981 and 2002, the US Food and Drug Administration (FDA) approved 1031 new small-molecule drugs, of which 5% were natural products and 23% were derived from natural products. In addition, 60% of anticancer drugs and about 75% of antiinfective drugs were found to be derived from natural products or natural product leads. Because of its unprecedented historical success, an increased focus on natural medicine-based drug discovery and development is warranted.

Because of the natural biological and biochemical diversity of herbs, they are essentially naturally occurring chemical libraries composed of vast numbers of potential therapeutically effective phytochemicals. However, effective compound discovery is a painstakingly long and difficult process that depends heavily on an element of serendipity.[172]

The rapid development of systems biology provides an efficient tool to address some of the limitations of natural medicine-based drug discovery. Systems biology has already entered into nearly all areas of new drug development. Various mathematical simulation models have been established based on drug-gene-disease networks, and a series of platforms, including the BioMAP System, BioMAP Database, Connectivity Map, Ingenuity Pathway Analysis, and PhysioLab, have been constructed for new pharmaceutical discovery and development.

Target discovery is one of the most important aims of systems biology research. Microarray mRNA analysis can simultaneously screen and identify drug or disease-related genes by comparing expression data between disease and control groups, which can be used to predict relevant biomarkers and potential drug targets. However, microarray analysis requires complex data processing procedures and extensive validation studies, and can sometime produce less than clear results. One reason for this is because mRNA expression does not necessary correlate with target protein expression and/or function. This can be a limitation for the widespread application of microarrays in drug target discovery and validation. Nevertheless, many successful examples exist,[173] especially in the drug target evaluation of AD,[174] Parkinson's disease,[175] and cancer.[176] Proteomics also can easily distinguish disease-related proteins by comparative analysis of the proteome from normal and diseased cells, and these proteins may lead to potential targets for drug development. Fong et al.[177] found that the cell-surface glycoprotein, TROP2, is a potential diagnostic marker for oral squamous cell carcinoma, and it is anticipated to be used as a target for the discovery of new drugs to treat oral squamous cell carcinoma.

Chemoproteomics is a promising approach that can specifically identify potential drug targets through the observation of protein-biochemical interactions. Small-molecule drugs are used as chemical probes to capture potential target-related proteins that are specifically bound to the probe drug. Through biological functional analysis, these proteins can then be established as probable targets for new drug development. For example, using chemoproteomics, YA29.Eps was discovered as a potential target for an anti-*Plasmodium* drug,[85] and PML-RAR was found to be a target for the treatment of APL.[86]

Toxicology plays a vital role in drug development. Indeed, toxicity is one of the most common reasons for the termination of the drug development process. Pharmaceutical toxicology assessment can guide clinical medication and reduce adverse drug reactions. Over the past 20 years, a series of "omics" technologies have been applied to drug toxicology and this work has promoted the development of various areas for TCM toxicology research.

Bioinformatics and network biology are also widely applied to drug target discovery and development. In a systematic perspective, a protein in a cellular context conducts its function through interaction with other molecules, and therefore a drug may not necessarily have a single molecular target as multiple molecular targets may be involved. Therefore, it is necessary to study drug targets and protein function in a molecular network. Currently, the PPI network is the most common molecular network, which involves complex information on the biological function of proteins. Based on omics analysis and data from related databases, disease-related networks and drug-action networks can be constructed. Comparison of domain-domain interactions and interfaces across an interactome can then guide the identification of selective drug targets or differentiate drugs that target multiple proteins (by blocking parallel pathways within a network).[134] In particular, compounds that interact within core nodes in two separate networks may represent most important molecules that are highly related to disease or drug administration, and may be considered as potential targets.

With growing understanding of disease pathogenesis, multitarget drug design has become an essential component of modern drug development. Scientists increasingly pay more and more attention to the multicomponent and multitargeted aspects of TCM. Systematic pharmacological evaluation of the active compounds in Chinese herbal formulae and the identification of the corresponding drug targets have become critical issues in modern Chinese materia medica and TCM research. However, the TCM drug discovery concepts and strategies that were once used no longer meet the growing demands of current TCM development. The rapid development of systems biology and its associated new technologies are now widely used in Chinese medicine research and development. Computer-aided drug design (CADD) technology shows unique advantages in active ingredients selection, target detection, toxicity prediction, and in clarifying the mechanistic principles of TCM.[178].

REFERENCES

1. Cavalli-Sforza LL. The human genome diversity project: past, present and future. *Nat Rev Genet* 2005;**6**(4):333–40.
2. Kandpal RP, Saviola B, Felton J. The era of 'omics unlimited. *Biotechniques* 2009;**46**(5):351.
3. Wang L. Pharmacogenomics: a systems approach. *Wiley Interdiscip Rev Syst Biol Med* 2010;**2**(1):3–22.
4. D'Alessandro A, Zolla L. Pharmacoproteomics: a chess game on a protein field. *Drug Discov Today* 2010;**15**(23–24):1015–23.
5. Beijer HJ, de Blaey CJ. Hospitalisations caused by adverse drug reactions (ADR): a meta-analysis of observational studies. *Pharm World Sci* 2002;**24**(2):46–54.
6. Garnett MJ, Edelman EJ, Heidorn SJ, et al. Systematic identification of genomic markers of drug sensitivity in cancer cells. *Nature* 2012;**483**(7391):570–5.
7. Visscher H, Ross CJ, Rassekh SR, et al. Pharmacogenomic prediction of anthracycline-induced cardiotoxicity in children. *J Clin Oncol* 2012;**30**(13):1422–8.
8. Qin J, Li R, Raes J, et al. A human gut microbial gene catalogue established by metagenomic sequencing. *Nature* 2010;**464**(7285):59–65.
9. Poinar HN, Schwarz C, Qi J, et al. Metagenomics to paleogenomics: large-scale sequencing of mammoth DNA. *Science* 2006;**311**(5759):392–4.
10. Ley RE, Backhed F, Turnbaugh P, et al. Obesity alters gut microbial ecology. *Proc Natl Acad Sci U S A* 2005;**102**(31):11070–5.
11. Turnbaugh PJ, Ley RE, Mahowald MA, et al. An obesity-associated gut microbiome with increased capacity for energy harvest. *Nature* 2006;**444**(7122):1027–31.
12. Le Chatelier E, Nielsen T, Qin J, et al. Richness of human gut microbiome correlates with metabolic markers. *Nature* 2013;**500**(7464):541–6.
13. Manichanh C, Rigottier-Gois L, Bonnaud E, et al. Reduced diversity of faecal microbiota in Crohn's disease revealed by a metagenomic approach. *Gut* 2006;**55**(2):205–11.
14. Siggers RH, Siggers J, Boye M, et al. Early administration of probiotics alters bacterial colonization and limits diet-induced gut dysfunction and severity of necrotizing enterocolitis in preterm pigs. *J Nutr* 2008;**138**(8):1437–44.
15. Scanlan PD, Shanahan F, Clune Y, et al. Culture-independent analysis of the gut microbiota in colorectal cancer and polyposis. *Environ Microbiol* 2008;**10**(3):789–98.
16. Larsen N, Vogensen FK, van den Berg FW, et al. Gut microbiota in human adults with type 2 diabetes differs from non-diabetic adults. *PLoS One* 2010;**5**(2). e9085.
17. Laird PW. Principles and challenges of genome-wide DNA methylation analysis. *Nat Rev Genet* 2010;**11**(3):191–203.
18. Jenuwein T, Allis CD. Translating the histone code. *Science* 2001;**293**(5532):1074–80.
19. Hake SB, Allis CD. Histone H3 variants and their potential role in indexing mammalian genomes: the "H3 barcode hypothesis" *Proc Natl Acad Sci U S A* 2006;**103**(17):6428–35.
20. Grewal SI, Elgin SC. Transcription and RNA interference in the formation of heterochromatin. *Nature* 2007;**447**(7143):399–406.
21. Fraser P, Bickmore W. Nuclear organization of the genome and the potential for gene regulation. *Nature* 2007;**447**(7143):413–7.
22. Sandoval J, Esteller M. Cancer epigenomics: beyond genomics. *Curr Opin Genet Dev* 2012;**22**(1):50–5.
23. Bradbury J. Human epigenome project—up and running. *PLoS Biol* 2003;**1**(3). e82.
24. Kulis M, Esteller M. DNA methylation and cancer. *Adv Genet* 2010;**70**:27–56.
25. Strahl BD, Allis CD. The language of covalent histone modifications. *Nature* 2000;**403**(6765):41–5.
26. Maskos U, Southern EM. Oligonucleotide hybridizations on glass supports: a novel linker for oligonucleotide synthesis and hybridization properties of oligonucleotides synthesised in situ. *Nucleic Acids Res* 1992;**20**(7):1679–84.
27. Velculescu VE, Zhang L, Vogelstein B, et al. Serial analysis of gene expression. *Science* 1995;**270** (5235):484–7.
28. Brenner S, Johnson M, Bridgham J, et al. Gene expression analysis by massively parallel signature sequencing (MPSS) on microbead arrays. *Nat Biotechnol* 2000;**18**(6):630–4.
29. Morin R, Bainbridge M, Fejes A, et al. Profiling the HeLa S3 transcriptome using randomly primed cDNA and massively parallel short-read sequencing. *Biotechniques* 2008;**45**(1):81–94.

30. Chu Y, Corey DR. RNA sequencing: platform selection, experimental design, and data interpretation. *Nucleic Acid Ther* 2012;**22**(4):271–4.

31. Wang Z, Gerstein M, Snyder M. RNA-Seq: a revolutionary tool for transcriptomics. *Nat Rev Genet* 2009;**10**(1):57–63.

32. Sutherland GT, Janitz M, Kril JJ. Understanding the pathogenesis of Alzheimer's disease: will RNA-Seq realize the promise of transcriptomics? *J Neurochem* 2011;**116**(6):937–46.

33. Fehlbaum-Beurdeley P, Sol O, Desire L, et al. Validation of AclarusDx, a blood-based transcriptomic signature for the diagnosis of Alzheimer's disease. *J Alzheimers Dis* 2012;**32**(1):169–81.

34. Voineagu I, Wang X, Johnston P, et al. Transcriptomic analysis of autistic brain reveals convergent molecular pathology. *Nature* 2011;**474**(7351):380–4.

35. Heidecker B, Hare JM. The use of transcriptomic biomarkers for personalized medicine. *Heart Fail Rev* 2007;**12**(1):1–11.

36. Cui Y, Paules RS. Use of transcriptomics in understanding mechanisms of drug-induced toxicity. *Pharmacogenomics* 2010;**11**(4):573–85.

37. Kandoth C, Schultz N, Cherniack AD, et al. Integrated genomic characterization of endometrial carcinoma. *Nature* 2013;**497**(7447):67–73.

38. Curtis C, Shah SP, Chin SF, et al. The genomic and transcriptomic architecture of 2,000 breast tumours reveals novel subgroups. *Nature* 2012;**486**(7403):346–52.

39. Labbé RM, Irimia M, Currie KW, et al. A comparative transcriptomic analysis reveals conserved features of stem cell pluripotency in planarians and mammals. *Stem Cells* 2012;**30**(8):1734–45.

40. Wilkins MR, Pasquali C, Appel RD, et al. From proteins to proteomes: large scale protein identification by two-dimensional electrophoresis and amino acid analysis. *Biotechnology* 1996;**14**(1):61–5.

41. Anderson NL, Anderson NG. Proteome and proteomics: new technologies, new concepts, and new words. *Electrophoresis* 1998;**19**(11):1853–61.

42. Blackstock WP, Weir MP. Proteomics: quantitative and physical mapping of cellular proteins. *Trends Biotechnol* 1999;**17**(3):121–7.

43. Marouga R, David S, Hawkins E. The development of the DIGE system: 2D fluorescence difference gel analysis technology. *Anal Bioanal Chem* 2005;**382**(3):669–78.

44. Tannu NS, Hemby SE. Two-dimensional fluorescence difference gel electrophoresis for comparative proteomics profiling. *Nat Protoc* 2006;**1**(4):1732–42.

45. Bennett KL, Funk M, Tschernutter M, et al. Proteomic analysis of human cataract aqueous humour: comparison of one-dimensional gel LCMS with two-dimensional LCMS of unlabelled and iTRAQ (R)-labelled specimens. *J Proteome* 2011;**74**(2):151–66.

46. Irar S, Brini F, Masmoudi K, et al. Combination of 2DE and LC for plant proteomics analysis. *Methods Mol Biol* 2014;**1072**:131–40.

47. Stalmach A, Albalat A, Mullen W, et al. Recent advances in capillary electrophoresis coupled to mass spectrometry for clinical proteomic applications. *Electrophoresis* 2013;**34**(11):1452–64.

48. Asara J, Christofk H, Freimark L, et al. A label-free quantification method by MS/MS TIC compared to SILAC and spectral counting in a proteomics screen. *Proteomics* 2008;**8**(5):994–9.

49. Gygi SP, Rist B, Gerber SA, et al. Quantitative analysis of complex protein mixtures using isotope-coded affinity tags. *Nat Biotechnol* 1999;**17**(10):994–9.

50. Zieske LR. A perspective on the use of iTRAQ reagent technology for protein complex and profiling studies. *J Exp Bot* 2006;**57**(7):1501–8.

51. Schwanhäusser B, Gossen M, Dittmar G, et al. Global analysis of cellular protein translation by pulsed SILAC. *Proteomics* 2009;**9**(1):205–9.

52. Chen J, Kähne T, Röcken C, et al. Proteome analysis of gastric cancer metastasis by two-dimensional gel electrophoresis and matrix assisted laser desorption/ionization-mass spectrometry for identification of metastasis-related proteins. *J Proteome Res* 2004;**3**(5):1009–16.

53. Ping S, Wang S, Zhang J, et al. Effect of all-*trans*-retinoic acid on mRNA binding protein p62 in human gastric cancer cells. *Int J Biochem Cell Biol* 2005;**37**(3):616–27.

54. Poon TC, Sung JJ, Chow SM, et al. Diagnosis of gastric cancer by serum proteomic fingerprinting. *Gastroenterology* 2006;**130**(6):1858–64.

55. AK M, Chan YS, Kang SS, et al. Detection of host-specific immunogenic proteins in the saliva of patients with oral squamous cell carcinoma. *J Immunoass Immunochem* 2014;**35**(2):183–93.

56. Kubota D, Yoshida A, Kikuta K, et al. Proteomic approach to gastrointestinal stromal tumor identified prognostic biomarkers. *J Proteomics Bioinform* 2014;**7**(1):10–6.

57. Lim YP. Mining the tumor phosphoproteome for cancer markers. *Clin Cancer Res* 2005;**11**(9):3163–9.

58. LR Y, Issaq HJ, Veenstra TD. Phosphoproteomics for the discovery of kinases as cancer biomarkers and drug targets. *Proteomics Clin Appl* 2007;**1**(9):1042–57.

59. Bolger SJ, Hurtado PA, Hoffert JD, et al. Quantitative phosphoproteomics in nuclei of vasopressin-sensitive renal collecting duct cells. *Am J Phys Cell Physiol* 2012;**303**(10):1006–20.

60. Rinschen MM, MJ Y, Wang G, et al. Quantitative phosphoproteomic analysis reveals vasopressin V2-receptor- dependent signaling pathways in renal collecting duct cells. *Proc Natl Acad Sci U S A* 2010;**107**(8):3882–7.

61. Zhao B, Knepper MA, Chou CL, et al. Large-scale phosphotyrosine proteomic profiling of rat renal collecting duct epithelium reveals predominance of proteins involved in cell polarity determination. *Am J Phys Cell Physiol* 2012;**302**(1):27–45.

62. Feric M, Zhao B, Hoffert JD, et al. Large-scale phosphoproteomic analysis of membrane proteins in renal proximal and distal tubule. *Am J Phys Cell Physiol* 2011;**300**(4):755–70.

63. Gonzales PA, Pisitkun T, Hoffert JD, et al. Large-scale proteomics and phosphoproteomics of urinary exosomes. *J Am Soc Nephrol* 2009;**20**(2):363–79.

64. Hoffert JD, Pisitkun T, Wang G, et al. Quantitative phosphoproteomics of vasopressin-sensitive renal cells: regulation of aquaporin-2 phosphorylation at two sites. *Proc Natl Acad Sci U S A* 2006;**103**(18):7159–64.

65. Tissot B, North SJ, Ceroni A, et al. Glycoproteomics: past, present and future. *FEBS Lett* 2009;**583**(11):1728–35.

66. Hagglund P, Bunkenborg J, Elortza F, et al. A new strategy for identification of N-glycosylated proteins and unambiguous assignment of their glycosylation sites using HILIC enrichment and partial deglycosylation. *J Proteome Res* 2004;**3**(3):556–66.

67. Yang Z, Hancock WS. Approach to the comprehensive analysis of glycoproteins isolated from human serum using a multi-lectin affinity column. *J Chromatogr A* 2004;**1053**(1–2):79–88.

68. Hirabayashi J, Hayama K, Kaji H, et al. Affinity capturing and gene assignment of soluble glycoproteins produced by the nematode *Caenorhabditis elegans*. *J Biochem* 2002;**132**(1):103–14.

69. Madera M, Mechref Y, Klouckova I, et al. Semiautomated high-sensitivity profiling of human blood serum glycoproteins through lectin preconcentration and multidimensional chromatography/tandem mass spectrometry. *J Proteome Res* 2006;**5**(9):2348–63.

70. Kameyama A, Kikuchi N, Nakaya S, et al. A strategy for identification of oligosaccharide structures using observational multistage mass spectral library. *Anal Chem* 2005;**77**(15):4719–25.

71. Yen TY, Haste N, Timpe LC, et al. Using a cell line breast cancer progression system to identify biomarker candidates. *J Proteome* 2014;**96**:173–83.

72. Ahn JM, Sung HJ, Yoon YH, et al. Integrated glycoproteomics demonstrates fucosylated serum paraoxonase 1 alterations in small cell lung cancer. *Mol Cell Proteomics* 2014;**13**(1):30–48.

73. Bones J, Byrne JC, O'Donoghue N, et al. Glycomic and glycoproteomic analysis of serum from patients with stomach cancer reveals potential markers arising from host defense response mechanisms. *J Proteome Res* 2011;**10**(3):1246–65.

74. Wu J, Xie X, Liu Y, et al. Identification and confirmation of differentially expressed fucosylated glycoproteins in the serum of ovarian cancer patients using a lectin array and LC-MS/MS. *J Proteome Res* 2012;**11**(9):4541–52.

75. Ito K, Kuno A, Ikehara Y, et al. LecT-Hepa, a glyco-marker derived from multiple lectins, as a predictor of liver fibrosis in chronic hepatitis C patients. *Hepatology* 2012;**56**(4):1448–56.

76. Butterfield DA, Owen JB. Lectin-affinity chromatography brain glycoproteomics and Alzheimer disease: insights into protein alterations consistent with the pathology and progression of this dementing disorder. *Proteomics Clin Appl* 2011;**5**(1–2):50–6.

77. Strassberger V, Fugmann T, Neri D, et al. Chemical proteomic and bioinformatic strategies for the identification and quantification of vascular antigens in cancer. *J Proteome* 2010;**73**(10):1954–73.

78. Adam GC, Sorensen EJ, Cravatt BF. Chemical strategies for functional proteomics. *Mol Cell Proteomics* 2002;**1**(10):781–90.

79. Terstappen GC, Schlupen C, Raggiaschi R, et al. Target deconvolution strategies in drug discovery. *Nat Rev Drug Discov* 2007;**6**(11):891–903.

80. Lomenick B, Olsen RW, Huang J. Identification of direct protein targets of small molecules. *ACS Chem Biol* 2010;**6**(1):34–46.

81. Sato S-i, Murata A, Shirakawa T, et al. Biochemical target isolation for novices: affinity-based strategies. *Chem Biol* 2010;**17**(6):616–23.

82. Lomenick B, Hao R, Jonai N, et al. Target identification using drug affinity responsive target stability (DARTS). *Proc Natl Acad Sci U S A* 2009;**106**(51):21984–9.

83. Huang J, Zhu H, Haggarty SJ, et al. Finding new components of the target of rapamycin (TOR) signaling network through chemical genetics and proteome chips. *Proc Natl Acad Sci U S A* 2004;**101**(47):16594–9.

84. Barabasi A-L, Oltvai ZN. Network biology: understanding the cell's functional organization. *Nat Rev Genet* 2004;**5**(2):101–13.

85. Greenbaum DC, Baruch A, Grainger M, et al. A role for the protease falcipain 1 in host cell invasion by the human malaria parasite. *Science* 2002;**298**(5600):2002–6.

86. Zhang XW, Yan XJ, Zhou ZR, et al. Arsenic trioxide controls the fate of the PML-RARalpha oncoprotein by directly binding PML. *Science* 2010;**328**(5975):240–3.

87. Nicholson JK. Global systems biology, personalized medicine and molecular epidemiology. *Mol Syst Biol* 2006;**2**:52.

88. Trygg J, Holmes E, Lundstedt T. Chemometrics in metabonomics. *J Proteome Res* 2007;**6**(2):469–79.

89. Smith CA, Want EJ, O'Maille G, et al. XCMS: processing mass spectrometry data for metabolite profiling using nonlinear peak alignment, matching, and identification. *Anal Chem* 2006;**78**(3):779–87.

90. Tautenhahn R, Patti GJ, Rinehart D, et al. XCMS online: a web-based platform to process untargeted metabolomic data. *Anal Chem* 2012;**84**(11):5035–9.

91. Katajamaa M, Miettinen J, Orešič M. MZmine: toolbox for processing and visualization of mass spectrometry based molecular profile data. *Bioinformatics* 2006;**22**(5):634–6.

92. Lommen A. MetAlign: interface-driven, versatile metabolomics tool for hyphenated full-scan mass spectrometry data preprocessing. *Anal Chem* 2009;**81**(8):3079–86.

93. Baran R, Kochi H, Saito N, et al. MathDAMP: a package for differential analysis of metabolite profiles. *BMC Bioinformatics* 2006;**7**:530.

94. Robertson DG. Metabonomics in toxicology: a review. *Toxicol Sci* 2005;**85**(2):809–22.

95. Sabatine MS, Liu E, Morrow DA, et al. Metabolomic identification of novel biomarkers of myocardial ischemia. *Circulation* 2005;**112**(25):3868–75.

96. Zhang A, Sun H, Yan G, et al. Metabolomics in diagnosis and biomarker discovery of colorectal cancer. *Cancer Lett* 2014;**345**(1):17–20.

97. Denkert C, Budczies J, Weichert W, et al. Metabolite profiling of human colon carcinoma – deregulation of TCA cycle and amino acid turnover. *Mol Cancer* 2008;**7**(72):1476–4598.

98. Clayton TA, Lindon JC, Cloarec O, et al. Pharmaco-metabonomic phenotyping and personalized drug treatment. *Nature* 2006;**440**(7087):1073–7.

99. Wang X, Yan SK, Dai WX, et al. A metabonomic approach to chemosensitivity prediction of cisplatin plus 5-fluorouracil in a human xenograft model of gastric cancer. *Int J Cancer* 2010;**127**(12):2841–50.

100. Amacher DE. The discovery and development of proteomic safety biomarkers for the detection of drug-induced liver toxicity. *Toxicol Appl Pharmacol* 2010;**245**(1):134–42.

101. Klawitter J, Haschke M, Kahle C, et al. Toxicodynamic effects of ciclosporin are reflected by metabolite profiles in the urine of healthy individuals after a single dose. *Br J Clin Pharmacol* 2010;**70**(2):241–51.

102. Ichikawa W. Prediction of clinical outcome of fluoropyrimidine-based chemotherapy for gastric cancer patients, in terms of the 5-fluorouracil metabolic pathway. *Gastric Cancer* 2006;**9**(3):145–55.

103. Howells DW, Sena ES, O'Collins V, et al. Improving the efficiency of the development of drugs for stroke. *Int J Stroke* 2012;**7**(5):371–7.

104. Han X, Gross RW. Global analyses of cellular lipidomes directly from crude extracts of biological samples by ESI mass spectrometry: a bridge to lipidomics. *J Lipid Res* 2003;**44**(6):1071–9.

105. Wenk MR. The emerging field of lipidomics. *Nat Rev Drug Discov* 2005;**4**(7):594–610.

106. Watson AD. Thematic review series: systems biology approaches to metabolic and cardiovascular disorders. Lipidomics: a global approach to lipid analysis in biological systems. *J Lipid Res* 2006;**47**(10):2101–11.
107. Bligh EG, Dyer WJ. A rapid method of total lipid extraction and purification. *Can J Biochem Physiol* 1959;**37**(8):911–7.
108. Wenk MR. Lipidomics in drug and biomarker development. *Expert Opin Drug Discovery* 2006;**1**(7):723–36.
109. Marechal E, Riou M, Kerboeuf D, et al. Membrane lipidomics for the discovery of new antiparasitic drug targets. *Trends Parasitol* 2011;**27**(11):496–504.
110. Adibhatla RM, Hatcher JF, Dempsey RJ. Lipids and lipidomics in brain injury and diseases. *AAPS J* 2006;**8**(2):E314–321.
111. Bilder RM, Sabb FW, Cannon TD, et al. Phenomics: the systematic study of phenotypes on a genome-wide scale. *Neuroscience* 2009;**164**(1):30–42.
112. Joy T, Hegele RA. Genetics of metabolic syndrome: is there a role for phenomics? *Curr Atheroscler Rep* 2008;**10**(3):201–8.
113. Finkel E. With 'Phenomics', plant scientists hope to shift breeding into overdrive. *Science* 2009;**325**(5939):380–1.
114. Pizza M, Scarlato V, Masignani V, et al. Identification of vaccine candidates against serogroup B meningococcus by whole-genome sequencing. *Science* 2000;**287**(5459):1816–20.
115. Bambini S, Rappuoli R. The use of genomics in microbial vaccine development. *Drug Discov Today* 2009;**14**(5–6):252–60.
116. He Y. Omics-based systems vaccinology for vaccine target identification. *Drug Dev Res* 2012;**73**(8):559–68.
117. Bulman A, Neagu M, Constantin C. Immunomics in skin cancer-improvement in diagnosis, prognosis and therapy monitoring. *Curr Proteomics* 2013;**10**(3):202.
118. Haraguchi H. Metallomics as integrated biometal science. *J Anal At Spectrom* 2004;**19**(1):5–14.
119. Szpunar J. Advances in analytical methodology for bioinorganic speciation analysis: metallomics, metalloproteomics and heteroatom-tagged proteomics and metabolomics. *Analyst* 2005;**130**(4):442–65.
120. Chéry CC, Günther D, Cornelis R, et al. Detection of metals in proteins by means of polyacrylamide gel electrophoresis and laser ablation-inductively coupled plasma-mass spectrometry: application to selenium. *Electrophoresis* 2003;**24**(19–20):3305–13.
121. Carmona A, Cloetens P, Devès G, et al. Nano-imaging of trace metals by synchrotron X-ray fluorescence into dopaminergic single cells and neurite-like processes. *J Anal At Spectrom* 2008;**23**(8):1083–8.
122. González-Fernández M, García-Barrera T, Arias-Borrego A, et al. Metallomics integrated with proteomics in deciphering metal-related environmental issues. *Biochimie* 2009;**91**(10):1311–7.
123. Sun X, Tsang C-N, Sun H. Identification and characterization of metallodrug binding proteins by (metallo) proteomics. *Metallomics* 2009;**1**(1):25–31.
124. Yan XD, Pan LY, Yuan Y, et al. Identification of platinum-resistance associated proteins through proteomic analysis of human ovarian cancer cells and their platinum-resistant sublines. *J Proteome Res* 2007;**6**(2):772–80.
125. Schooley K, Zhu P, Dower SK, et al. Regulation of nuclear translocation of nuclear factor-kappaB relA: evidence for complex dynamics at the single-cell level. *Biochem J* 2003;**369**(Pt 2):331–9.
126. Valet G. Cytomics as a new potential for drug discovery. *Drug Discov Today* 2006;**11**(17):785–91.
127. Jang YJ, Jeon OH, Kim DS. Saxatilin, a snake venom disintegrin, regulates platelet activation associated with human vascular endothelial cell migration and invasion. *J Vasc Res* 2007;**44**(2):129–37.
128. Shanks RH, Rizzieri DA, Flowers JL, et al. Preclinical evaluation of gemcitabine combination regimens for application in acute myeloid leukemia. *Clin Cancer Res* 2005;**11**(11):4225–33.
129. Danku JM, Gumaelius L, Baxter I, et al. A high-throughput method for *Saccharomyces cerevisiae* (yeast) ionomics. *J Anal At Spectrom* 2009;**24**(1):103–7.
130. Young LW, Westcott ND, Attenkofer K, et al. A high-throughput determination of metal concentrations in whole intact *Arabidopsis thaliana* seeds using synchrotron-based X-ray fluorescence spectroscopy. *J Synchrotron Radiat* 2006;**13**(4):304–13.

131. Eide DJ, Clark S, Nair TM, et al. Characterization of the yeast ionome: a genome-wide analysis of nutrient mineral and trace element homeostasis in *Saccharomyces cerevisiae*. *Genome Biol* 2005;**6**(9):R77.

132. Ziegler G, Terauchi A, Becker A, et al. Ionomic screening of field-grown soybean identifies mutants with altered seed elemental composition. *Plant Genome* 2013;**6**(2):1–9.

133. Sanchez C, Lachaize C, Janody F, et al. Grasping at molecular interactions and genetic networks in *Drosophila melanogaster* using FlyNets, an internet database. *Nucleic Acids Res* 1999;**27**(1):89–94.

134. Keskin O, Gursoy A, Ma B, et al. Towards drugs targeting multiple proteins in a systems biology approach. *Curr Top Med Chem* 2007;**7**(10):943–51.

135. Wang L, Zhou GB, Liu P, et al. Dissection of mechanisms of Chinese medicinal formula Realgar-Indigo naturalis as an effective treatment for promyelocytic leukemia. *PNAS* 2008;**105**:4826–31.

136. Tao J, Hou YY, Ma XY, et al. An integrated global chemonics and system biology approach to analyze the mechanisms of the traditional Chinese medicinal preparation *Eriobotrya japonica* – *Fritillaria ussuriensis* dropping pills for pulmonary diseases. *BMC Complement Altern Med* 2016;**16**(1):4.

137. Huang L, Lv Q, Liu FF. A systems biology-based investigation into the pharmacological mechanisms of sheng-ma-bie-jia-tang acting on systemic lupus erythematosus by multi-level data integration. *Sci Rep* 2015;**5**(16):401.

138. Chen MJ, Zhao LP, Jia W. Metabonomic study on the biochemical profiles of a hydrocortisone-induced animal model. *J Proteome Res* 2005;**4**(6):2391–6.

139. Wang XY, MM S, Qiu YP, et al. Metabolic regulatory network alterations in response to acute cold stress and ginsenoside intervention. *J Proteome Res* 2007;**6**(9):3449–55.

140. Chen MJ, MM S, Zhao LP, et al. Metabonomic study of aristolochic acid-induced nephrotoxicity in rats. *J Proteome Res* 2006;**5**(4):995–1002.

141. Auffray C, Chen Z, Hood L. Systems medicine: the future of medical genomics and healthcare. *Genome Med* 2009;**1**(1):2.

142. Wang J, Qian X, Li X, Yang H, et al. Screening and cluster of differentially expressed MSCs genes induced by Shuanglong prescription. *World Sci Technol/Modern Tradit Chin Med* 2007;**9**(3):39–42.

143. G-A L, Q-L L, Y-M W, Q-F L, Li X. A perspective on the development of TCM systems biology. *Chin J Nat Med* 2009;**7**(4):242–8.

144. Zhao SW, Li S. Network-based relating pharmacological and genomic spaces for drug target identification. *PLoS One* 2010;**5**(7). e11764.

145. Zhu W, Qiu XH, XJ X, et al. Computational network pharmacological research of Chinese medicinal plants for chronic kidney disease. *Sci China Chem* 2010;**53**(11):2337–42.

146. Deng ZY. Discussion on the concept of syndrome. *Guangxi J Tradit Chin Med* 1992;**15**(5):35–7.

147. Shen ZY. System biology and research of TCM syndrome. *Chin J Integr Tradit Western Med* 2005;**25**(3):255–8.

148. Li L, Wang J, Ren J, et al. Metabonomics analysis of the urine of rats with Qi deficiency and blood stasis syndrome based on NMR techniques. *Chin Sci Bull* 2007;**52**(22):3068–73.

149. Wang X, Zhang A, Han Y, et al. Urine metabolomics analysis for biomarker discovery and detection of jaundice syndrome in patients with liver disease. *Mol Cell Proteomics* 2012;**11**(8):370–80.

150. Zhao HH, Hou N, Wang W, et al. Study on proteomic specificity of unstable angina with Qi deficiency and blood stasis syndrome. *Chin J Integr Tradit Western Med* 2009;**29**(6):489–92.

151. Jiang N, Liu HF, Li SD, et al. An integrated metabonomic and proteomic study on kidney-Yin deficiency syndrome patients with diabetes mellitus in China. *Acta Pharmacol Sin* 2015;**36**:689–98.

152. Zhai X, Feng XC, Liu JW, et al. Neuro-endocrine-immune biological network construction of Qi deficiency pattern and Qi stagnation pattern in traditional Chinese medicine. *J Biol Syst* 2015;**23**(2):305–21.

153. YY L, Chen QL, Guan Y, et al. Study of ZHENG differentiation in hepatitis B-caused cirrhosis: a transcriptional profilin g analysis. *BMC Complement Altern Med* 2014;**14**:371.

154. SL S, Duan JA, Cui WX, et al. Network-based biomarkers for cold coagulation blood stasis syndrome and the therapeutic effects of Shaofu Zhuyu decoction in rats. *Evid-Based Complalt* 2013;**2013**:901943. https://doi.org/10.1155/2013/901943.

155. Wang J, Yu G. A systems biology approach to characterize biomarkers for blood stasis syndrome of unstable angina patients by integrating microRNA and messenger RNA expression profiling. *Evid-Based Complalt* 2013;**2013**:510208. https://doi.org/10.1155/2013/510208.

156. Zhang AH, Sun H, Han Y, et al. Exploratory urinary metabolic biomarkers and pathways using UPLC-Q-TOF-HDMS coupled with pattern recognition approach. *Analyst* 2012;**137**:4200–8.

157. Wang XJ, Wang QQ, Zhang AH, et al. Metabolomics study of intervention effects of Wen-Xin formula using ultra high-performance liquid chromatography/mass spectrometry coupled with pattern recognition approach. *J Pharmaceut Biomed* 2013;**74**(23):22–30.

158. Q X, Wen G, Wang J, Xie S. Research on urine metabolomics of HIV/AIDS patients with spleen-lung Qi-deficiency based on H-NMR technique. *World Sci Technol/Modern Tradit Chin Med Mater Med* 2015;**17**(2):356–61.

159. X L, Liang H, Tian Z, et al. Comparative proteomic analysis of human kidney-Yang deficiency syndrome serum. *Chin J Biochem Mol Biol* 2007;**23**(7):592–9.

160. Liu JL, Song JN, Lei Y, et al. Differential plasma protein profiles in patients with hyperlipidemia & atherosclerosis of different patterns of phlegm-stasis syndrome. *Chin J Integr Tradit West Med* 2010;**30**(5):482–7.

161. Bo LJ, Jin GL. Bioinformatics analysis of differentially expressed fragments in hippocampus of rats with phlegm-stasis syndrome. *Jilin J Tradit Chin Med* 2012;**32**(5):507–9.

162. Zhang BL, Gao XM, Shang HC, et al. Study on pharmaceutical matters and functional mechanisms of complex prescriptions of Radix Salvial Milti Orrhizal. *World Sci Technol/Modern Tradit Chin Med Mater Med* 2003;**5**(5):14–7.

163. Shang HC, Zhang BL, Wang YY, et al. A method for proportion screening of TCM small prescriptions. *Chin J Exp Tradit Med Formulae* 2003;**9**(3):1–3.

164. Liu QL. Clinical application of *Salvia miltiorrhiza*. *Shanxi J Tradit Chin Med* 2004;**20**(1):51–2.

165. G C, B L, M J, A L. System analysis of the synergistic mechanisms between *Salvia miltiorrhiza* and *Panax notoginseng* in combination. *World Sci Technol/Modern Tradit Chin Med Mater Med* 2010;**12**(4):566–70.

166. Liu CX. Difficulty and hot-points on pharmacokinetics studies of traditional Chinese medicin. *Acta Pharm Sin* 2005;**40**(5):395–401.

167. Liu Y, Yang L. Early metabolism evaluation making traditional Chinese effective and safe therapeutics. *J Zhejiang Univ Sci B* 2006;**7**(2):99–106.

168. Chen QH, Gao SM, XF D, et al. A comprehensive study of Chinese rhubarb: absorption, distribution and excretionof anthraquinone derivatives in rhubarb. *Acta Pharm Sin* 1963;**10**(9):525–30.

169. Huang X, Zang YM, Xia T, et al. A new hypothesis of TCM therapeutic pharmacokinetics. *Pharmacol Clin Chin Mater Med* 1994;**6**:43–4.

170. Xue Y. The theory of traditional Chinese medicine formula. *Chin Pharm Sci* 1997;38–40.

171. Zhang AH, Sun H, Yan GL, Han Y, Wang XJ. Establishment of three-dimensional integrated "serum pharmacochemistry pharmacokinetics (pharmacodynamics)-systems biology" for research of traditional Chinese medicine prescription and its application in Yinchenhao Tang. *China J Chin Mater Med* 2013;**38**(21):3786–9.

172. Wong VK, Law BY, Yao XJ, Ch X, Xu SW, Liu L, et al. Advanced research technology for discovery of new effectivecompounds from Chinese herbal medicine and their molecular targets. *Pharmacol Res* 2016;**111**:546–55.

173. Jayapal M, Melendez AJ. DNA microarray technology for target identification and validation. *Clin Exp Pharmacol Physiol* 2006;**33**(5–6):496–503.

174. Ricciarelli R, d'Abramo C, Massone S, et al. Microarray analysis in Alzheimer's disease and normal aging. *IUBMB Life* 2004;**56**(6):349–54.

175. Grünblatt E, Mandel S, Maor G, et al. Gene expression analysis in N-methyl-4-phenyl-1,2,3,6-tetrahydropyridine mice model of Parkinson's disease using cDNA microarray: effect of R-apomorphine. *J Neurochem* 2001;**78**:1): 1–12.

176. Stam RW, den Boer ML, Meijerink JP, et al. Differential mRNA expression of Ara-C-metabolizing enzymes explains Ara-C sensitivity in MLL gene-rearranged infant acute lymphoblastic leukemia. *Blood* 2003;**101**(4):1270–6.

177. Fong D, Spizzo G, Gostner JM, et al. TROP2: a novel prognostic marker in squamous cell carcinoma of the oral cavity. *Mod Pathol* 2007;**21**(2):186–91.

178. Sun DM, Chen YX, Zeng XH, Huang DE. New model based on systems biology of computer aided drug design for research and development of traditional Chinese medicine. *Chin J Exp Tradit Med Formulae* 2014;**20**(17):223–7.

CHAPTER 4

Network Pharmacology in the Study of TCM Formulae

Jing Zhao*, Dale G. Nagle†, YuDong Zhou†, Weidong Zhang‡
*Shanghai University of Traditional Chinese Medicine, Shanghai, PR China
†University of Mississippi, University, MS, United States
‡Second Military Medical University, Shanghai, PR China

Abstract

To target complex, multifactorial diseases more effectively, a trend has emerged toward the use of multitarget drug development based on network biology as well as an increasing interest in traditional Chinese medicine (TCM) that applies a more holistic philosophy to the treatment to disease. Thousands of years of clinical practice in TCM has accumulated a considerable number of medicinal formulae that exhibit reliable in vivo efficacy and safety. However, for most of these agents, the molecular mechanisms responsible for their therapeutic effectiveness remain unclear. The development of network-based systems biology has provided considerable support for the understanding of the holistic, complementary, and synergic essence of TCM in the context of molecular networks. This chapter introduces available sources and methods that can be utilized for the network-based study of TCM pharmacology, proposes a workflow for network-based TCM pharmacology research, and presents two case studies where the application of these methods have helped to clarify the mode of action of TCM formulae.

Keywords: Network pharmacology, Molecular networks, Signaling pathways, Disease-associated networks, Drug-associated networks.

Traditional Chinese medicine (TCM) has a history that goes back thousands of years. Considerable knowledge has been accumulated concerning the in vivo efficacy and safety of TCM in treating complex chronic diseases. Compared with the often single drug to single target principle of many western medicines, TCM approaches the function and dysfunction of living organisms in a more holistic manner. In TCM theory, disease status is considered as the unbalance of the whole body system, and natural product-based concoctions are formulated to regain the overall system balance. Currently, due to the emerging acceptance of more systems-based multitarget drug development paradigms,[1–5] the field of drug discovery is showing increasing interest in TCM and considers it to be a new source of inspiration.[6–8] However, a huge obstacle for the advancement of TCM is that, in most cases, the mode of action of TCM related to its therapeutic effectiveness is often unknown.

TCM formulae are almost always a complex combination of many natural materials such as plants, animals, and minerals, each of which contains considerable numbers of chemical compounds. Its therapeutic effects primarily depend on the composition and

Systems Biology and Its Application in TCM Formulas Research
https://doi.org/10.1016/B978-0-12-812744-5.00004-7

content of its various effective substances. From the viewpoint of chemical structures, there is considerable overlap between TCM components and the often natural product-derived chemical constituents in western drugs.[9] Therefore, at the molecular level, TCM formulae are multicomponent and multitarget agents, essentially acting in the same way as a combination therapy of multicomponent drugs.[10] It could be deduced that the therapeutic effectiveness of a TCM formulae is achieved through collectively modulating the molecular network system of the body through the actions of its various active ingredients.

The rapid development in "omics" technologies and systems biology over the past decade has facilitated a more systems-level understanding of biological processes that involves the interactions of genes, proteins, and environmental factors. This increased understanding has highlighted new possibilities for the systematic discovery of the molecular mechanisms responsible for the therapeutic efficacy of TCM.[11] Systems biology depicts the complex interactions at multiple levels as various networks and can elucidate the underlying mechanisms of biological systems though the analysis of the networks.[12] Applying network-based systems biology to the study of TCM pharmacology is an exciting new way to help examine the explicit targets of active TCM ingredients and define their function in the context of molecular networks.

Because TCM formulae contain mixtures of complex components, unclear targets, and synergistically integrated regulatory interactions, our research program has proposed a workflow for the systematic network-based evaluation of TCM pharmacology (see Fig. 4.1), which includes four key steps: (1) identification of therapeutically effective TCM compounds; (2) identification of the targets of active TCM compounds; (3) identification of disease-associated genes and construction of disease-related networks; and (4) identification of TCM formulae-regulated signaling pathways and networks and the evaluation of TCM formulae on disease-related networks.[13] In this chapter, we illustrate the workflow according to these four steps and present two case studies.

4.1. IDENTIFICATION OF THERAPEUTICALLY EFFECTIVE TCM COMPOUNDS

While TCM formulae may contain hundreds of ingredients, only a handful of active ingredients truly play therapeutic roles. Therefore, identification of active TCM compounds is a key to understand their mechanisms of action.

To identify the bioactive compounds from the numerous constituents within a complex TCM formulation, the conventional method was to extract and separate its components directly from the TCM, and then to conduct a pharmacological evaluation of each separate component. In this way, the compound astragaloside IV (AGS-IV) was extracted from the TCM material *Astragalus membranaceus* and developed as a drug. *Astragalus membranaceus* has long been used in TCM for the treatment of cardiovascular diseases but its bioactive components remained unknown. Our laboratory isolated AGS-IV from the aqueous extract of *Astragalus membranaceus*, performed a series of

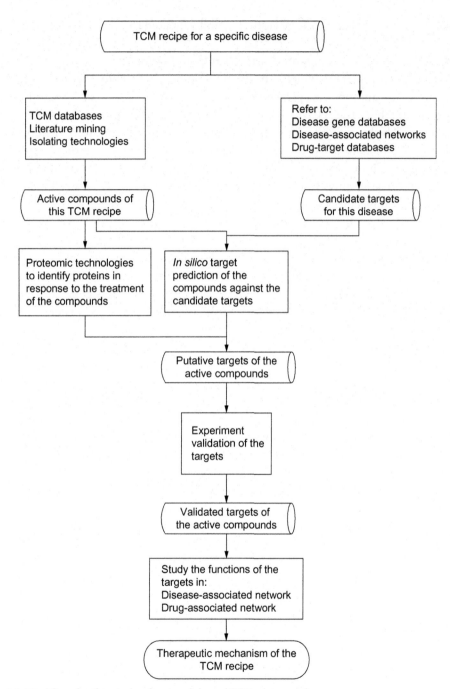

Fig. 4.1 Workflow for the study of network-based TCM pharmacology.

in vivo and in vitro pharmacological studies, and validated the cardioprotective effects of AGS-IV.[14,15]

Because only a few compounds may be responsible for the therapeutic effects of TCM, biochromatography, which is based on biological interactions between bioactive compounds and immobilized proteins, enzymes, and antibodies, has been applied to quickly identify bioactive TCM compounds and eliminate interference by nonbioactive components. The bioactive components in *Artemisia capillaris* Thunb were thereby identified based on their affinity with human serum albumin (HSA), which binds many synthetic drugs.[16] Those of *Radix Angelica Sinensis* were screened out by immobilized liposome chromatography (ILC) which mimics the filtering ability of a cell membrane system to drug molecules.[17]

As most TCM is taken orally, only the components that eventually appear in blood or their metabolites can generally be considered to have the greatest chance of exerting therapeutic effects. A serum-based pharmacological screening strategy was thus proposed to identify the primary components absorbed into the bloodstream following TCM administration.[18] Applying this methodology, we examined rat plasma chemistry after oral administration of the *Shexiang Baoxin Pill* (SBP), a Chinese traditional patent medicine for the treatment of cardiovascular diseases. Twenty-one components, including 17 SBP components and 4 SBP-derived metabolites, were observed from a comprehensive chromatographic analysis of the SBP-dosed plasma relative to control plasma samples. Fourteen of the identified compounds, which were present in high concentration, had previously been reported to have therapeutic effects on cardiovascular diseases.[19] Further studies are underway to identify their targets, investigate their mode(s) of action, and conduct comparative pharmacological evaluations of active compound combinations and with the SBP itself. Along these lines, it may be possible to develop a new multicomponent drug that consists of rational design-based therapeutically enhanced reformulated combination SBP active constituent formulation for the future treatment of cardiovascular diseases.

Databases have been constructed to provide information concerning herb constituents, bioactive compounds, and other aspects of TCM formulae, such as the TCM database,[20] 3D-MSDT,[21] TCMID,[22] and TCM Database@Taiwan.[23] The TCM database includes information about Chinese medicinal plants and 27,593 bioactive compounds.[20] The 3D-MSDT database provides the basic molecular properties and optimized three-dimensional structure of active compounds from 6500 TCM herbs.[21] The TCMID database (Traditional Chinese Medicine Information Database) collects comprehensive information on 46,914 TCM prescriptions, 8159 constituent herbs, and 25,210 herbal ingredients, including molecular structure and functional properties of active ingredients, therapeutic activities and side effects, clinical indications, and related information.[22] The TCM Database@Taiwan database contains information for 453 TCM herbs and >20,000 active compounds.[23] These databases can be data-mined to obtain valuable information about TCM chemistry and its potential therapeutic efficacy. Several reviews describe important approaches and strategies to screen bioactive compounds from TCM formulae.[24,25]

4.2. IDENTIFICATION OF THE TARGETS OF ACTIVE TCM COMPOUNDS

Small-molecule drugs generally perform their therapeutic functions by interacting with activity-associated binding sites on key proteins, thereby influencing their biological function. Therefore, the identification of protein-based molecular targets affected by active TCM components is an essential step to help understand the underlying mechanisms of TCM formulae. Herein, we survey methods used to identify protein-based drug targets.

4.2.1 Proteomic Technologies

The same proteomic methods used to profile drug treatment-induced changes in protein expression and differential patterns of protein expression have proven to be an effective means to identify the potential protein targets of active TCM compounds.[26] From a technological point of view, the most applied tools currently are two-dimensional gel electrophoresis (2-DE) for separation of proteome proteins, and mass spectrometry (MS) for protein identification.[27] Wong et al.[26] provide a detailed review of the use of proteomics to identify the targets of natural products.

4.2.2 Computational Predictions

In silico virtual screening approaches can provide rapid low-cost new ways to predict the targets of active TCM compounds. These methods apply computer-aided drug design technologies to predict potential drug targets through calculation-based simulations of three-dimensional drug molecules-proteins interactions. Inverse docking and chemical similarity searching are currently among the most popular drug target prediction methods.

Inverse docking uses a small-molecule compound as a probe to search possible binders in the candidate target database of known protein structures. It automatically searches for protein cavities derived from three-dimensional structures of all available candidate proteins. An energy value statistically derived from the analysis of a large number of PDB ligand-protein complexes can be used as a threshold for screening likely binders.[28] A protein is considered as a putative target of the compound if the molecule could be docked into the protein and the binding satisfies molecular mechanics-based criteria for chemical complementarity.

In 2013, Timothy Cardozo, a pharmacologist at New York University's Langone Medical Center, presented the "largest computational docking ever done by mankind" at the U.S. National Institutes of Health's High Risk—High Reward Symposium in Bethesda, Maryland. Cardozo's research team chose about 60 million compounds from PubChem and ChEMBL databases and evaluated the binding strength of these molecules with over 7000 distinct structural pockets of 570 proteins.[29] This work eventually created a public website called Drugable (www.drugable.com), which allows researchers to predict potential targets of a compound purely on the basis of chemical structure.

When studying the therapeutic effects of AGS IV on myocardial injury, our group applied INVDOCK inverse docking software to identify 39 potential AGS IV targets.[30] Three targets, calcineurin (CN), angiotensin-converting enzyme (ACE), and c-Jun N-terminal kinase (JNK), were selected for secondary molecular-level validation studies. Our results verified the activity of AGS-IV in these protein targets, but their potencies were weaker than relevant therapeutically used FDA-approved drugs. We further performed cellular level experiments to compare the protective function of AGS-IV and the CN inhibitor, cyclosporin A (CsA), on adriamycin-induced injury in cardiomyocytes. It was confirmed that both AGS-IV and CsA could enhance the repair of adriamycin-induced myocardial cell injury by inhibiting lactate dehydrogenase (LDH) activity. In addition, AGS-IV produced a greater effect at the cellular level. This phenomenon suggests that, at the cellular level, AGS-IV's action on multiple targets may act in a synergistic manner to enhance its effects.

Ganoderma lucidum is a medicinal mushroom used in TCM for the prevention or treatment of a variety of diseases including a number of forms of cancer.[31,32] Triterpenes in *Ganoderma lucidum* have been regarded as the main anticancer active ingredients due to their ability to inhibit growth, induce apoptosis, and cause cell cycle arrest of cancer cells.[33–35] In work by Yue and coworkers, a proteomic approach was applied to investigate the possible targets of the major *Ganoderma* triterpene, ganoderic acid D (GAD), in cancer cells; it identified 21 differentially expressed proteins following GAD exposure.[36] These possible GAD target-related proteins were evaluated using the in silico INVDOCK ligand-protein inverse docking software.[37] Seven of the 21 proteins were found to potentially bind with GAD. The protein-protein interaction (PPI) network between the 21 putative targets was constructed, and the enrichment of a group of proteins called 14-3-3 proteins and their central localizations in this network indicated that they could be important targets of GAD in cancer cells.

The basic assumption of chemical similarity search and screening strategies is that compounds with similar structures tend to target similar proteins.[38] Therefore, for a compound with no known targets, it is possible to consider its potential targets as those of structurally similar compounds.

In 2012, scientists at the Novartis Institute for Biomedical Research used a similarity ensemble approach (SEA) to predict the activity of 656 marketed drugs on 73 unintended potential side-effect-related targets.[39] Their computations predicted hundreds of previously unknown drug-protein interactions, of which nearly half were later confirmed.

When investigating pharmacological mechanisms of the TCM formulae known as Wu Tou Tang on rheumatoid arthritis (RA), Zhang and coworkers first searched the TCM Database@Taiwan database to obtain the chemical structures of 165 Wu Tou Tang-associated compounds. The therapeutic target database (TTD)[40] drug similarity searching tool identified 153 drugs of similar structure that were used to predict 56 potential Wu Tou Tang targets.[41] Li's team proposed an algorithm drugCIPHER to infer drug-target interactions in the context of PPI networks, which integrated drug therapeutic similarity information with chemical similarity data.[42] Applying the chemical similarity module in this algorithm, they predicted the potential targets of 235 active compounds in TCM formulae known as Qing-Luo-Yin.[43] In silico approaches to predict the putative protein targets of small molecules are further reviewed by Jenkins and coworkers.[44]

4.2.3 Database Searching

The DrugBank database,[45,46] TTD,[40,47] SuperTarget,[48,49] Matador,[48,50] and Potential Drug Target Database (PDTD)[51,52] have collected known information on thousands of potential drug targets. The search tool for interactions of chemicals (STITCH) database[53,54] integrates information about the interactions of chemicals with proteins from multiple databases. The information provided by each database has its own focus. Thus, they can add complementary information. For instance, our group searched the targets of the anticholesteremic agent simvastatin in each database with the primary target of simvastatin, HMG-CoA reductase (HMGCR), and produced different results (Table 4.1). The PDTD database focuses on targets with known three-dimensional structures and provides the web server TarFisDock to predict the potential binding targets of a drug

Table 4.1 Comparison of drug target databases

Database	Drug (chemical) no.	Target (protein) no.	Example targets of simvastatin (anticholesteremic agent)
DrugBank	4765	4566	AGT; BMP2; CASP3; CCL2; CD40; COL13A1; CYP3A3; F2; HLA-DRB5; **HMGCR**; ICAM1; IFNG; IL6; IL8; ITGB2; LTB; MAPK3; MMP3; MMP9; PPARA; RAC1; RHOA; SERPINE1; TNF; VEGF
TTD	4198	1675	**HMGCR**; PPARG
PDTD	–	841	–
Matador	801	2901	*Direct interaction*: CYP3A4; **HMGCR** *Indirect interaction*: APOE; COG2; LDL; ENSP00000352471; LDLR; Lipoprotein(a); LPA
STITCH	>68,000	$>1.5 \times 10^6$	LPA; CYP3A4; LDLR; ENSP00000352471; APOE; **HMGCR**; COG2

The primary target of simvastatin, HMG-CoA reductase (HMGCR), is bold and it appears in four databases.

in silico. The TTD databases also permit target similarity and drug similarity searches that enable a user to find potential targets by identifying drug structures that associate with particular protein sequences. These tools provided by the PDPD and TTD databases can be applied to predict the putative targets of the active compound found in TCM formulae. The Matador database is a manually annotated subset of SuperTarget that provides additional binding information and indirect interactions. The therapeutically relevant multiple-pathways (TRMP) database[55,56] integrates information on therapeutic targets and disease-associated signaling pathways.

Databases such as HIT (herbal ingredients' targets database),[57] TCM-PTD (the potential target database of TCM, http://tcm.zju.edu.cn/ptd/), and the TCM Database@Taiwan specifically collect targets of active TCM compounds. The HIT database includes 586 active compounds from 1300 herbs and their 1301 corresponding protein targets, which were manually assembled from relevant literature sources. The TCM-PTD database is a target prediction database for TCM that is based on multiple machine learning algorithms. The TCM Database@Taiwan database contains the structural information of >20,000 compounds from 453 herbs used in TCM.

In our previously described study of the antirheumatoid arthritis (anti-RA) effects of the TCM formulae Huang-Lian-Jie-Du-Tang (HLJDT), we searched the HIT database to yield 91 targets of 14 active compounds. We also searched the Drug-Bank database and extracted all the 32 FDA-approved antirheumatic arthritis drugs and their corresponding 51 protein targets. These drugs were categorized into four classes. We found that HLJDT shares five target proteins with three classes of anti-RA drugs. Such results may help explain the anti-RA effects of HLJDT.[58]

4.3. IDENTIFICATION OF DISEASE-ASSOCIATED GENES AND CONSTRUCTION OF DISEASE-RELATED NETWORKS

In cells, there are many distinct interactions at various levels between genes and gene products. These interactions are deeply linked to the pathogenesis of many diseases. Most diseases, especially complex chronic diseases, are not simply caused by changes in a single gene, but by an imbalance in regulatory networks that results from the dysfunctions of multiple genes or their products.[59–62] On one hand, genes associated with the same disorder tend to share common functional features and can be coexpressed in specific tissues, and their protein products also have a tendency to interact with each other.[62] On the other hand, different disorders are sometimes related to one another through shared disease-associated, genetically linked functional networks or pathways.[62–65] Like molecular network systems,[66–69] physiological and biochemical disease-associated networks also exhibit a certain level of redundancy and robustness.[70] Typically, simply interfering with one single target often cannot change the pathogenic phenotype.[3] Instead, alternative compensatory signaling routes can be activated to bypass the inhibition of a single target protein,[66,70] counteracting the efficacy of the drug and potentially causing undesired side effects. Thus it has come to be recognized that to treat many diseases, drugs must target disease-associated networks rather than disrupt the function of a single protein target.

From a pharmacological perspective, genes and proteins implicated in a pathophysiological process can also be potential drug targets for the therapeutic intervention of that disease process. On the other hand, genes associated with other diseases have little relationship in its treatment. Specifically, network analysis studies indicate a relatively high correlation exists between known drug targets and disease for some categories of diseases, such as endocrine, hematological, cardiovascular, and psychiatric disease, that are closely associated with specific genes. Whereas targets for other disease categories, such as cancer, muscular, skeletal, gastrointestinal, and dermatological diseases, are associated with fewer disease-specific genes.[71] For these latter conditions, other means of disease targeting may be needed.[72] Overall, the identification of disease-associated genes and the construction of disease-related networks have become very important aspects of disease network pharmacology.

4.3.1 Identification of Disease-Associated Genes

Information on specific disease-related genes can be obtained through database query and literature mining. There are many databases that record disease-related gene information, such as OMIM (online Mendelian inheritance in man),[73,74] GAD (genetic association database),[75] and GeneCard.[76] The OMIM[73,74] database contains data on known Mendelian genetic diseases, genetically determined traits, and corresponding disease genes. It also provides information such as linkage, chromosomal localization, structure, and function of disease genes. Unlike Mendelian genetic disorders, complex pathological conditions such as cardiovascular disease, cancers, autoimmune diseases, and metabolic diseases are multifactorial disease processes. They often do not have clear specific genetic disease-associated genes. In these conditions, alteration of specific genes exhibits only a minor contribution to the overall disease process. The GAD database focuses on the information of common complex disease processes with no known gene-specific associations. The information in this database is primarily derived from literature sources. The DisGeNET database[77] is a collection of gene-associated diseases for Mendelian diseases and other more complex diseases. The database is an integration of several expert-annotated databases and literature mining tools. These databases are good resources for obtaining disease-associated genetic information.

4.3.2 Construction of Disease Networks

Within a specific disease process, proteins encoded by multiple genes associated with that disease often interact with each other to form a disease-related network. However, because our understanding of complex diseases is far from complete, we are often unable to identify and assemble the subnetwork processes that may link many of these to disease etiologies within human genomic networks.

Because within a given network, any specific node will first affect its immediate neighbors, the most intuitive way to extract known disease-related genes is to examine their immediate neighbors, together with all interactions between these genes in the network, in order to construct a disease-associated network. For example, when studying asthma, Hwang and coworkers obtained 606 asthma-associated genes by searching the OMIM database and analyzing asthma microarray data from the GEO (gene expression omnibus) database.[78] Extracting these genes and their interactions from the human genomic PPI network constructed from the HPRD database,[79] they assembled an unconnected subnetwork that consisted of 297 separately connected components, 269 of which were single nodes. They then constructed another subnetwork that included the 606 asthma-associated gene nodes and their immediate neighbors. This network contained 2438 nodes, 2256 of which were linked together. Obviously, such networks best reflect interactions between asthma-associated genes. However, immediate neighbors of the same disease gene may have different associations with the corresponding disease. For example, if genes A and B are direct neighbors of one and five disease genes of the same disease, respectively, it becomes obvious that gene B may have a greater degree of association with the disease. Even if both gene B and C have five immediate neighbors of the same disease, if gene B has more direct neighbors than gene C, these two genes exhibit a different level of association with the disease. Therefore, when constructing disease networks, we need to further analyze the topological relationships between disease genes and other nodes within the background networks.

In recent years, many algorithms have been proposed to predict an increasing number of genes that are associated with disease processes. Among them, the basic idea of network-based algorithms is to use known disease genes as "seeds" to score and rank other nodes in the human genome network background, according to their proximity to the "seeds." Higher-ranking genes are predicted as disease-related genes. These network-based algorithms can then be used to construct disease networks. Known disease genes, predicted disease-associated genes, and the interactions between all these genes can be extracted to construct an overall disease network.

Disease gene prediction algorithms quantify network proximity of a given node with seed nodes from multiple perspectives. Earlier approaches, such as the nearest neighbor method[80] and the shortest path method[81], used information of local proximity; whereas later algorithms, such as random walk with restart,[82] PageRank,[83] k-step Markov,[83] network propagation,[84] and Katz-centrality[85] methods applied global network proximity information. Navlakha and coworkers[86] compared multiple prediction methods and showed that the results of the globally based approaches are significantly better than earlier used locally based network algorithms.

Li's team proposed an algorithm called "CIPHER" to predict disease genes that integrated disease similarity information with network node proximity data.[87] Using disease genes that were known to be related to RA in the OMIM database as seeds, they applied this method to predict an expanded number of other potential RA-associated genes so as to construct an RA disease network.[43] To understand the pathogenesis of the disease known as axial spondyloarthropathy (SpA), our group identified 168 SpA-associated genes from the OMIM database as well as proteomic and microarray data. Using these 168 genes as seeds, we utilized the Katz-centrality method to predict other potential SpA-associated genes. Based on a priority ranking of SpA-related genes, we constructed an SpA-specific PPI network, identified potential pathways associated with SpA, and eventually outlined an overview of the biological processes involved in the development of SpA. The PPI network and pathways reflected the interplay between two distinct pathological SpA processes, one involving immune-mediated inflammation and another related to an imbalance in bone remodeling, particularly with respect to new bone formation and bone loss.[88]

4.4. IDENTIFICATION OF TCM FORMULAE-REGULATED SIGNALING PATHWAYS AND THE EVALUATION OF THE TCM FORMULAE ON DISEASE-RELATED NETWORKS

Small-molecule drugs generally perform their therapeutic functions by binding to binding pockets within the structures of proteins, thereby influencing their biological activities. To understand the therapeutic mechanisms of a drug, it is critical to identify the biological processes its targets may participate in, the mechanisms of its drug-target interactions, and its specifically associated target-target interactions. Using network biology methods and techniques to identify signaling pathways and subnetworks regulated by active ingredients in TCM formulae and to examine the interactions between target proteins and the status/role of target proteins within networks can help illustrate the potential impact of TCM-based therapy and better elucidate its mechanisms of action.

4.4.1 Identification of Drug Target-Rich Pathways

Signaling pathways are biomolecule subsystems or subnetworks that perform important biological tasks and process complex signals between molecules. Existing signaling pathway databases such as KEGG[89] and Biocarta contain known signaling pathway information, the constitutive genes, and their recognized interactions. For example, the KEGG database assembles data on >500 signaling pathways with attention to six key aspects, that is, metabolism, genetic information processing, environmental information processing, cellular processes, organismal systems, and human diseases. By simply mapping drug target proteins onto these signaling pathways, we can identify pathways that contain these target proteins. Typically, pathways significantly enriched with drug target proteins are believed to be most likely to be regulated by the drug.

Statistical methods can be used to identify drug target protein-enriched pathways. Hypergeometric cumulative probability distribution is a simple and practical method to quantitatively measure whether a pathway is more enriched with targets that are associated with a particular drug than would be expected by chance.[90] Specifically, if we randomly draw n-samples from a finite set, the probability of getting i-samples with the desired feature by chance obeys hypergeometric distribution:

$$f(i) = \frac{\left(\dfrac{K}{i}\right)\left(\dfrac{N-K}{n-i}\right)}{\left(\dfrac{N}{n}\right)}$$

where N is the size of the set and K is the number of items with the desired feature in the set. Then the probability of getting at least k-samples with the desired feature by chance can be represented by hypergeometric cumulative distribution defined as P-value:

$$P = 1 - \sum_{i=0}^{k-1} f(i) = \sum_{i=0}^{k-1} \frac{\left(\dfrac{K}{i}\right)\left(\dfrac{N-K}{n-i}\right)}{\left(\dfrac{N}{n}\right)}$$

Given the significance level defined as "α," a P-value smaller than α demonstrates a low probability that the items with the desired feature were selected by chance. In our case, if all pathways under study include N distinct genes, in which K genes are the targets of this drug, for a pathway with n genes, a P-value $<\alpha$ implies a low probability that the k targets will appear in the pathway by chance. Thus, the pathway can be regarded as significantly regulated by the drug.

In the study of the mechanisms responsible for the anti-RA of the TCM formula known as HLJDT,[58] our group applied the hypergeometric cumulative distribution method to identify 32 pathways enriched with potential HLJDT targets, including immune system-associated pathways, proinflammatory molecule-related pathways, and osteoclast metabolism pathways. Based on the functions of these pathways and molecular network-based research results related to TCM "cold" and "hot" syndromes,[91] we inferred that HLJDT primarily regulates immune system and bone formation/degradation balance to achieve its therapeutic effects on the hot syndrome RA.

Gene set enrichment analysis (GSEA) defined more specific statistical measures, including enrichment score (ES), normalized enrichment score (NES), false-positive discovery ratio (FDR), and nominal P-value for the identification of pathways enriched with a gene set.[92] The GSEA software that integrates data of common pathway databases is available for free download.

4.4.2 Construction of Subnetworks Influenced by Drugs and Evaluation of the Effects of TCM Formulae

PPI networks between drug target proteins are considered to be a component of drug-affected subnetworks. Similar to the construction of disease networks, target proteins are not necessarily linked together in the genome-wide background network; thus we need to establish reasonable algorithms to determine the nodes and edges within their subnetworks. Herein, we briefly describe several commonly used algorithms.

4.4.2.1 Heuristic Algorithm

The Heuristic algorithm is a class of simple and intuitive methods for the construction of networks, including top-down and bottom-up methods. The top-down method first extracts all target proteins, their immediate neighbors (called bridge nodes), and interactions between all these proteins to build a subnetwork. Then two steps are performed to simplify the network: remove the links between the bridge nodes, and if there are multiple bridge nodes between two target proteins, remove nodes with smaller node degrees. Ultimately, a simplified interaction network between target proteins is constructed. Huang and coworkers applied this approach to build a protein-protein network affected by the active TCM compound artemisinin.[93]

The bottom-up algorithm works from the target proteins. It first calculates the shortest distance of each pair of the target proteins in the background network, and then gradually connects the target proteins by their shortest paths until getting a connected network. The steps are as follows: 1. Connect neighbored target proteins to form a subnetwork; and 2. if the current subnetwork is not connected, starting from the largest connected component, connect it with another component with a length-two path between a pairs of targets. This process is repeated until there is no longer a length-two path between target nodes in different components, and then follows with length-three and length-four paths connecting pairs of target nodes in different connected components. Antonov used this algorithm to make a software PPI spider, which is available for free download.[94]

4.4.2.2 Steiner Minimum Tree Algorithm

The Steiner minimum tree problem is to construct a minimum spanning tree of a network that contains a specific set of seed nodes. Many practical problems can be considered as solving the Steiner tree problem, such as the shortest path between cities, power grid layout planning, and optimal node connection in networks. When the seed node set is taken as the target protein set of a drug, a Steiner minimum tree can be considered as a minimum interaction network between target proteins. Finding a Steiner minimum tree is an NP-complete problem. That is, the time required to solve such a problem using any currently known algorithm increases very quickly as the size of the network grows. Generally, some suboptimal heuristic algorithms are used for generating approximate solutions.

When our group tried to construct a PPI network between the targets of the active TCM compound AGS-IV, we applied the Steiner minimum tree algorithm[57] to identify a minimum subnetwork, which included as many targets of AGS-IV and as few other proteins as possible. Each potential AGS-IV target protein was allowed to interact with other target proteins through no more than one nontarget protein.[30,95]

4.4.2.3 Network Proximity Scoring Algorithm

As previously mentioned, the principle of the network-based disease gene prediction method is to quantify the degree of proximity of a node to disease gene seed nodes, which can be used to construct disease networks. Similarly, when the target proteins associated with a drug are taken as seed nodes, such methods can be used to construct drug-affected networks. An advantage of such a method is that it can use scores given by the prediction algorithm to approximately quantify the impact of the targets on other proteins within the network. In this way, we can get approximate scores that describe the extent of the effects of a drug on all proteins in the network.[58] By extracting proteins whose impact scores are higher than a given threshold and their interactions, we can build a probable drug-affected network.

Most TCM formulae are presumed to exhibit their therapeutic potential through synergistic effects achieved by their diverse components acting on multiple targets. How best to quantitatively verify such synergy and evaluate the ultimate therapeutic effects of TCM formulae are still highly challenging problems in TCM pharmacology research. Li's team[96] proposed a network target-based algorithm NIMS to prioritize synergistic agent combinations in a high-throughput manner. They defined topology scores and agent scores to evaluate the synergistic relationships between each given agent in combinations and applied the algorithm to prioritize potential synergistic agent pairs from 63 agents on a pathological process characterized by alterations in angiogenesis. In our previous study, we applied the inner product between the score vectors of disease effect and drug effect to measure how the drug impacts the human interactome under the influence of the disease. Using this method, we quantitatively analyzed the anti-RA effect of HLJDT and compared it with those of FDA approved anti-RA drugs.[58] It is found that the anti-RA effect score of each HLJDT component was very low, while the whole HLJDT combination achieves a much higher effect score, which is comparable to that of FDA approved antiinflammatory agents. These methods represent the emerging potential of network-based TCM pharmacology to evolve from simple qualitative studies to more definable quantitative research.

4.5. CASE STUDIES

In this section, we present two case studies that use network pharmacology methods to characterize the potential TCM formulae modes in action.

4.5.1 Case Study 1: Antidepressant Activity of St. John's Wort

St. John's Wort (SJW) is prepared as an extract from the plant *Hypericum perforatum* L. Clinical trials have demonstrated that SJW has significant antidepressant efficacy and reduced occurrence of side effects relative to standard pharmaceutically based antidepressants.[97–100] In many countries, SJW is widely used for the treatment of mild to moderate forms of depression and it has been included in the German and US pharmacopoeias.

The main active ingredients of SJW are considered to be hyperforin (HP), hypericin (HY), pseudohypericin (pH), amentoflavone (AF), and several flavonoids (FL).[101] Experimental results have suggested that HP, HY, pH, and AF are able to pass the blood-brain barrier.[102–104] Furthermore, the antidepressant activity of SJW is highly associated with these active compounds.[101,105–109]

We conducted a comprehensive literature search and identified the neurotransmitter receptors, transporter proteins, and ion channels by which the SJW active compounds have been shown to have an effect (see Table 4.2). By mapping these proteins onto

Table 4.2 Effects of single SJW compounds on different neurotransmitter receptors and protein targets

Protein	Gene name	HP	HY	PH	FL	AF
NMDA-receptor	NMDAR	↓[106]				
CRF1 receptor	CRHR1		↓[110]	↓[107]		
5-Hydroxytryptamine receptor 1D	HTR1D					↓[101]
Dopamine receptor D1	DRD1	↓[101]				
Dopamine receptor D5	DRD5	↓[101]				
Dopamine receptor D3	DRD3		↓[101]	↓[101]		↓[101]
Dopamine receptor D4	DRD4		↓[101]	↓[101]	↓[101]	
Delta-type opioid receptor	OPRD1					↓[101]
Alpha-2A adrenergic receptor	ADRA2A				↓[101]	
Alpha-2C adrenergic receptor	ADRA2C				↓[101]	
Beta-1 adrenergic receptor	ADRB1		↓[101]			
Beta-2 adrenergic receptor	ADRB2		↓[101]			
Muscarinic acetylcholine receptor M2	CHRM2				↓[101]	
Muscarinic acetylcholine receptor M5	CHRM5				↓[101]	
Benzodiazapine receptor	TSPO					↓[101]
Sodium-dependent noradrenaline transporter	SLC6A2	↓[101]				
Sodium-dependent dopamine transporter	SLC6A3					↓[101]
Transient receptor potential cation channel	TRPV1	↓[108]				
MAO type A	MAOA				↓[105,109]	

↓ represents the inhibition effect.

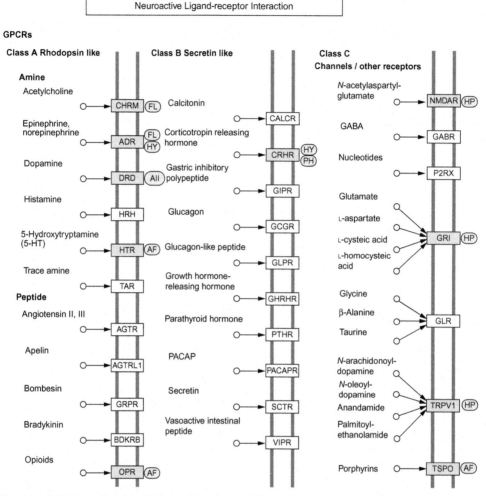

Fig. 4.2 Inhibitions of single SJW compounds on different neurotransmitter receptors. *This plot is modified from the KEGG pathway map.*

KEGG pathways, it was found that SJW intervenes in primarily three pathways, neuro-active ligand–receptor interactions, the calcium-signaling pathway, and the gap junction-related pathway. In Fig. 4.2 we show the effects of the SJW active compounds on the system of neuroactive ligand-receptor interaction. It can be seen that the SJW active compounds act on different receptors respectively so as to regulate the uptake and transport systems of neurotransmitters in a multitargeted pattern. In this way, SJW blocks the reuptake of multiple neurotransmitters such as serotonin, norepinephrine, and dopamine and stimulates the release of these neurotransmitters. We then extracted all the FDA-approved antidepressants, that is, the drugs with the first four ATC code (anatomical therapeutic chemical code) of N06A, and their targets from the DrugBank database. Integrating these data with information in Table 4.2, we constructed the drug-target network for FDA-approved antidepressants and SJW compounds, as shown in Fig. 4.3. This network shows that the active compounds of SJW share the same targets with different types of antidepressants such as monoamine oxidase (MAO) inhibitors and monoamine reuptake inhibitors, respectively, suggesting that the effect of SJW is similar to that of a combination of different classes of antidepressants.

However, the inhibitory effects of the active SJW compounds on each of the targets was lower than individual therapeutic dosages, thus the results were inadequate to fully explain the antidepressant effect of the herb only from the inhibition of any single

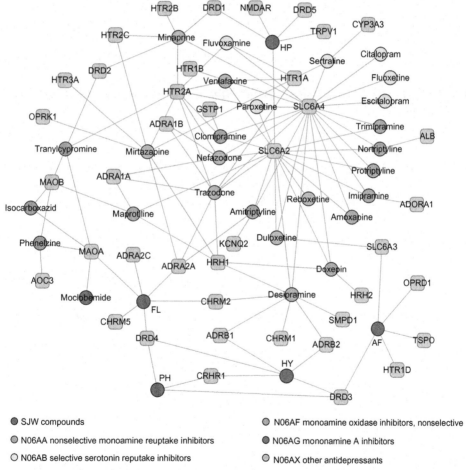

Fig. 4.3 Drug-target network of FDA approved antidepressants and SJW compounds. *Circle*: drugs; *box*: targets. A target protein node and a drug node are linked if the protein is targeted by the corresponding drug. This graph is drawn with Cytoscape software.[111]

target.[101] For instance, SJW compounds inhibit MAO only at millimolar concentrations, effects that are much weaker than conventional antidepressant MAO inhibitors.[109,112] Therefore, it is likely that the actions of multiple active SJW compounds result in an additive or synergistic antidepressant effect,[113,114] making SJW produce a similar antidepressant effect as normal lower dose monotherapy with separate compounds.

In fact, many potential targets for central nervous system (CNS) drugs participate in multiple signaling pathways that maintain the normal physiological cell function. Only in overactive or unbalanced conditions do they disrupt nerve cell function.[115] Many CNS drugs that work by specific high-affinity binding to their targets can potentially block all activity including normal cellular processes. Thus, they are often associated with intolerable side effects. Therefore, in the treatment of CNS diseases, low-affinity binding agents[115] and drug combination strategies have been proven useful in reinforcing efficacy, limiting side effects, and improving compliance.[116] Accordingly, the significant antidepressant efficacy and lower side effects of SJW could be attributable to the synergetic actions of the low-dose combination of multiple active compounds.

4.5.2 Case Study 2: The Effect of Realgar-Indigo Naturalis Formula on Acute Promyelocytic Leukemia

Acute promyelocytic leukemia (APL) is a subtype of acute myeloid leukemia (AML) caused by a specific chromosome translocation t(15;17). It is a malignancy of the bone marrow in which there is an excess of immature cells (called promyelocytes) and a deficiency of mature blood cells in the myeloid line of cells. APL can be effectively controlled by the differentiating agent all-*trans*'retinoic acid (ATRA), which activates the retinoid receptor RAR and induces the promyeloctes to differentiate toward mature granulocytes.[117] The TCM formula, Realgar-Indigo naturalis formula (RIF), has been applied in China to treat APL since the 1980s. Clinical trials have shown that 60-day RIF treatment of APL patients resulted in a complete remission (CR) rate of 98.3%[118]; a CR rate of 95% for relapsed APL[119] and 5 year survival rate of 86.88%[120] were achieved following RIF treatment.

The RIF TCM formulae consists of four kinds of materials: realgar, *Indigo naturalis*, *Salvia miltiorrhiza*, and *Radix pseudostellariae*. In TCM theory, multiple agents contained in one formula are believed to work synergistically. Realgar is regarded as the principal component of the formula RIF, and the other three thought of as adjuvant components that assist the effect of realgar. Studies in recent years have shown that the main active compounds of realgar, *Indigo naturalis* and *Salvia miltiorrhiza*, are tetra'arsenic tetra-sulfide (As_4S_4, A),[121] indirubin (I),[122], and tanshinone IIA (T),[123] respectively. Applying approaches of modern biological research, a group of Chinese scientists investigated the multitarget, synergetic actions of the three active compounds in RIF and successfully illustrated the therapeutic mechanism of the TCM formulae at the molecular level.[124] Their in vivo experiments in a murine APL model showed that monotherapy with

Table 4.3 Effects of As$_4$S$_4$ (A), indirubin (I), and tanshinone IIA (T) on APL-associated proteins[124]

Protein	Gene name	A	T	I	AT	AI	TI	ATI
PML-RARα	PML-RARA	↓	N	N	⇓	⇓	N	⇓⇓
C/EBPa	CEBPA	↑	–	–	–	–	–	⇑
C/EBPb	CEBPB	↑	N	N	⇑	⇑	N	⇑⇑
C/EBPe	CEBPE	↑	↑	N	⇑	⇑	⇑	⇑⇑
c-Myc	MYC	↓	↓	↓	⇓↓	⇓	⇓	⇓⇓
PU.1	SPI1	N	↑	↑	⇑	⇑	↑	⇑
RARB2	RARB	↑	↑	N	⇑	N	⇑	⇑
CDK2	CDK2	↓	N	↓	↓	↓	↓	⇓
P27	CDKN1B	↑	↑	↑	⇑	⇑	↑	⇑⇑
Rb	RB1	N	↑	N	↑	N	↑	↑
AQP9	AQP9	N	N	N	↑	↑	N	⇑

The primary target of simvastatin, HMG-CoA reductase (HMGCR), is bold and it appears in four databases.
↓, ↑, and "N" represents downregulation, upregulation, and no effect, respectively. Double and triple arrows represent that the regulation effect is strengthened.

A significantly prolonged the overall survival, while the ATI combination exhibited the most potent therapeutic efficacy compared with mono- or bitherapy of A, T, and I. In vitro experiments showed that A or T alone induced a certain degree of differentiation of APL cells, and the ATI combination resulted in synergistic effects that caused APL cells to differentiate toward mature cell types. At the molecular level, the ATI combination strengthened the regulation on APL-associated proteins such as PML-RARα and c-Myc.

To understand the therapeutic mechanism of RIF in the context of network regulation, our group collected the results from Wang and coworkers[124] concerning the effects of A, T, and I alone and their different combinations on APL-associated proteins and listed them in Table 4.3. We also searched the OMIM database and found six APL-associated disease genes. We now refer to the proteins in Table 4.3 and those encoded by the six APL genes as "RIF-associated proteins."

We first constructed a PPI network for the human genome based on the HPRD[79] data and mapped the RIF-associated proteins onto this network. Then we adopted the Steiner minimal tree algorithm[125] to identify a minimum subnetwork, which includes as many RIF-associated proteins and as few other proteins as possible while allowing each RIF-associated protein to interact with others through at most one bridge protein. We used the P-value[51] to quantitatively measure whether a network is more enriched with proteins of a specific gene ontology (GO) term than what would be expected by chance. Given significance level $\alpha = 0.05$, a P-value smaller than α demonstrates a low probability that the proteins of the same GO term appear in the network by chance. As can be seen in Fig. 4.4A, the RIF-associated proteins are tightly connected together due to their direct interactions while the network is significantly enriched with

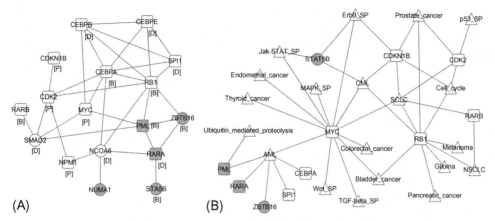

(A)   (B)

Fig. 4.4 Functional networks of APL disease gene-encoded proteins and RIF-targeted proteins. (A) Protein interaction network. (B) Protein-pathway association network. *Box*: RIF-targeted proteins; *circle*: other proteins; *triangle*: pathways. *Gray nodes*: APL disease gene-encoded proteins; *white circular* nodes: proteins which are neither APL disease gene-encoded proteins nor RIF-targeted proteins but bridges that link them together. [D]: Gene ontology (GO) of the protein: regulation of cell differentiation; [P]: GO: regulation of cell proliferation; [B]: GO: regulation of cell differentiation, and regulation of cell proliferation. This graph was drawn with Cytoscape software.[111]

proteins whose GO terms are regulation of cell differentiation and cell proliferation (P-value $= 1.26 \times 10^{-6}$, 1.09×10^{-10}, respectively), two biological processes highly associated with the progress of cancers. Specifically, the GO suggests that five of the proteins (CEBPA, CEBPB, PML, RB1, and NCOA6) are involved in the biological process of myeloid cell differentiation (P-value $= 1.72 \times 10^{-9}$). This PPI network indicates a possible concerted functional mechanism of RIF on the APL-associated proteins.

We also mapped the RIF-associated proteins onto KEGG pathways and generated a bipartite graph of protein-pathway association, in which a protein and a pathway were linked if the protein appeared in the pathway. Fig. 4.4B shows that the RIF-targeted proteins are involved in a series of cancer pathways, five of which participate in the AML pathway, suggesting that the pathway is the important pathway modulated by RIF. In Fig. 4.5 we show the targets of RIF on the AML pathway and the effects of RIF on the targets. It can be seen that, on one hand, by upregulating C/EBPa and PU.1 proteins and downregulating PML-RARα oncoprotein, RIF stimulates APL cell differentiation; on the other hand, by inhibiting PML-RARα and c-Myc, RIF deters the promyelocte proliferation. In conclusion, RIF intervenes in the AML pathway by targeting multiple proteins localized at its two associated—but distinct—branches, resulting in a synergetic anticancer action on APL.

Fig. 4.4B shows that RIF also targets multiple proteins at the pathways of chronic myeloid leukemia (CML) and small-cell lung cancer (SCLC), indicating that RIF may also be efficacious against these cancers. More research is needed to clarify the meanings of these interactions.

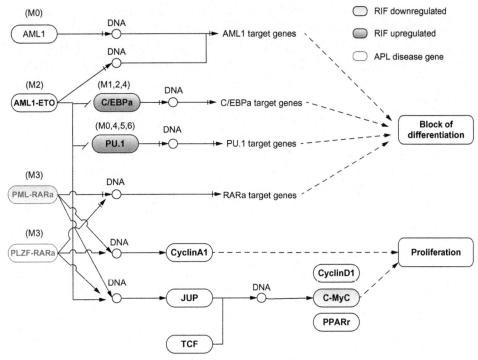

Fig. 4.5 Regulation of single RIF compounds on AML pathway proteins. M0: acute myeloblastic leukemia with minimal differentiation; M1: acute myeloblastic leukemia without maturation; M2: acute myeloblastic leukemia with maturation; M3: acute promyelocytic leukemia; M4: acute myelomonocytic leukemia; M5: acute monocytic leukemia; M6: erythroleukemia; M7: acute megakaryocytic leukemia. Oncogenes: AML1-ETO, PML-RARα, PLZF-RARα; tumor suppressors: AML1, C/EBPa, PU.1. *This plot is modified from a KEGG pathway map.*

4.6. PERSPECTIVES

Network-based TCM pharmacology seeks to develop a systematic understanding of the actions of TCM by considering their targets in the context of molecular networks. The sources and methods of molecular networks introduced here may facilitate the network-based study of TCM pharmacology. The examples in this chapter suggest that by integrating information from different sources, network-based TCM pharmacology provides a perspective for a better understanding of the holistic, complementary, and synergic essence of TCM at a molecular level. In essence, TCM is a combination therapy by multiple active compounds. Considerable experience with the combinatorial use of natural products has been accumulated in TCM to achieve synergetic therapeutic efficacy with reduced side effects. By a combination of multiple chemical ingredients, TCM remedies elicit their beneficial effects by gently affecting specific proteins within networks, achieving a similar degree of therapeutic efficacy monoingredient based agents at much lower doses of separate compounds. Thus, it is believed that this suppresses the occurrence of TCM side effects relative to the use of high concentrations of weaker monotherapy agents in western medicine. One great value of TCM is in its application for thousands of years and considerable knowledge accumulated concerning in vivo efficacy and safety, two of the confounding problems facing newly designed drugs. Thus, drug discovery starting with well-validated TCM remedies shows promise in developing new multitarget agents, or potent drug combinations that may be individually less therapeutic but potently efficacious in combination. This approach also has the advantage of controlling the pharmacokinetics and drug-drug interactions of multiple components. We expect that, along this reverse drug discovery path, it is possible to more rapidly develop new-entity drugs or efficient drug combinations at a lower cost.

REFERENCES

1. Keith CT, Borisy AA, Stockwell BR. Multicomponent therapeutics for networked systems. *Nat Rev* 2005;**4**:1–8.
2. Korcsmáros T, Szalay MS, Böde C, Kovács IA, Csermely P. How to design multi-target drugs: target search options in cellular networks. *Expert Opin Drug Discovery* 2007;**2**:1–10.
3. Csermely P, Agoston V, Pongor S. The efficiency of multi-target drugs: the network approach might help drug design. *Trends Pharmacol Sci* 2005;**26**(4):178–82.
4. Hopkins AL. Network pharmacology: the next paradigm in drug discovery. *Nat Chem Biol* 2008;**4** (11):682–90.
5. Pawson T, Linding R. Network medicine. *FEBS Lett* 2008;**582**:1266–70.
6. Kong D-X, Li X-J, Zhang H-Y. Where is the hope for drug discovery? Let history tell the future. *Drug Discov Today* 2009;**14**(3–4):115–9.
7. Verpoorte R, Crommelin D, Danhof M, Gilissen LJWJ, Schuitmaker H, van der Greef J, et al. Commentary: "A systems view on the future of medicine: inspiration from Chinese medicine?" *J Ethnopharmacol* 2009;**121**(3):479–81.
8. Qiu J. Back to the future' for Chinese herbal medicines. *Nat Rev Drug Discov* 2007;**6**(7):506–7.
9. Kong D-X, Li X-J, Tang G-Y, Zhang H-Y. How many traditional Chinese medicine components have been recognized by modern western medicine? A chemoinformatic analysis and implications for finding multicomponent drugs. *ChemMedChem* 2008;**3**:233–6.
10. Herrick T, Million R. Tapping the potential of fixed-dose combinations. *Nat Rev Drug Discov* 2007;**6**:513–4.
11. Verpoorte R, Choi YH, Kim HK. Ethnopharmacology and systems biology: a perfect holistic match. *J Ethnopharmacol* 2005;**100**(1–2):53–6.
12. Barabasi AL, Oltvai ZN. Network biology: understanding the cells's functional organization. *Nat Rev Genet* 2004;**5**:101–13.
13. Zhao J, Jiang P, Zhang WD. Molecular networks for the study of TCM pharmacology. *Brief Bioinform* 2010;**11**:417–30.
14. Zhang WD, Chen H, Zhang C, Liu RH, Li H, Chen HZ. Astragaloside IV from *Astragalus membranaceus* shows cardioprotection during myocardial ischemia *in vivo* and *in vitro*. *Planta Med* 2006;**72** (1):4–8.
15. Zhang WD, Zhang C, Wang XH, Gao PJ, Zhu DL, Hong C, et al. Astragaloside IV dilates aortic vessels from normal and spontaneously hypertensive rats through endothelium-dependent and endothelium-independent ways. *Planta Med* 2006;**72**:621–6.
16. Wang H, Zou H, Ni J, Kong L, Gao S, Guo B. Fractionation and analysis of *Artemisia capillaris* Thunb. By affinity chromatography with human serum albumin as stationary phase. *J Chromatogr A* 2000;**870**:501–10.

17. Mao X, Kong L, Luo Q, Li X, Zou H. Screening and analysis of permeable compounds in Radix Angelica Sinensis with immobilized liposome chromatography. *J Chromatogr B* 2002;**779**:331–9.

18. Homma M, Oka K, Yamada T, Niitsuma T, Ihto H, Takahashi N. A strategy for discovering biologically active compounds with high probability in traditional Chinese herb remedies: an application of Saiboku-To in bronchial asthma. *Anal Biochem* 1992;**202**(1):179–87.

19. Jiang P, Liu R, Dou S, Liu L, Zhang W, Chen Z, et al. Analysis of the constituents in the rat plasma after oral administration of Shexiang Baoxin Pill by HPLC-ESI-MS/MS. *Biomed Chromatogr* 2009;**23**(12):1333–43. https://doi.org/10.1002/bmc.1258.

20. Yan X, Zhou J, Xie G. Traditional Chinese medicine database and application on the web. *J Chem Inf Comput Sci* 2001;**41**(2):273–7.

21. Qiao X, Hou T, Zhang W, Guo S, Xu X. A 3D structure database of components from Chinese traditional medicinal herbs. *J Chem Inf Comput Sci* 2002;**42**:481–9.

22. Chen X, Zhou H, Liu Y, Wang J, Li H, Ung C, et al. Database of traditional Chinese medicine and its application to studies of mechanism and to prescription validation. *Br J Pharmacol* 2006;**149**:1092–103.

23. Chen CY-C. TCM Database@ Taiwan: the world's largest traditional Chinese medicine database for drug screening in silico. *PLoS One* 2011;**6**(1):e15939.

24. Huang X, Kong L, Li X, Chen X, Guo M, Zou H. Strategy for analysis and screening of bioactive compounds in traditional Chinese medicines. *J Chromatogr B* 2004;**812**(1–2):71–84.

25. Liu S, Yi L-Z, Liang Y-Z. Traditional Chinese medicine and separation science. *J Sep Sci* 2008;**31**:2113–37.

26. Wong CC, Cheng KW, He Q-Y, Chen F. Unraveling the molecular targets of natural products: insights from genomic and proteomic analyses. *Proteomics Clin Appl* 2008;**2**:338–54.

27. Burbaum J, Tobal G. Proteomics in drug discovery. *Curr Opin Chem Biol* 2002;**6**:427–33.

28. Lybrand TP. Ligand-protein docking and rational drug design. *Curr Opin Struct Biol* 1995;**5**(2):224–8.

29. Reardon S. Project ranks billions of drug interactions. *Nature* 2013;**503**:449–50.

30. Zhao J, Yang P, Li F, Tao L, Ding H, Rui Y, et al. Therapeutic effects of astragaloside IV on myocardial injuries: multi-target identification and network analysis. *PLoS One* 2012;**7**(9):e44938.

31. Yuen JW, Gohel MD. Anticancer effects of Ganoderma lucidum: a review of scientific evidence. *Nutr Cancer* 2005;**53**:11–7.

32. Sliva D. Ganoderma lucidum in cancer research. *Leuk Res* 2006;**30**:767–8.

33. Kimura Y, Taniguchi M, Baba K. Antitumor and antimetastatic effects on liver triterpenoid fractions of Ganoderma lucidum: mechanism of action and isolation of active substance. *Anticancer Res* 2002;**22**:3309–18.

34. Yang HL. Ganoderic acid produced from submerged culture of Ganoderma lucidum induces cell cycle arrest and cytotoxicity in human hepatoma cell line BEL7402. *Biotechnol Lett* 2005;**27**:835–8.

35. Yeung WH, QL L, Zhang Q, Go VLW. Chemical and biochemical basis of the potential anti-tumor properties of *Ganoderma lucidum*. *Curr Top Nutraceutical Res* 2004;**2**:67–77.

36. Yue Q-X, Cao Z-W, Guan S-H, Liu X-H, Tao L, W-Y W, et al. Proteomics characterization of the cytotoxicity mechanism of ganoderic acid D and computer-automated estimation of the possible drug target network. *Mol Cell Proteomics* 2008;**7**(5):949–61.

37. Chen YZ, Zhi DG. Ligand–protein inverse docking and its potential use in the computer search of protein targets of a small molecule. *Proteins Struct Funct Genet* 2001;**43**:217–26.

38. Willett P, Barnard JM, Downs GM. Chemical similarity searching. *J Chem Inf Comput Sci* 1998;**38**(6):983–96.

39. Lounkine E, Keiser M, Whitebread S, Mikhailov D, Hamon J, Jenkins J, et al. Large-scale prediction and testing of drug activity on side-effect targets. *Nature* 2012;**486**:361–7.

40. Chen X, Ji ZL, Chen YZ. TTD: therapeutic target database. *Nucleic Acids Res* 2002;**30**:412–5.

41. Zhang Y, Wang D, Tan S, Xu H, Liu C, Lin N. A systems biology-based investigation into the pharmacological mechanisms of Wu Tou Tang acting on rheumatoid arthritis by integrating network analysis. *Evid Based Complement Alternat Med* 2013;**2013**:548498.

42. Zhao S, Li S. Network-based relating pharmacological and genomic spaces for drug target identification. *PLoS One* 2010;**5**(7):e11764.

43. Zhang B, Wang X, Li S. An integrative platform of TCM network pharmacology and its application on a herbal formula, Qing-Luo-Yin. *Evid Based Complement Alternat Med* 2013;**2013**:456747.
44. Jenkins JL, Bender A, Davies JW. In silico target fishing: predicting biological targets from chemical structure. *Drug Discov Today Technol* 2006;**3**(4):413–21.
45. Wishart DS, Knox C, Guo AC, Shrivastava S, Hassanali M, Stothard P, et al. Drug Bank: a comprehensive resource for in silico drug discovery and exploration. *Nucleic Acids Res* 2006;**34**:D668–672.
46. DrugBank: http://www.drugbank.ca/.
47. TTD: http://bidd.nus.edu.sg/group/cjttd/ttd.asp.
48. Gunther S, Kuhn M, Dunkel M, Campillos M, Senger C, Petsalaki E, et al. SuperTarget and Matador: resources for exploring drug-target relationships. *Nucleic Acids Res* 2007;**36**(Database issue):D919–922.
49. SuperTarget: http://insilico.charite.de/supertarget/.
50. MATADOR: http://matador.embl.de/.
51. Gao Z, Li H, Zhang H, Liu X, Kang L, Luo X, et al. PDTD: a web-accessible protein database for drug target identification. *BMC Bioinformatics* 2008;**9**:104.
52. PDTD: http://www.dddc.ac.cn/pdtd/.
53. Kuhn M, von Mering C, Campillos M, Jensen LJ, Bork P. STITCH: interaction networks of chemicals and proteins. *Nucleic Acids Res* 2008;**36**(Suppl. 1):D684–688.
54. STITCH: http://stitch/embl.de.
55. Zheng C, Zhou H, Xie B, Han L, Yap C, Chen Y. TRMP: a database of therapeutically relevant multiple pathways. *Bioinformatics* 2004;**20**:2236–41.
56. TRMP: http://bidd.nus.edu.sg/group/trmp/trmp.asp.
57. Ye H, Ye L, Kang H, Zhang D, Tao L, Tang K, et al. HIT: linking herbal active ingredients to targets. *Nucleic Acids Res* 2011;**39**(Suppl. 1):D1055–9.
58. Fang H, Wang Y, Yang T, Ga Y, Zhang Y, Liu R, et al. Bioinformatics analysis for the Antirheumatic effects of Huang-Lian-Jie-Du-Tang from a network perspective. *Evid Based Complement Alternat Med* 2013;**2013**:245357.
59. Hornberg JJ, Bruggeman FJ, Westerhoff HV, Lankelm J. Cancer: a systems biology disease. *Biosystems* 2006;**83**:81–90.
60. Leonard BE. Inflammation, depression and dementia: are they connected? *Neurochem Res* 2007;**32**:1749–56.
61. Jones D. Pathways to cancer therapy. *Nat Rev Drug Discov* 2008;**7**:1–2.
62. Goh K-I, Cusick ME, Valle D, Childs B, Vidal M, Barabási A-L. The human disease network. *Proc Natl Acad Sci U S A* 2007;**104**:8685–90.
63. Lee D, Park J, Kay K, Christakis N, Oltvai Z, Barabási A. The implications of human metabolic network topology for disease comorbidity. *Proc Natl Acad Sci U S A* 2008;**105**:9880–5.
64. Li Y, Agarwal P. A pathway-based view of human diseases and disease relationships. *PLoS One* 2009;**4**(2):e4346.
65. Oti M, Brunner HG. The modular nature of genetic diseases. *Clin Genet* 2007;**71**(1):1–11.
66. Kitano H. Biological robustness. *Nat Rev Genet* 2004;**5**(11):826–37.
67. Zhao J, Yu H, Luo J, Cao Z, Li Y. Complex networks theory for analyzing metabolic networks. *Chin Sci Bull* 2006;**51**(13):1529–37.
68. Zhao J, Tao L, Yu H, Luo J-H, Cao ZW, Li Y. Bow-tie topological features of metabolic networks and the functional significance. *Chin Sci Bull* 2007;**52**:1036–45.
69. Zhao J, Yu H, Luo J, Cao Z, Li Y. Hierarchical modularity of nested bow-ties in metabolic networks. *BMC Bioinformatics* 2006;**7**:386.
70. Kitano H, Oda K, Kimura T, Matsuoka Y, Csete M, Doyle J, et al. Metabolic syndrome and robustness tradeoffs. *Diabetes* 2004;**53**(Suppl. 3):S6–15.
71. Yıldırım MA, Goh K-I, Cusick ME, Barabási A-L, Vidal M. Drug-target network. *Nat Biotechnol* 2007;**25**(10):1119–26.
72. Vassilev L, Vu B, Graves B, Carvajal D, Podlaski F, Filipovic Z, et al. In vivo activation of the p53 pathway by small-molecule antagonists of MDM2. *Science* 2004;**303**:844–8.

73. Hamosh A, Scott AF, Amberger JS, Bocchini CA, McKusick VA. Online Mendelian Inheritance in Man (OMIM), a knowledgebase of human genes and genetic disorders. *Nucleic Acids Res* 2005;**33**(Suppl. 1):D514–517.
74. OMIM: http://www.ncbi.nlm.nih.gov/omim/.
75. Becker KG, Barnes KC, Bright TJ, Wang SA. The genetic association database. *Nat Genet* 2004;**36**:431–2.
76. Safran M, Dalah I, Alexander J, Rosen N, Iny Stein T, Shmoish M, et al. GeneCards version 3: the human gene integrator. *Database* 2010. https://doi.org/10.1093/database/baq020.
77. Bauer-Mehren A, Bundschus M, Rautschka M, Mayer MA, Sanz F, Furlong LI. Gene-disease network analysis reveals functional modules in Mendelian, complex and environmental diseases. *PLoS One* 2011;**6**(6):e20284.
78. Hwang S, Son S-W, Kim SC, Kim YJ, Jeong H, Lee D. A protein interaction network associated with asthma. *J Theor Biol* 2008;**252**(4):722–31.
79. Keshava Prasad TS, Goel R, Kandasamy K, Keerthikumar S, Kumar S, Mathivanan S, et al. Human protein reference database—2009 update. *Nucleic Acids Res* 2009;**37**(Suppl. 1):D767–772.
80. Oti M, Snel B, Huynen MA, Brunner HG. Predicting disease genes using protein-protein interactions. *J Med Genet* 2006;**43**(8):691–8.
81. Krauthammer M, Kaufmann CA, Gilliam TC, Rzhetsky A. Molecular triangulation: bridging linkage and molecular-network information for identifying candidate genes in Alzheimer's disease. *Proc Natl Acad Sci U S A* 2004;**101**(42):15148–53.
82. Kohler S, Bauer S, Horn D, Robinson PN. Walking the interactome for prioritization of candidate disease genes. *Am J Hum Genet* 2008;**82**(4):949–58.
83. Chen J, Aronow B, Jegga A. Disease candidate gene identification and prioritization using protein interaction networks. *BMC Bioinformatics* 2009;**10**(1):73.
84. Vanunu O, Magger O, Ruppin E, Shlomi T, Sharan R. Associating genes and protein complexes with disease via network propagation. *PLoS Comput Biol* 2010;**6**(1):e1000641.
85. Zhao J, Yang T-H, Huang Y, Holme P. Ranking candidate disease genes from gene expression and protein interaction: a Katz-centrality based approach. *PLoS One* 2011;**6**(9):e24306.
86. Navlakha S, Kingsford C. The power of protein interaction networks for associating genes with diseases. *Bioinformatics* 2010;**26**(8):1057 63.
87. Wu X, Jiang R, Zhang MQ, Li S. Network-based global inference of human disease genes. *Mol Syst Biol* 2008;**4**:189.
88. Zhao J, Chen J, Yang T-H, Holme P. Insights into the pathogenesis of axial spondyloarthropathy from network and pathway analysis. *BMC Syst Biol* 2012;**6**(Suppl. 1):S4.
89. Kanehisa M, Goto S. KEGG: Kyoto encyclopedia of genes and genomes. *Nucleic Acids Res* 2000;**28**(1):27–30.
90. Zhao J, Ding G-H, Tao L, Yu H, ZH Y, Luo JH, et al. Modular co-evolution of metabolic networks. *BMC Bioinformatics* 2007;**8**:311.
91. Li S, Zhang Z, Wu L, Zhang X, Li Y, Wang Y. Understanding ZHENG in traditional Chinese medicine in the context of neuro-endocrine-immune network. *IET Syst Biol* 2007;**1**(1):51–60.
92. Subramanian A, Tamayo P, Mootha VK, Mukherjee S, Ebert BL, Gillette MA, et al. Gene set enrichment analysis: a knowledge-based approach for interpreting genome-wide expression profiles. *Proc Natl Acad Sci U S A* 2005;**102**(43):15545–50.
93. Huang C, Ba Q, Yue Q, Li J, Li J, Chu R, et al. Artemisinin rewires the protein interaction network in cancer cells: network analysis, pathway identification, and target prediction. *Mol BioSyst* 2013;**9**(12):3091–100.
94. Antonov AV, Dietmann S, Rodchenkov I, Mewes HW. PPI spider: a tool for the interpretation of proteomics data in the context of protein–protein interaction networks. *Proteomics* 2009;**9**(10):2740–9.
95. Lu B, Zhao J, Xu L, Xu Y, Wang X, Peng J. Identification of molecular target proteins in berberine-treated cervix adenocarcinoma HeLa cells by proteomic and bioinformatic analyses. *Phytother Res* 2011;**26**(5):646–56.

96. Li S, Zhang B, Zhang N. Network target for screening synergistic drug combinations with application to traditional Chinese medicine. *BMC Syst Biol* 2011;**5**(1):1–13.

97. Harrer G, Schulz V. Clinical investigation of the antidepressant effectiveness of hypericum. *J Geriatr Psychiatry Neurol* 1994;**7**(1):S6–8.

98. Volz HP. Controlled clinical trials of hypericum extracts in depressed patients: an overview. *Pharmacopsychiatry* 1997;**30**(Suppl. 2):72–6.

99. Philipp M, Kohnen R, Hiller K. Hypericum extract versus imipramine or placebo in patients with moderate depression: randomised multicentre study of treatment for eight weeks. *BMJ* 1999;**319**:1534–8.

100. Woelk H. Comparison of St John's wort and imipramine for treating depression: randomised controlled trial. *BMJ* 2000;**321**:536–9.

101. Butterweck V, Nahrstedt A, Evans J, Hufeisen S, Rauser L, Savage J, et al. In vitro receptor screening of pure constituents of St. John's wort reveals novel interactions with a number of GPCRs. *Psychopharmacology* 2002;**162**:193–202.

102. Ostrowski ED. *Investigational analysis, 14C labeling and pharmacokinetics of phenolic contents of Hypericum perforatum L.* [Dissertation]. Germany: University of Marburg; 1988.

103. Gutmann H, Bruggisser R, Schaffner W, Bogman K, Botomino A, Drewe J. Transport of amentoflavone across the blood-brain barrier in vitro. *Planta Med* 2002;**68**:804–7.

104. Stock S, Holzl J. Pharmacokinetic tests of [14C]-labeled hypericin and psudohypericin from *Hypericum perforatum* and serum kinetics of hypericin in man. *Planta Med* 1991;**57**(Suppl. 2):A61.

105. Bladt S, Wagner H. Inhibition of MAO by fractions and constituents of hypericum extract. *J Geriatr Psychiatry Neurol* 1994;**7**:S57–9.

106. Kumar V, Mdzinarishvili A, Kiewert C, Abbruscato T, Bickel U, van der Schyf C, et al. NMDA receptor-antagonistic properties of hyperforin, a constituent of St. John's wort. *J Pharmacol Sci* 2006;**102**:47–54.

107. Simmen U, Bobirnac I, Ullmer C, Lübbert H, Berger BK, Schaffner W, et al. Antagonist effect of pseudohypericin at CRF1 receptors. *Eur J Pharmacol* 2003;**458**(3):251–6.

108. Treiber K, Singer A, Henke B, Müller W. Hyperforin activates nonselective cation channels (NSCCs). *Br J Pharmacol* 2005;**145**(1):75–83.

109. Thiede H-M, Walper A. Inhibition of MAO and COMT by hypericum extracts and hypericin. *J Geriatr Psychiatry Neurol* 1994;**7**:S54–6.

110. Simmen U, Higelin J, Berger-Büter K, Schaffner W, Lundstrom K. Neurochemical studies with St. John's wort in vitro. *Pharmacopsychiatry* 2001;**34**(1):S137–42.

111. Shannon P, Markiel A, Ozier O, Baliga N, Wang J, Ramage D, et al. Cytoscape: a software environment for integrated models of biomolecular interaction networks. *Genome Res* 2003;**13**(11):2498–504.

112. Jürgenliemk G, Nahrstedt A. Phenolic compounds from *Hypericum perforatum*. *Planta Med* 2002;**68**:88–91.

113. Jia J, Zhu F, Ma X, Cao ZW, Li YX, Chen YZ. Mechanisms of drug combinations: interaction and network perspectives. *Nat Rev Drug Discov* 2009;**8**(2):111–28.

114. Ma XH, Zheng CJ, Han LY, Xie B, Jia J, Cao ZW, et al. Synergistic therapeutic actions of herbal ingredients and their mechanisms from molecular interaction and network perspectives. *Drug Discov Today* 2009;**14**(11–12):579–88.

115. Lipton SA. Turning down, but not off. Neuroprotection requires a paradigm shift in drug development. *Nature* 2004;**428**:473.

116. Millan MJ. Multi-target strategies for the improved treatment of depressive states: conceptual foundations and neuronal substrates, drug discovery and therapeutic application. *Pharmacol Ther* 2006;**110**:135–370.

117. Huang ME, Ye YC, Chen SR, Chai JR, JX L, Zhoa L, et al. Use of all-trans retinoic acid in the treatment of acute promyelocytic leukemia. *Blood* 1988;**72**(2):567–72.

118. Huang S, Guo A, Xiang Y, Wang X, Lin H, Fu L. Clinical study on the treatment of acute promyelocytic leukemia with composite indigo Naturalis tablets. *Chin J Hematol* 1995;**16**:26–8.

119. Chen Y, Huang S, Xiang Y, Chen N, Sun F, Guo A, et al. The clinical study of relapsed acute promyelocytic leukemia treated with compound Huangdai tablets. *JETCM* 2007;**16**:1066–71.

120. Sun F, Chen N, Chen Y. Compound realgar and natural indigo tablets in treatment of acute promye-locytic leukemia: a summary of experience in 204 cases. *Chin J Integr Med* 2008;**6**:639–42.
121. Zhu J, Chen Z, Lallemand-Breitenbach V, de Thé H. How acute promyelocytic leukaemia revived arsenic. *Nat Rev Cancer* 2002;**2**(9):705–14.
122. Hoessel R, Leclerc S, Endicott J, Nobel M, Lawrie A, Tunnah P, et al. Indirubin, the active constituent of a Chinese antileukaemia medicine, inhibits cyclin-dependent kinases. *Nat Cell Biol* 1999;**1**:60–7.
123. Sung H, Choi S, Yoon Y, An K. Tanshinone IIA, an ingredient of salvia miltiorrhiza BUNGE, induces apoptosis in human leukemia cell lines through the activation of caspase-3. *Exp Mol Med* 1999;**31**:174–8.
124. Wang L, Zhou G-B, Liu P, Song J-H, Liang Y, Yan X-J, et al. Dissection of mechanisms of Chinese medicinal formula Realgar-Indigo naturalis as an effective treatment for promyelocytic leukemia. *Proc Natl Acad Sci U S A* 2008;**105**:4826–31.
125. Klein P, Ravi R. A nearly best-possible approximation algorithm for node-weighted steiner trees. *J Algoritm* 1995;**19**(1):104–14.

CHAPTER 5

Application of Intestinal Flora in the Study of TCM Formulae

Xianpeng Zu*, Dale G. Nagle[†], YuDong Zhou[†], Weidong Zhang*
*Second Military Medical University, Shanghai, PR China
[†]University of Mississippi, University, MS, United States

Abstract

The human gastrointestinal tract is colonized by a large number of diverse microorganisms that constitute the intestinal microecological system. Mutualistic intestinal microflora regulate a series of functions essential to life, including digestion and nutrient absorption, immune regulation, and biological antagonism. Disruption of the intestinal flora is closely associated with the occurrence and development of many human diseases. Therefore, it is critical to maintain a healthy intestinal microecological environment. Following oral traditional Chinese medicine (TCM) administration, human intestinal bacteria can metabolize or biotransform its active metabolites to increase their activities, facilitate their intestinal absorption, and detoxify substances that produce undesired side effects or toxicities. Aspects of synergistic TCM formulae compatibility can be established from the perspective of the intestinal flora metabolism. Similarly, ingredients found in TCM formulae can also regulate intestinal flora composition and protect intestinal mucosal barrier function so as to restore intestinal microecology homeostasis. Herein, we discuss gut microflora classification, the relationships between intestinal dysbacteriosis and disease, the important roles of gut microflora in TCM metabolism and the effects of TCM on modulating intestinal dysbacteriosis. Finally, future prospects for multiomics technique-based TCM mechanism of action studies are discussed.

Keywords: Intestinal microbiota, Gut microbial ecology, Gastrointestinal microflora, Traditional Chinese medicine, Effective ingredients, Disease, Metabolism, Interaction.

Many pathogenic microorganisms including bacteria, fungi, parasites, and viruses can act against human skin, the digestive tract, and the respiratory and urinary tracts; most of these can be found within the digestive tract.[1] The vast majority of mutualistic and symbiotic bacteria are also found in the human gut microflora. There are more than 1000 types of bacteria that comprise a mass of about 1.5 kg in the human gastrointestinal tract.[2,3] About 10^{14} (ten trillion) bacteria colonize the intestinal tract of the average adult, approximately 10 times the number of human cells in the body.[4,5] Simply stated, the eukaryotic cells only account for 10% of the total cells of a human while smaller microorganism cells account for 90%. Some scholars have pointed out that such a large bacterial community could be considered to be a postnatally acquired "super organ".[6] From the perspective of the gene level, the human genome carries approximately 23,000 genes[7] while the total number of microbial genes in the gastrointestinal tract is at least 150 times that of the human genes.[8,9] Thus, as proposed by Joshua Lederberg, the human body could be considered as a "super-organism" composed of eukaryotic cells and symbiotic microbial communities.[10] The sum of the microbial genetic information is known as the gut metagenome, also called the second genome in the human body, which affects nearly all pathophysiological processes and alters drug metabolism along with an individual's own genome.[11,12]

Chinese medicine and its traditional Chinese medicine (TCM) formulae constitute a rich cultural treasure for the Chinese nation; its use in the prevention and treatment of diseases goes back thousands of years. Most TCM products (i.e., liquids, pills, powders) are primarily administered orally. Effective components in these oral dosage forms inevitably interact with the intestinal flora after entering the gastrointestinal tract. These components are absorbed and only play a pharmacological role following interaction/ metabolism by the intestinal flora.[13] Other metabolites generated by the medicine enter the enterohepatic circulation and, together with bile acids, are secreted into the intestinal tract after detoxification by the liver. They are also capable of interacting with the intestinal flora and can be subject to further metabolism and biotransformation.[14] Therefore, like the liver, the intestinal flora plays an important role in the metabolic conversion of TCM components. The gut microflora can improve active ingredient absorption and bioavailability as well as increase TCM efficacy. Moreover, the flora also can even decrease or increase the toxicity of TCM formulae. At the same time, TCM can protect the barrier function of gastrointestinal mucosa, promote probiotic colonization, and inhibit the growth of pathogenic bacteria, which all play key roles in maintaining normal intestinal microecosystem balance that contributes to good health.

5.1. CLASSIFICATION OF INTESTINAL FLORA

Numerous research programs in many countries have begun to examine the composition of the intestinal flora from subjects with different genetic backgrounds and differing dietary habits. Studies show that despite their complex composition of more than thousands of types of the human intestinal flora, there are 30–40 types of dominant bacteria that account for 99% of the total bacterial flora in the gastrointestinal tract.[4] At the phylum level, nine phyla have been identified, including seven commonly occurring phyla: Firmicutes, Bacteriodetes, Proteobacteria, Actinobacteria, Fusobacteria, Verrucomicrobia, and Cyanobacteria,[3] and two lesser frequency, Spirochaeates and VadinBE97.[15] Approximately 70%–75% of the intestinal bacteria belong to the two dominant phyla, Firmicutes and Bacteroidetes,[3,16] while the number and variety of Proteobacteria, Actinobacteria, Fusobacteria, and Verrucomicrobia are much fewer and may be less physiologically significant.[3]

According to their relationships with the host, the intestinal flora can be roughly classified into three categories. The first type is the physiological bacteria that act symbiotically with the host, also known as symbiotic bacteria or beneficial bacteria. These are primarily obligate anaerobic bacteria such as *Bifidobacteria*, *Lactobacillus*, and *Peptococcus*;

they are dominant bacteria in the intestine, comprising nearly 99% of the gut microflora. They are important to the host's bacterial metabolism and immunoregulation. The second microflora class is that of conditioned pathogens that are commensal with the host, also known as neutral bacteria. They are mainly nondominantly intestinal facultative anaerobes such as *Enterococcus* and *Enterobacteria*. They are harmless when the intestinal microecosystem is in balance. However, these bacteria can grow rapidly and become the dominant flora, producing severe illness when the body resistance decreases or broad-spectrum antibiotics disrupt the normal physiological flora. The third class of gut microflora is the pathogenic or harmful bacteria. They are primarily transient flora (i.e., *Proteus*, *Pseudomonas*, and *Staphylococcus*) that exist in low numbers but can cause illness to the host when their numbers exceed certain critical levels.[16,17]

5.2. THE RELATIONSHIP BETWEEN INTESTINAL DYSBACTERIOSIS AND DISEASE

The intestinal flora is an important component of the intestinal microecosystem, which has formed a mutualistic relationship with human beings in a long-term evolutionary process. However, once affected by changes in the host or external environment, the equilibrium between the host and the intestinal flora can be disturbed, resulting in an imbalance of the intestinal microecosystem and dysfunction within the human body that can lead to disease. Many factors can cause intestinal dysbacteriosis, including host genetic factors,[18] diet,[19] age,[20] antibiotic intake,[21] patient morbidity, and the introduction of exotic bacteria. Recent research indicates that intestinal dysbacteriosis is closely related to the occurrence and development of many diseases (Table 5.1 and Fig. 5.1). Despite

Table 5.1 Changes in the gut microbiota associated with disease

Human system	Disease	Association of gut microbiota with disease[a]
Digestive system	Periodontitis	*Porphyromonas gingivalis* could be a keystone pathogen of the disease-provoking periodontal microbiota[b]
	Diarrhea	*Escherichia/Shigella*, *Granulicatella* species and *Streptococcus mitis*/pneumoniae groups are positively associated with moderate to severe diarrhea[c]
	Irritable bowel syndrome (IBS)	Small intestinal bacterial overgrowth can occur in patients with IBS. *Veillonella* ↑; *Lactobacillus* ↑[d]
	Inflammatory bowel disease (IBD)	Roseburia ↓; Ruminococcaceae ↓; Enterobacteriaceae ↑[e]
	Colorectal cancer	*Bacteroides fragilis* ↑; Streptococcus ↑; Peptostreptococcus ↑; butyrate-producing bacteria of the family Lachnospiraceae ↓[f]

Continued

Table 5.1 Changes in the gut microbiota associated with disease—cont'd

Human system	Disease	Association of gut microbiota with disease
Metabolic disease	Cirrhosis	*Streptococcus* ↑; *Veillonella* ↑; *Clostridium* ↑; *Prevotella* ↑[g]
	Hepatic carcinoma (HCC)	Intestinal colonization by *Helicobacter hepaticus* is sufficient to promote aflatoxin- and hepatitis C virus transgene-induced HCC[h]
	Obesity	Monoassociation of germfree C57BL/6J mice with strain *Enterobacter cloacae* B29 isolated from the volunteer's gut induced fully developed obesity[i]
	Type II diabetes	*Akkermansia muciniphila* ↓[j]
	Nonalcoholic fatty liver disease (NAFLD)	Gut microbiota (Lachnospiraceae *bacterium* 609, *Barnesiella intestinihominis*, *Bacteroides vulgatus*) contributes to the development of NAFLD[k]
Immune system	Rheumatoid arthritis	Potentially harmful microorganisms (such as segmented filamentous bacteria or *Lactobacillus*) are key to the development of joint inflammation[l]
Respiratory system	Asthma	Chronic infection with *Aspergillus fumigatus* can lead to bronchiectasis, a disease that can occur in parallel with asthma[m]
Circulatory system	Atherosclerosis	*Collinsella* ↑; *Eubacterium* ↓; *Roseburia* ↓[n]
Nervous system	Depression	Spore-forming bacteria from gut microbiota modulate host serotonin levels[o]
	Autism	*Bacteroides fragilis* treatment corrects autism spectrum disorder (ASD)-related behavioral abnormalities[p]

[a]Changes relative to healthy subjects. Increase: ↑, decrease: ↓. Reference are exemplary rather than exhaustive and focus on studies that compare healthy versus diseased individuals.

[b]Hajishengallis G, Darveau RP, Curtis MA. The keystone pathogen hypothesis. *Nat Rev Microbiol* 2012;**10**:717–25.

[c]Pop M, Walker AW, Paulson J, Lindsay B, Antonio M, Hossain MA, et al. Diarrhea in young children from low-income countries leads to large-scale alterations in intestinal microbiota composition. *Genome Biol* 2014;**15**:1–12.

[d]Dupont AW, Dupont HL. The intestinal microbiota and chronic disorders of the gut. *Nat Rev Gastroenterol Hepatol* 2011;**8**:523–31.

[e]Morgan XC, Tickle TL, Sokol H, Gevers D, Devaney KL, Ward DV, et al. Dysfunction of the intestinal microbiome in inflammatory bowel disease and treatment. *Genome Biol* 2012;**13**:1–18.

[f]Wang TT, Cai GX, Qiu YP, Fei N, Zhang MH, Pang XY, et al. Structural segregation of gut microbiota between colorectal cancer patients and healthy volunteers. *ISME J* 2012;**6**:320–29.

[g]Qin N, Yang F, Li A, Prifti E, Chen Y, Shao L, et al. Alterations of the human gut microbiome in liver cirrhosis. *Nature* 2014;**513**:59–64.

[h]Fox JG, Feng Y, Theve EJ, Raczynski AR, Fiala JLA, Doernte AL, et al. Gut microbes define liver cancer risk in mice exposed to chemical and viral transgenic hepatocarcinogens. *Gut* 2010;**59**:88–97.

[i]Fei N, Zhao L. An opportunistic pathogen isolated from the gut of an obese human causes obesity in germfree mice. *ISME J* 2013;**7**:880–84.

[j]Everard A, Belzer C, Geurts L, Ouwerkerk JP, Druart C, Bindels LB, et al. Cross-talk between *Akkermansia muciniphila* and intestinal epithelium controls diet-induced obesity. *Proc Natl Acad Sci U S A* 2013;**110**:9066–71.

[k]Roy TL. Intestinal microbiota determines development of non-alcoholic fatty liver disease in mice. *Gut* 2013;**62**:1787–94.

[l]Scher JU, Abramson SB. The microbiome and rheumatoid arthritis. *Nat Rev Rheumatol* 2011;**7**:569–78.

[m]Edwards MR, Bartlett NW, Hussell T, Openshaw P, Johnston SL. The microbiology of asthma. *Nat Rev Microbiol* 2012;**10**:459–71.

[n]Karlsson FH, Fåk F, Nookaew I, Tremaroli V, Fagerberg B, Petranovic D, et al. Symptomatic atherosclerosis is associated with an altered gut metagenome. *Nat Commun* 2011;**3**:1245.

[o]Yano JM, Yu K, Donaldson GP, Shastri GG, Ann P, Ma L, et al. Indigenous bacteria from the gut microbiota regulate host serotonin biosynthesis. *Cell* 2015;**161**:264–76.

[p]Hsiao EY, Mcbride SW, Hsien S, Sharon G, Hyde ER, Mccue T, et al. Microbiota modulate behavioral and physiological abnormalities associated with neurodevelopmental disorders. *Cell* 2013;**155**:1451–63.

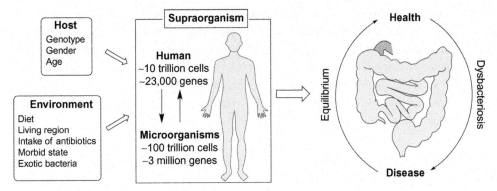

Fig. 5.1 Effect of interactions among the host, environment, and gut microbiota in human health and disease.

the encouraging progress, much work is needed to further characterize these complex physiological phenomena that have only recently begun to be recognized.

5.3. INFLUENCE OF INTESTINAL BACTERIAL METABOLISM ON EFFECTIVE TCM INGREDIENTS

The chemical composition of TCM formulae is often extremely complex. They not only contain directly acting effective ingredients such as flavonoids, terpenes, anthraquinones, alkaloids, and steroids, but also nutrients such as proteins, carbohydrates, lipids, trace elements, vitamins, and so on. This means that TCM, especially TCM formulae, have an affect on both nutritional and pharmacological systems. Generally, TCM is administrated orally and impacted by direct interaction with the gut microbial community and its metabolic enzymes, thus resulting in a series of metabolic or bioconversion reactions. These process results from intracellular or extracellular microbial enzyme reactions that selectively and specifically catalyze certain chemical reactions on orally consumed foods and TCM products.[22,23]

Intestinal bacteria can produce various glycosidases,[24] nitroreductases,[25] azoreductases[26], and carbohydrate metabolizing enzymes in the process of growth and reproduction,[27] which take part in the degradation of many TCM components. The primary metabolic pathway involves substrate hydrolysis,[28] and secondary processes include substrate oxidation[29] and reduction.[30] It has been found that metabolites with strong pharmacological activities are produced after a variety of effective TCM ingredients, especially glycosides that are made up of sugar, and nonsugar parts are metabolically converted or "activated" by the intestinal flora. Numerous pharmacokinetic studies have shown that glycosides cannot be readily absorbed and have low bioavailability; they can be stable for extended periods in the gut, but are vulnerable to "activation" by intestinal flora. Such compounds are less likely to play a pharmacological role in the body in their naturally occurring prototype glycoside form and are effective only once enzymatically converted into their corresponding aglycone form.[31,32] In conclusion, active TCM ingredients can be converted into new effective metabolites after the metabolism of specific enzymes produced by intestinal flora, which exert a diversity of biological effects on the body. In addition, increasing our understanding of the intestinal tract microflora metabolism can lead to new insights into the synergistic components of TCM component efficacy and compatibility.

5.3.1 Enhanced Absorption and Elevated Efficacy of Intestinal Flora Metabolism on TCM Ingredients

Both rhubarb and senna leaves contain sennosides and anthrone glycosides, which, on their own, have no purgative activity and are not readily absorbed by the small intestine following oral administration. The real active ingredients are senna aglycones, which are produced through the hydrolysis of sennoside by enzymes known as β-D-glucosidases, which are secreted by intestinal *Bifidobacteria*. Together, they can play a purgative role after being absorbed by the small intestine. And among them, rhein anthrone has potent purgative activity[33] (Fig. 5.2). Likewise, compounds like aloe-emodin glycoside that contain an anthrone skeleton have no purgative effect. Studies have found that the bacterium *Eubacterium* sp. BAR in human feces can hydrolyze the carbon-carbon (C—C) glycosidic bond in aloe-emodin glycoside to release the aglycone aloe rhein anthrone as the metabolite that has the potent purgative effect.[34] Baicalin, the main active ingredient of *Scutellaria baicalensis*, has been shown to have multiple pharmalogical effects such as being antibacterial, antiinflammatory and antiinfective. Trinh and coworkers[35] found that baicalin is primarily converted by the human intestinal flora into deglycosylated baicalein and the methylated aglycone oroxylin A, which more effectively treat inflammation-mediated itching responses in mouse models than the natural product baicalin (Fig. 5.3). Ginseng saponins, the main active ingredient in ginseng, produce various pharmacological effects such as inhibiting inflammation, tumor suppression, reducing blood sugar, cholesterol reduction, and so on. Studies have demonstrated that ginsenosides cannot be absorbed directly or metabolized in the liver but are degraded in the

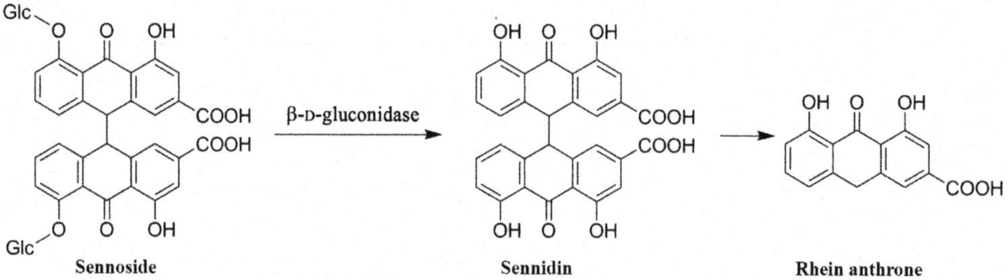

Fig. 5.2 Metabolic pathway of sennoside by gut microbiota.

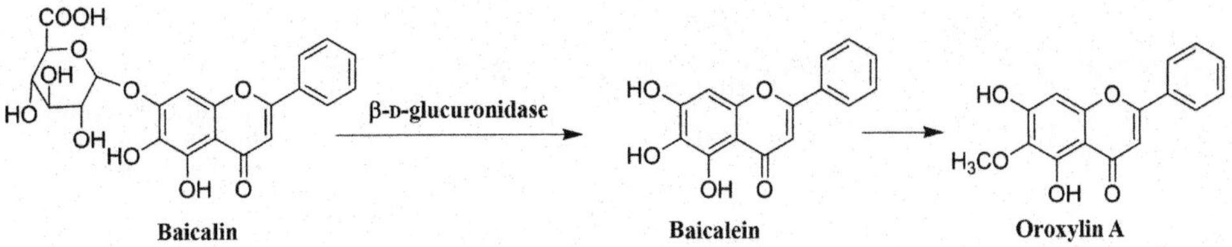

Fig. 5.3 Metabolic pathway of baicalin by intestinal microbiota.

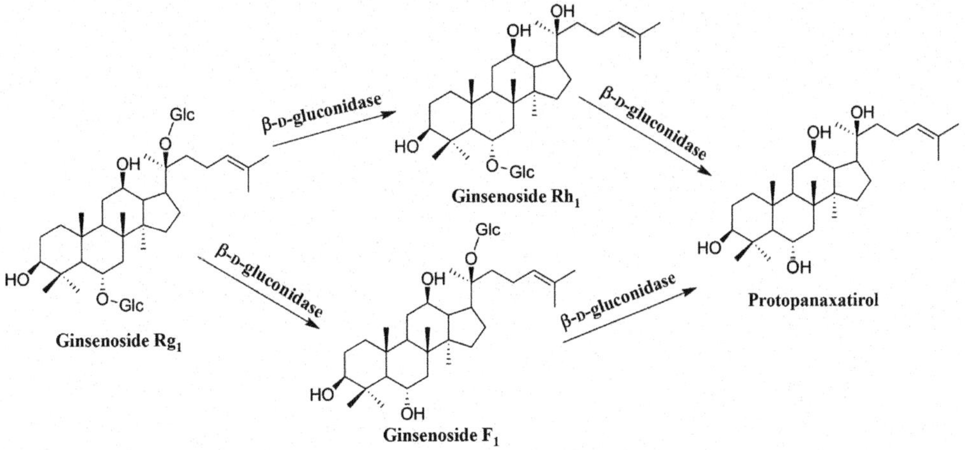

Fig. 5.4 Metabolic pathway of ginsenoside Rg1 by gut microbiota.

intestine. Wang et al.[36] found that ginsenoside Rg_1 can be metabolized by both human and rat intestinal bacteria but through different metabolic pathways in vitro and in vivo. Its metabolites persist as the primary active ingredients in the bloodstream and are believed to constitute the effective bioactive ingredients in the body (Fig. 5.4).

5.3.2 Attenuated or Increased Toxicity of Intestinal Flora on TCM Ingredients

In addition to biological conversion of active TCM ingredients and metabolizing TCM components into new effective metabolites, intestinal flora can also play a role in either decreasing or increasing the toxicity of TCM formulae.

Aconitine, the main toxic ingredient of medicinal plants like *Aconitum carmichaeli*, is capable of easing pain, diminishing inflammation, and exerting antitumor effects. However, it can also cause some toxicological effects to the central nervous and cardiovascular systems.[37] Zhao[38] studied the bioconversion of aconitine by human intestinal bacteria with the help of soft ionization tandem mass spectrometry. Aconitine was found to be metabolized through the processes of deacylation and esterification by the intestinal microbiota into less toxic metabolites, including various monoesters, diesters, and

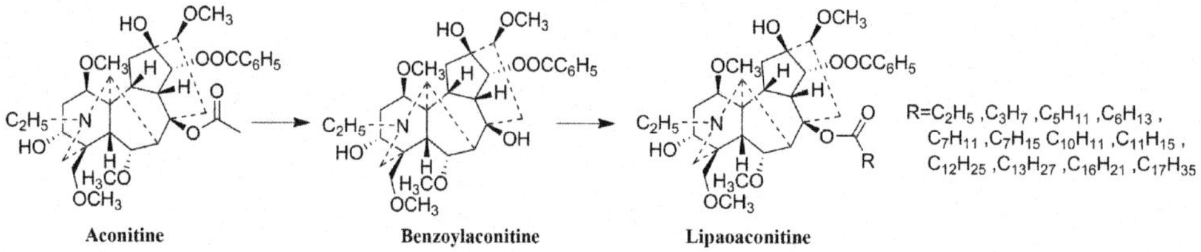

Fig. 5.5 Metabolic processes of aconitine by intestinal bacteria.

lipoaconitine (Fig. 5.5). Lipoaconitine produces similar pharmacological effects but with a much lower level of toxicity relative to aconitine.[39]

The toxicity of some TCM ingredients can even increase during intestinal flora metabolism. One example is amygdalin, the active ingredient in Semen Armeniacae Amarae. Amygdalin is widely used to treat asthma, bronchitis, emphysema, and constipation, and is used as an alternative or adjuvant in cancer therapy.[40,41] However, many cases of Semen Armeniacae Amarae poisoning have been reported.[42] Animal studies have shown that among an intravenous (IV) injection group and antibiotic-treated group, no significant toxic reactions and only minimal cyanide concentrations were detected in plasma as compared with a group administered with the drug by oral gavage.[43] In addition, the amygdalin was excreted unchanged from the rats given the drug by IV injection. However, following intragastric administration, amygdalin is first metabolized to prunasin and then converted into mandelonitrile (phenylacetonitrile) after deglycosylation, and further decomposed to benzaldehyde and prussic acid; it can release cyanide, which can cause toxic effects[44,45] (Fig. 5.6). Thus, intestinal flora plays a major role in amygdalin toxicity.

5.3.3 Confirmation of the Rationality of TCM Synergy and Compatibility

The concept of TCM formulae compatibility and potential synergy is a traditionally accepted component of Chinese medicine and embodies the holistic features of TCM-based therapy. Studies indicate that interactions between TCM components produce distinctly different effects from those observed through the action of single herbs and differ in both chemistry and pharmacology. Hence, these products do not just represent the addition of different materials and activities, but they work in concert to

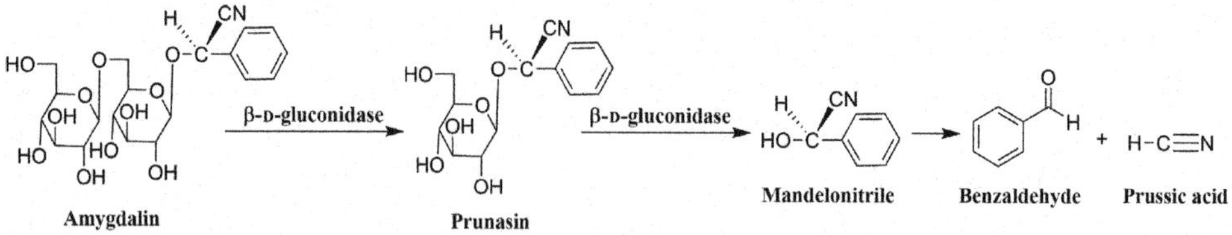

Fig. 5.6 Metabolic pathway of amygdalin by intestinal bacteria.

produce a combined synergistically enhanced effect.[46] From the perspective of the metabolism, various herbs in TCM formula go through distinctly different biotransformation processes under the effect of intestinal flora.

Tetrahydropalmatine, an isoquinoline alkaloid that is considered the active ingredient of *Corydalis yanhusuo*, has significant analgesic effects. It is often prescribed with other drugs in the clinical treatment of pain. For example, it can be compatible with *Angelica dahurica* to form the prescription known as Yuanhu Zhitong for the treatment of stomach pains, headache, and dysmenorrhea.[47] Liang et al.[48] explored the metabolism of tetrahydropalmatine by the intestinal flora in rats and the effects of the metabolism of extracts, coumarins, and essential oils from *A. dahurica* in combination and *Corydalis* alkaloids on the metabolism of tetrahydropalmatine in rats. It is concluded that, under in vitro conditions, tetrahydropalmatine is vulnerable to degradation by the rat intestinal flora, and as incubation time prolongs, the content of tetrahydropalmatine in the incubation buffer decreases. The metabolic characteristics of the coumarins and essential oils from *A. dahurica* are similar to that of *Corydalis* alkaloids. But the *A. dahurica* coumarins slow the metabolism of tetrahydropalmatine, which confirms the synergistic compatibility of *Corydalis* from the perspective of the intestinal flora metabolism.

Wuji Pills, which are composed of *Coptidis chinensis*, *Tetradium ruticarpum*, and fried *Radix Paeoniae alba*, is the commonly used formula to treat intestinal diseases such as irritable bowel syndrome and peptic ulcers. Men and coworkers[49] studied the human intestinal flora metabolism of berberine and palmatine in Wuji Pills. It is concluded that, among the *C. chinensis* components, the metabolic rate of berberine is positively correlated with the dose while it is opposite for palmatine. On one hand, the combination compatibility accelerates the metabolic rate of berberine in low doses and positively correlates with the dose of *T. ruticarpum* and fried *R. Paeoniae alba*. On the other hand, it reduces the metabolic rate of berberine at high doses and negatively correlates with the dose of *T. ruticarpum*. The TCM compatibility increases the metabolism of palmatine at high doses but reduces it in low doses. Its metabolic rate is negatively correlated with the dose of *T. ruticarpum* and fried *R. paeoniae alba*. The above results demonstrate the effect of Wuji Pill compatibility from the perspective of intestinal flora metabolism.

5.4. MODULATION OF THE INTESTINAL FLORA BY TCM

Under normal conditions, beneficial bacteria and pathogens coexist in the digestive tract and form a microbial community. When the body is infected with pathogenic bacteria or other diseases, the microecological balance of the organisms changes from a physiological combination to a more pathological combination. The intestinal dysbacteriosis can also affect nutrient absorption, weaken the barrier function of the gut, reduce immunity, further aggravate the disease, and result in a vicious pathogenic circle.[50] Increasingly, people have become aware of the importance of maintaining a balanced intestinal microecosystem and pay attention to the effects of TCM on this system. Following oral administration, TCM formulae interact with and affect the gastrointestinal tract flora, thus affecting the host's health. Studies have examined the impact of TCM on regulating intestinal disorders.[51] TCM helps keep the intestinal microecosystem balanced through both acting directly or indirectly to regulate intestinal dysbacteriosis.

5.4.1 Regulation of Intestinal Flora Composition by TCM

Both single herb/extract and combined TCM formulae studies have examined the effects of TCM on the composition of intestinal flora.

5.4.1.1 Effects of a Single Herb or Single Extract on Intestinal Flora Composition

Chang et al.[52] conducted research on the effect of the *Ganoderma lucidum* extract added to a high-fat diet in mice, and discovered that the extract not only reduced the elevated ratio of Firmicutes/Bacteroidetes and the level of endotoxin-producing *Proteobacteria* that were induced by the high-fat diet, but also maintained the intestinal barrier integrity and reduced endotoxemia. It was also observed that if the feces of the treated mice were transplanted to other obese mice, the beneficial metabolic effects were the same as those produced by *G. lucidum*. Guo and coworkers[53] found that both extracts from Red Ginseng and Semen Coix could promote the growth of probiotics such as *Lactobacillus* and *Bifidobacterium* and inhibit pathogens such as *Escherichia coli*, *Staphylococcus*, and *Salmonella* in vitro. The trinitrobenzene sulfonic acid-induced ulcerative colitis model was used to evaluate the efficacy. They found that both extracts could ameliorate intestinal dysbacteriosis and relieve the symptoms of colitis, which was especially obvious in the Red Ginseng extract treated group. Most TCM formulae contain carbohydrate constituents that can promote the growth of beneficial intestinal bacteria and inhibit the reproduction of the harmful ones. Veereman[54] found that if a proper proportion of inulin and fructo-oligo saccharide was added to the nutritional formula, the composition of an infant's intestinal microorganism flora was significantly adjusted, resulting in a reduced intestinal permeability and improved stool consistency. Concurrently, if the infant is fed with food containing fructo-oligo saccharide, the numbers of *Bifidobacterium* and *Lactobacillus* increase and intestinal *Clostridium* numbers decrease. Wang[55] studied the effects of the *Ophiopogon japonicus* polysaccharide MDG-1 on the intestinal flora of KKay diabetic mice and confirmed that high doses of MDG-1 can significantly reduce the number of intestinal *E. coli* and *Streptococcus*, and at the same time promote the proliferation of *Bifidobacterium* and *Lactobacillus*.

5.4.1.2 Effects of TCM Formulae on Intestinal Flora Composition

Chen and others[56] studied the regulation effect of the TCM formulae composed of *Codonopsis*, *Poria*, *Atractylodes*, White Paeony Root, and tangerine peel on the intestinal flora in mice, and found that after feeding, the intestinal probiotics *Lactobacillus* and *Bifidobacterium* dramatically increased and *Enterococcus* significantly decreased. Feng et al.[57] used a linco-mycin hydrochloride-induced intestinal flora disorder mouse model to establish that antibiotic-associated intestinal flora disruption significantly decreased the numbers of the probiotics *Lactobacillus* and *Bifidobacterium*. Following treatment with the modified Buzhong Yiqi Decoction (MBD), the numbers of those same probiotics recovered back to relatively normal levels. Thus the conclusion could be drawn that MBD can regulate the intestinal probiotics levels in mice following antibiotic-induced disruption. Luo[58] evaluated the Huang Lian Jie Du decoction (HLJDD) on intestinal flora in an antibiotic-induced intestinal flora disorder mouse model and compared antibiotic-induced groups with mice treated with various doses of HLJDD by gavage. They found that the group treated with low HLJDD doses had no observed flora disorder but that mice fed chronically with high doses of HLJDD suffered destructive effects such as a decrease in the intestinal probiotics *Lactobacillus* and *Bifidobacteria*, similar to the effects caused by antibiotics. Spleen-deficient diarrhea syndrome can generate composition changes in the intestinal flora while the Sijunzi decoction can cure spleen–deficient diar-rhea syndrome in rats, not only by increasing the proportion of intestinal probiotics but also by the diversity of the intestinal flora.[59]

5.4.2 Protecting the Intestinal Mucosa Barrier Function and Preventing the Intestinal Bacteria Translocation Penetration

In addition to direct protective effects, based on the composition and number of intestinal flora, TCM can indirectly protect the intestinal mucosal barrier. The barrier function of the intestinal mucosa is an important feature of the intestine that is essential for defending against the effects of exogenous materials. The intestinal mucosal barrier consists of four parts, including a mechanical barrier formed by intestinal epithelial cells, tight intercel-lular junctions and biofilms, an immune barrier formed by gut-associated lymphoid tis-sues and their active metabolites, a chemical barrier formed by chemical substances such as gastric acid, mucus and digestive enzymes secreted by the gastrointestinal tract, and a critical biological barrier formed by normal intestinal flora.[60] The normal intestinal mucosal barrier can protect against exogenous infection, the occurrence of systemic inflammation response syndrome, and multiple organ and system failure by effectively preventing intestinal bacteria and endotoxins from entering the intestinal mucosa. It has been discovered that a variety of single TCM herbs, TCM formulae, and various TCM preparations can protect the intestinal mucosal barrier.

5.4.2.1 Single TCM Herbs

Zhang and coworkers[61] studied the protective effects of rhubarb on the intestinal barriers of piglets with sepsis and found that intestinal epithelial cell apoptosis was significantly reduced in the rhubarb treatment group and the expressions of the tight junction protein occludin ZO-1 and occludin mRNA were significantly enhanced relative to the control animals. The tight junctions were relatively compact as observed by an electron micrograph. TNF-α mRNA expression was reduced while IL-10 mRNA expression was increased. The level of malondialdehyde decreased and superoxide dismutase activity increased. Taken together, these data suggest that rhubarb can protect the intestinal mucosal barrier of piglets with sepsis by relieving intestinal epithelial cell apoptosis through antiinflammation and antioxidant effects and by increasing the expression of tight junction proteins. Xie and Tang[62] found that *Patchouli* essential oil can protect the intestinal barrier in ischemia-reperfusion rats. The protection mechanism may be related to the significant increase in the intestinal mucus level, a significant reduction in mast cell numbers, a decrease in the activity of diamine oxidase in plasma, and alleviation of injuries in the epithelial structure on the intestinal mucosa.

5.4.2.2 TCM Formulae

Lu and Xie[63] explored the influence of the TCM formulae Qingchang Suppository on the colon mucosa permeability of trinitrobenzene sulfonic acid-induced ulcerative colitis. They used fluorescein isothiocyanate-dextran 4000 as the marker and determined the colon mucosa permeability of rats through in vitro and in vivo experiments. It was established that the Qingchang Suppository can effectively inhibit the increase in permeability of rat colon mucosa, improve intestinal mucosa barrier function, and promote ulcer healing. Modified Zhishu Decoction can promote intestinal motility, maintain normal intestinal locomotor function, improve the excretion of intestinal bacteria and endotoxin, and reduce toxin absorption. It can also inhibit the penetration of intestinal bacteria and reduce the permeability of the intestinal mucosa.[64] Therefore, it can provide a better protective effect to the intestinal mucosal barrier function.

5.4.2.3 Other TCM Preparations

The Shenfu injection can protect the rat intestinal mucosa barrier in acute necrotizing pancreatitis through inhibiting the expression of NF-κB in the intestine and reducing the generation of proinflammatory regulators (i.e., TNF-α, ICAM-1, and iNOS).[65] Zhao[66] established a rat model of severe acute pancreatitis (SAP) by retrograde injection of 3.5% sodium taurocholate through the cholangio-pancreatic duct. Using this model, this group found that Qingyi particles can reduce pancreatic injury and the permeability of the intestinal mucosa as well as protect the intestinal mucosal barrier of rats with SAP.

Mutualistic and symbiotic intestinal microorganisms and their hosts have been involved in coevolution processes for millennia. These microorganisms continuously exchange material and information with the host, resulting in the formation of an interdependent and tightly controlled intestinal microecosystem. With the development of methods to examine interplay between this microecology and modern Chinese medicine, there is growing recognition of the close relationship between the intestinal flora and the corresponding health or illness of the host. Once the dynamic equilibrium of the intestinal microecosystem is broken, the intestinal flora will lose balance and allow the entry of pathogenic disease-associated organisms. The traditional medicines of China have gradually gained worldwide acceptance because of their reduced incidence of adverse reactions and lack of drug resistance or tolerance with long-term use. The theory of TCM emphasizes understanding the human body at the integral level and carrying out treatment based on physiological syndromes with treatments guided to a holistic approach to medicine in order to prevent and treat disease. The intestinal flora, the biggest microecosystem in the superorganism of the human body, has been found to have an inevitable connection with TCM. Therefore some scholars have suggested that the intestinal flora may be the potential target for many of the effects of TCM on disease.

The recent rapid development of various omics technologies, such as transcriptomics, proteomics, metabolomics, and metagenomics provides great convenience for researchers to study the interactions of effective TCM ingredients and intestinal flora. It is estimated that 99% of nature's bacteria cannot be readily cultured in vitro. However, metagenome sequencing techniques can not only acquire the composition and genetic functioning information of the flora but also identify specific bacteria associated with diseases.[67] Metabolomic technologies can help reveal the close relationships between the intestinal flora and the TCM metabolism, find potential metabolic markers, and identify key functional bacteria required for the TCM metabolism. These methods can provide valuable clues to increase our understanding of the mechanistic basis action of TCM at the multiingredient, multitarget, and multilevels. However, metagenomics analysis does not easily distinguish between those genes that are expressed and nonexpressed genes. Therefore, the application of transcriptomics and proteomics becomes necessary to provide additional context. Eventually, the combined use of multiple "omics" technologies will be needed to further clarify the material basis of TCM's efficacy and distinguish the potential role(s) of the intestinal bacteria-mediated molecular mechanisms associated with TCM use (Fig. 5.7).

The intestinal flora is composed of a large number of microorganisms that are indispensable to the human body; it dramatically affects or may even determine the efficacy and toxicity of TCM. Components in TCM formulae function, at least in part, by regulating the balance of the intestinal microecosystem. In-depth research on the

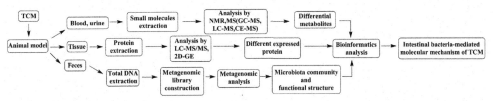

Fig. 5.7 Research strategies for studying the mechanism of action of TCM based on multiomics techniques.

interactions of TCM with the intestinal bacteria will contribute to our appreciation of the metabolism, absorption, and toxic effects following oral TCM administration as well as help us clarify the functional material basis of TCM mechanisms. Such research can also guide the development of intestinal flora-oriented personalized medicine preparations and rationally designed clinical medication combinations, thus providing new research ideas and methods for modern TCM research and new drug development.

REFERENCES

1. Kamada N, Seo SU, Chen GY, Núñez G. Role of the gut microbiota in immunity and inflammatory disease. *Nat Rev Immunol* 2013;**13**:321–35.
2. Nicholson JK, Holmes E, Wilson ID. Gut microorganisms, mammalian metabolism and personalized health care. *Nat Rev Microbiol* 2005;**3**:431–8.
3. Eckburg PB, Bik EM, Bernstein CN, Purdom E, Dethlefsen L, Sargent M, et al. Diversity of the human intestinal microbial flora. *Science* 2005;**308**:1635–8.
4. Guarner F, Malagelada J. Gut flora in health and disease. *Lancet* 2003;**361**:512–9.
5. Rabiu BA, Gibson GR. Carbohydrates: a limit on bacterial diversity within the colon. *Biol Rev* 2002;**77**:443–53.
6. O'Hara AM, Shanahan F. The gut flora as a forgotten organ. *EMBO Rep* 2006;**7**:688–93.
7. Yang X, Xie L, Li Y, Wei C. More than 9,000,000 unique genes in human gut bacterial community: estimating gene numbers inside a human body. *PLoS One* 2009;**4**:e6074.
8. Qin J, Li R, Raes J, Arumugam M, Burgdorf KS, Manichanh C, et al. A human gut microbial gene catalog established by metagenomic sequencing. *Nature* 2010;**464**:59–65.
9. Gill SR, Pop M, Deboy RT, Eckburg PB, Turnbaugh PJ, Samuel BS, et al. Metagenomic analysis of the human distal gut microbiome. *Science* 2006;**312**:1355–9.
10. Lederberg J. Infectious history. *Science* 2000;**288**:287–93.
11. Zhao L. Genomics: the tale of our other genome. *Nature* 2010;**465**:879–80.
12. Wei J, Li H, Zhao L, Nicholson JK. Gut microbiota: a potential new territory for drug targeting. *Nat Rev Drug Discov* 2008;**7**:123–9.
13. Park EK, Shin J, Bae EA, Lee YC, Kim DH. Intestinal bacteria activate estrogenic effect of main constituents puerarin and daidzin of *Pueraria thunbergiana*. *Biol Pharm Bull* 2007;**29**:2432–5.
14. T S PR, Moore V, Carlsson A, Abrahamsson B, Basit AW. The gastrointestinal microbiota as a site for the biotransformation of drugs. *Int J Pharm* 2008;**363**:1–25.
15. Bäckhed F, Ley RE, Sonnenburg JL, Peterson DA, Gordon JI. Host-bacterial mutualism in the human intestine. *Science* 2005;**307**:1915–20.
16. Diamant M, Blaak EE, de Vos WM. Do nutrient-gut-microbiota interactions play a role in human obesity, insulin resistance and type 2 diabetes? *Obes Rev* 2011;**12**:272–81.
17. Bäckhed F, Manchester JK, Semenkovich CF, Gordon JI. Mechanisms underlying the resistance to diet-induced obesity in germ-free mice. *Proc Natl Acad Sci U S A* 2007;**104**:979–84.
18. Zoetendal EG, Akkermans ADL, Akkermans-van Vliet WM, de Visser JAGM, de Vos WM. The host genotype affects the bacterial community in the human gastronintestinal tract. *Microb Ecol Health Dis* 2000;**13**:129–34.
19. Filippo CD, Cavalieri D, Paola MD, Ramazzotti M, Poullet JB, Massart S, et al. Impact of diet in shaping gut microbiota revealed by a comparative study in children from Europe and rural Africa. *Proc Natl Acad Sci U S A* 2010;**107**:S445–6.
20. Mueller S, Saunier K, Hanisch C, Norin E, Alm L, Midtvedt T, et al. Differences in fecal microbiota in different European study populations in relation to age, gender, and country: a cross-sectional study. *Appl Environ Microbiol* 2006;**72**:1027–33.
21. Jernberg C, Löfmark S, Edlund C, Jansson JK. Long-term ecological impacts of antibiotic administration on the human intestinal microbiota. *ISME J* 2007;**1**:56–66.

22. Jin JS, Zhao YF, Nakamura N. Enantioselective dehydroxylation of enterodiol and enterolactone precursors by human intestinal bacteria. *Biol Pharm Bull* 2007;**30**:2113–9.

23. Jin JS, Hattori M. Human intestinal bacterium, strain END-2 is responsible for demethylation as well as lactonization during plant lignan metabolism. *Biol Pharm Bull* 2010;**33**:1443–7.

24. Miwa M, Horimoto T, Kiyohara M, Katayama T, Kitaoka M, Ashida H, et al. Cooperation of β-galactosidase and β-*N*-acetylhexosaminidase from Bifidobacteria in assimilation of human milk oligosaccharides with type 2 structure. *Glycobiology* 2010;**20**:1402–9.

25. de Oliveira IM, Henriques JA, Bonatto D. In silico identification of a new group of specific bacterial and fungal nitroreductases-like proteins. *Biochem Biophys Res Commun* 2007;**355**:919–25.

26. Chen H, Wang RF, Cerniglia CE. Molecular cloning, overexpression, purification, and characterization of an aerobic FMN-dependent azoreductase from *Enterococcus faecalis*. *Protein Expr Purif* 2004;**34**:302–10.

27. Turnbaugh PJ, Quince C, Faith JJ, Mchardy AC, Yatsunenko T, Niazi F, et al. Organismal, genetic, and transcriptional variation in the deeply sequenced gut microbiomes of identical twins. *Proc Natl Acad Sci U S A* 2010;**107**:7503–8.

28. Kim YS, Kim JJ, Cho KH, Jung WS, Moon SK, Park EK, et al. Biotransformation of ginsenoside Rb1, crocin, amygdalin, geniposide, puerarin, ginsenoside Re, hesperidin, poncirin, glycyrrhizin, and baicalin by human fecal microflora and its relation to cytotoxicity against tumor cells. *J Microbiol Biotechnol* 2008;**18**:1109–14.

29. Wang LQ, Meselhy MR, Li Y, Nakamura N, Min BS, Qin GW, et al. The heterocyclic ring fission and dehydroxylation of catechins and related compounds by *Eubacterium* sp. strain SDG-2, a human intestinal bacterium. *ChemInform* 2002;**33**:1640–3.

30. Jin JS, Nishihata T, Kakiuchi N, Hattori M. Biotransformation of C-glucosylisoflavone puerarin to estrogenic (3S)-equol in co-culture of two human intestinal bacteria. *Biol Pharm Bull* 2008;**31**:1621–5.

31. Kanaze F, Bounartzi MI, Georgarakis M, Niopas I. Pharmacokinetics of the citrus flavanone aglycones hesperetin and naringenin after single oral administration in human subjects. *Eur J Clin Nutr* 2007;**61**:472–7.

32. Liu ZQ, Jiang ZH, Liu L, Hu M. Mechanisms responsible for poor oral bioavailability of paeoniflorin: role of intestinal disposition and interactions with sinomenine. *Pharm Res* 2006;**23**:2768–80.

33. Matsumoto M, Ishige A, Yazawa Y, Kondo M, Muramatsu K, Watanabe K. Promotion of intestinal peristalsis by *Bifidobacterium* spp. capable of hydrolysing sennosides in mice. *PLoS One* 2012;**7**:e31700.

34. Akao T, Che QM, Kobashi K, Hattori M, Namba T. A purgative action of barbaloin is induced by *Eubacterium* sp. strain BAR, a human intestinal anaerobe, capable of transforming barbaloin to aloe-emodin anthrone. *Biol Pharm Bull* 1996;**19**:136–8.

35. Trinh HT, Joh EH, Kwak HY, Baek NI, Kim DH. Anti-pruritic effect of baicalin and its metabolites, baicalein andoroxylin A, in mice. *Acta Pharmacol Sin* 2010;**31**:718–24.

36. Wang Y, Liu TH, Wang W, Wang BX. Research on the transformation of ginsenoside Rg1 by intestinal flora. *China J Chin Mater Med* 2001;**26**:188–90.

37. Wu KH, Tang LY, Wang ZJ, Xu YL, Zhou XD. Advances in studies on chemical constituents and bioactivities of *Aconitum carmichaeli*. *Chin J Exp Tradit Med Formulae* 2014;**20**:212–20.

38. Zhao YF, Song FR, Guo XH, Liu SY. Studies on the biotransformation of aconitine in human intestinal bacteria using soft-ionization mass spectrometry. *Chem J Chin Univ* 2008;**29**:55–9.

39. Kawata Y, Ma CM, Meselhy MR, Nakamura N, Wang H, Hattori M, et al. Conversion of aconitine lipoaconitine by human intestinal bacteria and their antinociceptive effects in mice. *J Trad Med* 1999;**16**:15–23.

40. Chang HK, Yang HY, Lee TH, Shin MC, Lee MH, Shin MS, et al. Armeniacae semen extract suppresses lipopolysaccharide-induced expressions of cycloosygenase-2 and inducible nitric oxide synthase in mouse BV2 microglial cells. *Biol Pharm Bull* 2005;**28**:449–54.

41. Lv JZ, Deng JG. Research progress in pharmacological effects of amygdalin. *Drugs Clin* 2012;**27**:530–5.

42. Akyildiz BN, Kurtoğlu S, Kondolot M, Tunç A. Cyanide poisoning caused by ingestion of apricot seeds. *Ann Trop Paediatr* 2010;**30**:39–43.

43. Carter JH, Mclafferty MA, Goldman P. Role of the gastrointestinal microflora in amygdalin (laetrile)-induced cyanide toxicity. *Biochem Pharmacol* 1980;**29**:301–4.

44. Fang MF, Fu ZL, Wang QL, Zhen XH. Effect of cream processing on metabolism and tissue distribution of bitter almond in rat. *Chin J Exp Tradit Med Formulae* 2011;**17**:132–7.

45. Fu ZL, Zheng XH, Fang MF. Effect of defatted method on metabolism and excretion of bitter almond in rat urine. *Chin Tradit Pat Med* 2011;**33**:1202–5.

46. Men W, Chen Y, Li YJ, Yang Q, Weng XG, Gong ZP, et al. Research progress of biotransformation on effective ingredients of Chinese medicine via intestinal bacteria. *Chin J Exp Tradit Med Formulae* 2015;**21**:229–34.

47. Zhu YY. Comparative studies on chemistry and pharmacodynamics of the compatibility of Yuanhu Zhitong prescription. *J China Pharm Univ* 2003;**34**:461–4.

48. Liang XL, Zhu QY, Liao ZG, Zhao GW, Wang GF. Effect of the compatibility of *Corydalis yanhusuo* and *Angelicae dahuricae* on metabolism of tetrahydropalmatine in intestinal flora. *Chin J Exp Tradit Med Formulae* 2010;**16**:92–4.

49. Men W, Chen Y, Yang Q, Li YJ, Gong ZP, Weng XG, et al. Study on metabolism of *Coptis chinensis* alkaloids from different compatibility of Wuji Wan in human intestinal flora. *China J Chin Mater Med* 2013;**38**:417–21.

50. Ao MY, Wang MJ, Jiang SY, Xiong SQ, Li ZX, Wu QL, et al. Research progress on the effect of Chinese herbal medicine on intestinal probiotics. *Chin J Microecol* 2011;**23**:475–8.

51. Li G, Xiao XH, Jin C. Chinese medicinal compound and modulation of intestinal microecology. *Chin J Integr Tradit West Med* 2007;**27**:466–9.

52. Chang CJ, Lin CS, CC L, Martel J, Ko YF, Ojcius DM, et al. *Ganoderma lucidum* reduces obesity in mice by modulating the composition of the gut microbiota. *Nat Commun* 2015;**6**:7489.

53. Guo M, Ding S, Zhao C, Gu X, He X, Huang K, et al. Red Ginseng and Semen Coicis can improve the structure of gut microbiota and relieve the symptoms of ulcerative colitis. *J Ethnopharmacol* 2014;**162**:7–13.

54. Veereman G. Pediatric applications of inulin and oligofructose. *J Nutr* 2007;**137**:2585–9.

55. Wang LY. Effect of MDG-1 on oral glucose tolerance and intestinal microecological balance in diabetic mice. *World Chin J Digestol* 2011;**19**:2058–62.

56. Chen C, Jiang ZY, Song KY, Shi SS, Yan QC, Sa WU, et al. The effect of Chinese herbal medicine on mouse intestinal flora. *Chin J Microecol* 2011;**23**:15–7.

57. Feng XZ, Zhang YN, Jiang X, Wang HG. Research of modified Bu zhongyiqitang on promote the growth of intestinal probiotics. *Chin J Microecol* 2008;**20**:159–60.

58. Luo HH, Dong S, Zhang S, Li D, Shi Q, Zhou H, et al. Effects of Coptidis Decoction on the intestinal flora of mice. *J Trop Med* 2009;**9**:369–71.

59. Meng LY, Chen XQ, Shi DY, Huang HD, Guo SN. Influence of Sijunzi Decoction on intestinal flora diversity in spleen-deficient rats. *Acta Vet Zootech Sin* 2013;**44**:2029–35.

60. Hu YY, Peng JH, Feng Q. The key target of Chinese medicine treatment on alcoholic and nonalcoholic fatty liver disease: the gut. *Chin J Integr Tradit West Med* 2011;**31**:1269–72.

61. Zhang YQ, Liu JH, Li DG, Sun B. Study on protective effect and mechanism of rhubarb on intestinal barrier of piglet with sepsis. *China J Tradit Chin Med Pharm* 2007;**22**:843–7.

62. Xie SC, Tang F. Protective effect of volatile oil from pogostemon cablin on intestinal barrier function. *Chin Tradit Herb Drugs* 2009;**40**:942–4.

63. Lu L, Xie JQ. Effect of Qingchang suppository on intestinal permeability in rats with ulcerative colitis. *Chin J Integr Tradit West Med* 2010;**30**:1087–90.

64. Zhang JH, Chen Q, Luo D, You-Li KE, Yang Y. Effect of the Zhishu Decoction on the permeability of rat intestinal mucosal barrier. *Chin J Integr Tradit West Med Dig* 2009;**17**:227–9.

65. Hu ZL, Lv ZW, Zhang XY, Jiang MS, Han DE. Effects of Shenfu on the damage of intestinal mucosa with acute necrotizing pancreatitis in rats. *Chin J Pancreatol* 2008;**8**:24–7.

66. Zhao G, Zhang S, Cui N. Protective effect of Qing Yi particles on intestinal mucosa barrier in rats with severe acute pancreatitis. *Chin J Surg Integr Tradit West Med* 2010;**16**:323–6.

67. Hess M, Rubin EM. Metagenomic discovery of biomass-degrading genes and genomes from cow rumen. *Science* 2011;**331**:463–7.

CHAPTER 6

Application of Connectivity Map (CMAP) Database to Research on Traditional Chinese Medicines (TCMs)

Chao Lv*, Dale G. Nagle[†], YuDong Zhou[†], Weidong Zhang*
*Second Military Medical University, Shanghai, PR China
[†]University of Mississippi, University, MS, United States

Abstract

The connectivity map (CMAP) database is established initially to connect biology, chemistry, and clinical conditions, which helps to discover the connections between disease-gene-drug. The CMAP approach has been applied in the widely recognized field of drug discovery and development. In recent years, CMAP analysis has also been applied to research on traditional Chinese medicine (TCM). The study of TCM is facing a wide range of challenges such as complicated ingredients, multiple targets, multiple pathways of action, and complex functioning mechanisms. The idea of employing CMAP in TCM research has brought a new perspective for researchers while providing a systematic method for elucidating the mechanisms of TCM and TCM formulae.

Keywords: Connectivity map, Establishing CMAP database, Mechanism, Traditional Chinese medicine, TCM formulae.

Since the first piece of the DNA chip was made by Stanford University in 1995,[1] the development of such technology and the concept of fast and comprehensive characterizing DNA on a chip have been broadly extended. In biological chips, the DNA chip was one of the earliest and most widely used, able to detect changes in the whole genome of drug-treated cells and disease tissues.[2] A study conducted by Hughes et al.[3] on using chip technology was used to establish a gene expression profile database from 300 different yeast mutants in response to small molecules, and to predict the function of the small molecule by the phenotypical change of yeast transcriptomes. .

Based on previous studies, a novel analysis database employing gene expression profiles was developed by Lamb et al.,[4] which resulted in the establishment of the connectivity map (CMAP) database. Researchers used small-molecule compounds to treat human cell lines, obtaining gene expression profile data that was then included in the CMAP database. By exploiting gene expression profiling as a common "language" to associate biology, chemistry, and clinical conditions, the CMAP database connected the disease-gene-drug network regardless of the microarray platforms used.[5,6] This remarkable work has brought convenience to scientific researchers by helping them find

Systems Biology and Its Application in TCM Formulas Research
https://doi.org/10.1016/B978-0-12-812744-5.00006-0

the biological significance from the CMAP database. In the analysis, researchers could find out the potential correlation of compounds and their inferred mechanisms, which provided a new and reliable way for drug development.

Traditional Chinese medicine (TCM) has a long history in China; it also has good efficacy in the prevention and treatment of a variety of diseases. With TCM receiving more and more attention, the method of TCM research has also diversified. Due to the complex mechanism of TCM caused by multiple components and multiple targets, previous methods offered the limited capacity to acquire comprehensive knowledge for incorporating the clinical level to the cell level and even the molecular level.[7] However, the CMAP approach, by analyzing the gene expression profiles of small molecules and TCM, could discover the new function of components of TCM and elucidate the mechanism of TCM. Therefore, such an effective research approach of CMAP applied in the field of TCM brought a new perspective for researchers and provided a systematic method for the study of the mechanisms of TCM and TCM formulae.

6.1. ESTABLISHING THE CMAP DATABASE

6.1.1 Molecules Treating Cell Lines

Lamb et al.[4] established the CMAP database, and the result was published in Science. In the early stage of establishing the CMAP database, researchers selected 164 distinct small-molecule compounds representing different biological activities that had been approved by the FDA. The selection of cell lines was limited by the experimental requirements such as whether they could be stably grown over long periods of time, whether they were able to culture in microplates, and whether they were used as reference cell lines in laboratories across the world. In compliance with such requirements, researchers chose four cell lines: breast cancer epithelial cells (MCF7), prostate cancer cells (PC3), leukemia cells (HL60), and melanoma cells (SKMEL5). The concentration and treatment time of the small-molecule compounds were also important factors in the experiment. A relatively high concentration of $10\ \mu mol/L$, which was commonly used in high-throughput screening-based cell assays, was selected as the initial treatment concentration. On top of that, researchers also conducted an extra experiment using a subset of compounds across a range of concentrations to explore the sensitivity of results to the dose. The selection of the small molecule compounds treating cells was proven to have an effect on the gene expression profiles. Therefore, 6 and 12 h treatment time were selected as the two time points for small-molecule compounds treating cells in the experiment. In the latter part of the work, researchers aimed at improving the CMAP database. The initial profiles of 164 drugs were expanded to 1309 FDA-approved small molecules; the cell lines increased to five human cell lines (adding the ssMCF7 cell line), generating over 7000 expression profiles in the CMAP database.[6] All data were included in the site (http://www.broadinstitute.org/cmap), which could be queried and downloaded for free.

6.1.2 The CMAP Concept

The analytic method of CMAP adopts a nonparametric, rank-based, pattern-matching strategy akin to the well-known approach of Gene Set Enrichment Analysis.[8] In the query process, the gene expression profile data are divided into lists of upregulated genes and downregulated genes for input to the CMAP database. The analysis results are presented with a connectivity score ranging from +1 to −1. A positive connectivity score indicates the degree of similarity and a negative score indicates an inverted similarity (Fig. 6.1).

6.2. APPLICATION IN TCM

Since the establishment of the CMAP database, it has been widely used in the field of drug discovery and development. So far, numerous achievements have been obtained in many research areas such as drug repurposing,[9–14] lead discovery,[15–18] and elucidating the mode of action.[19–23] In recent years, the CMAP database has been increasingly used in the field of TCM, achieving remarkable outcomes.

6.2.1 Application in Components of TCM

TCM contains diverse ingredients, which addresses a large part of the current TCM research. Recently, research by Ozcan and coworkers[24] using the CMAP database found that celastrol isolated from *Tripterygium wilfordii* has significant efficacy against obesity. Researchers obtained the corresponding differentially expressed genes from cells of the liver and hypothalamus in mice and analyzed them in CMAP. The resulting scores

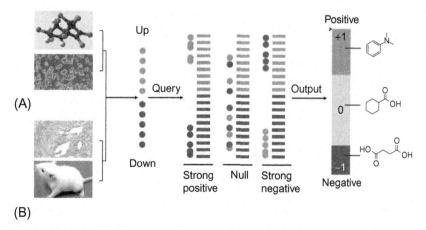

Fig. 6.1 Schematic view of CMAP analysis. Two sets of gene expression data were obtained: (A) gene expression data of compounds treating cells; (B) gene expression data of disease and disease model. After scoring using a pattern-matching algorithm, compounds were ranked by their "connectivity score."Fig. 6.1

were converted to absolute enrichment scores for the next analysis. Finally, researchers used all absolute enrichment scores to discover the small-molecule celastrol with the highest score to all the other molecules in the CMAP database. Furthermore, the experiment confirmed that celastrol increased leptin sensitivity to suppress food intake and dramatically reduced the body weight of obese mice in vivo. This work finds the drug celastrol as a candidate for the treatment of obesity, and provides a new method for the discovery of new drugs in TCM.

A recent study conducted by Lee et al.[25] mined the CMAP database to explore the molecular mechanisms of berberine. Berberine, a component of traditional Chinese herbal medicine, is isolated from various medicinal herbs such as *Coptis chinensis* and has a wide range of pharmacological actions including anticancer, antimicrobial, antiinflammatory, and antidiabetic effects.[26] In this study, researchers obtained berberine-induced differentially expressed genes from the Gene Expression Omnibus (GEO) at the National Center for Biotechnology Information (NCBI). Then, they analyzed the gene expression signatures of berberine by the CMAP database to compare similarities of gene expression profiles between berberine and compounds included in the CMAP database. The results showed that the gene expression signatures of berberine were positively correlated with protein synthesis, AKT/mTOR, and HDAC inhibitors, which were subsequently verified by experiments.

6.2.2 Application in TCM Formulae

In some occasions, TCM formulae have better therapeutic effects than single compounds alone in clinical practice, due to the multiple active phytochemical components and multiple targets/pathways therapeutic approach.[27] At present, the research of TCM formulae is hindered by the lack of suitable methods to tackle such complex mechanisms. However, the CMAP database applied to research TCM formulae provided a useful tool and received some achievements.

An impressive piece of work employing the CMAP approach was conducted by Zhou et al.,[28] which aimed at the identification of effective components in the TCM formula known as Danshen Dripping Pills. In this study, the gene expression data of atherosclerotic carotid artery tissues and histologically normal tissues in the human body were collected from GEO. The differentially expressed genes screened by significance analysis of the microarray (SAM) were imported to the CMAP database for analysis. The results showed seven compounds with a significant negative enrichment score, which indicated that these compounds could reversely regulate the gene expression profiles of pathological tissues. Then, based on the hypotheses that the similar chemical structures had similar activities, 10 candidate active ingredients of Danshen Dripping Pills were obtained by comparison with seven compounds in two-dimensional molecular fingerprints. Yu et al.[29] elucidated the effect of the Fuzheng Huayu Capsule (FHC) and its potential multiple target molecular pharmacology. The gene expression profile data was obtained from cells of patients with *Qi*-deficiency and blood-stasis (Qixu Xueyu) syndrome who were treated with FHC. Afterward, the differentially expressed genes were analyzed in the CMAP database to match compounds with similar effects. According to the analysis results, FHC showed antihyperglycemic, antihyperlipidemic, antihypotensive, and antiinflammatory effects. The potential mechanism may involve the Ca^{2+} related pathway. Another study using CMAP analysis was conducted by Wen et al.[30] to study the TCM formula known as the Siwu Decoction (SWD). In the study, the gene expression profiles of SWD-treated MCF7 cells were used for analysis in the CMAP database. The results showed that most of the compounds with strong positive correlation were estrogen drugs such as butyl hydroxybenzoate, alpha-estradiol, and genistein. Among the negatively correlated compounds, fulvestrant was a pure estrogen receptor antagonist with a significant negative score. These results were consistent with SWD's previously recognized use as a TCM formula for gynecologic diseases and proved the reliability of the CMAP application in TCM.

6.3. PERSPECTIVES

TCM has a thousand years of clinical practice and has undergone modern research for decades, which can lead to new drug discoveries. The constituents of TCM are complex and the mode of action is diverse. The multiple targets, the relative instability, and the complexity of the dose effect are especially challenging.[31] These factors contributed to a great challenge to the research of TCM, which obstructed understanding the mechanism of TCM, leaving little significant progress until now. With the development of new techniques, lots of new approaches have been applied in the field of TCM such as network biology and network pharmacology.[32] Since the emergence of the CMAP database, it has been widely applied in TCM research. In previous works, researchers used the CMAP database to identify the active ingredients in TCM, reveal the mechanism and efficacy of TCM, and find candidate drugs from TCM.

Although the application of CMAP is increasingly exploited and recognized, lots of challenges need to be addressed. For instance, in the case of removing batch effects in the analysis of microarray data, Chen et al.[33] systematically evaluated six algorithms using multiple measures of precision, accuracy, and overall performance. The results suggested that ComBat, an Empirical Bayes method, outperformed the other five programs by most metrics in removing batch effects. Also, Wang et al.[34] measured the gene expression similarity by calculating the Bridge Adjusted Expression Similarity (BAES) to adjust the batch effect in CMAP data. In addition, Li et al.[35] established a gene ontology module (GOM) approach based on the CMAP database, which integrated the expression pattern comparison into every GOM. Through the modularization of expression patterns, the GOM analysis method reduced experimental noises and marginal effects and directly correlated small chemical molecules with gene function modules. The methods above have improved the reliability of the analysis results using the CMAP database.

The previous studies demonstrated that the CMAP data-mining approach might be a new way to study TCM. In future studies, such an approach is promising in resolving the major challenges in current TCM research, such as elucidating the mechanism of multiple components and multiple targets of TCM formulae, synergistic effects and reduced toxicity, the theory of Chinese herbal nature, and discovering new therapeutic effect of TCM ingredients. Furthermore, employing the CMAP database in the study of TCM can prevent unnecessary animal experiments, reduce experimental costs, shorten the development cycle, and improve research efficiency. With further development, CMAP as a new weapon will have a more profound application and implication in the field of TCM research.

REFERENCES

1. Schena M, Shalon D, Davis RW, Brown PO. Quantitative monitoring of gene expression patterns with a complementary DNA microarray. *Science* 1995;**270**(5235):467–70.
2. Zhang Q, Sheng J. Development and application of gene chip technology. *Acta Acad Med Sin* 2008;**30**(3):344–7.
3. Hughes TR, Marton MJ, Jones AR, Roberts CJ, Stoughton R, Armour CD, et al. Functional discovery via a compendium of expression profiles. *Cell* 2000;**102**(1):109–26.
4. Lamb J, Crawford ED, Peck D, Modell JW, Blat IC, Wrobel MJ, et al. The connectivitiy map: using gene-expression signatures to connect small molecules, genes, and disease. *Science* 2006;**313**(5795):1929–35.
5. Justin L. The connectivity map: a new tool for biomedical research. *Nat Rev Cancer* 2007;**7**(1):54–60.
6. XA Q, Rajpal DK. Applications of connectivity map in drug discovery and development. *Drug Discov Today* 2012;**17**(23):1289–98.
7. Sun D, Shu Q. Gene expression profile—thinking of TCM functional genomics research. *J Zhejiang College TCM* 2002;**26**(1):5–9.
8. Subramanian A, Tamayo P, Mootha VK, Mukherjee S, Ebert BL, Gillette MA, et al. Gene set enrichment analysis: a knowledge-based approach for interpreting genome-wide expression profiles. *Proc Natl Acad Sci U S A* 2005;**102**(43):15545–50.
9. Zhang M, Luo H, Xi Z, Rogaeva E. Drug repositioning for diabetes based on 'Omics' data mining. *PLoS One* 2015;**10**(5). e0126082.
10. Ishimatsu YT, Soma TJ. Identification of novel hair-growth inducers by means of connectivity mapping. *FASEB J* 2010;**24**(5):1489–96.
11. Chang M, Smith S, Thorpe A, Barratt MJ, Karim F. Evaluation of phenoxybenzamine in the CFA model of pain following gene expression studies and connectivity mapping. *Mol Pain* 2010;**6**(1):1–13.
12. Marina S, Dudley JT, Jeewon K, Chiang AP, Morgan AA, Alejandro SC, et al. Discovery and preclinical validation of drug indications using compendia of public gene expression data. *Sci Transl Med* 2011;**3**(96). 96ra77.
13. Cheng HW, Liang YH, Kuo YL, Chuu CP, Lin CY, Lee MH, et al. Identification of thioridazine, an antipsychotic drug, as an antiglioblastoma and anticancer stem cell agent using public gene expression data. *Cell Death Dis* 2015;**6**(5). e1753.
14. Chiena W, Sun QY, Lee KL, Ding LW, Wuensche P, Lucia AT, et al. Activation of protein phosphatase 2A tumor suppressor as potential treatment of pancreatic cancer. *Mol Oncol* 2015;**9**(4):889–905.

15. Kumar RA, Kuick R, Kurapati H, Standiford TJ, Omenn GS, Keshamouni VG. Identifying inhibitors of epithelial-mesenchymal transition by connectivity-map based systems approach. *J Thorac Oncol* 2011;**6** (11):1784–92.

16. Wang G, Ye Y, Yang Y, Liao H, Zhao C, Liang S. Expression-based in silico screening of candidate therapeutic compounds for lung adenocarcinoma. *PLoS One* 2011;**6**(1). e14573.

17. Boyle JO, Gümüs ZH, Kacker A, Choksi VL, Bocker JM, Zhou XK. Effects of cigarette smoke on the human oral mucosal transcriptome. *Cancer Prev Res* 2010;**3**(3):266–78.

18. Babcock JJ, Du F, Xu K, Wheelan SJ, Li M. Integrated analysis of drug-induced gene expression profiles predicts novel hERG inhibitors. *PLoS One* 2013;**8**(7). e69513.

19. Seung-Bae R, Boh-Ram K, Sokbom K. A gene signature-based approach identifies thioridazine as an inhibitor of phosphatidylinositol-3-kinase (PI3K)/AKT pathway in ovarian cancer cells. *Gynecol Oncol* 2011;**120**(1):121–7.

20. Gheeyaa J, Johanssona P, Chena QR, Dexheimer T, Metaferiaa B, Songa YK, et al. Expression profiling identifies epoxy anthraquinone derivative as a DNA topoisomerase inhibitor. *Cancer Lett* 2010;**293** (1):124–31.

21. Zhang XZ, Yin AH, Lin DJ, Zhu XY, Ding Q, Wang CH, et al. Analyzing gene expression profile in K562 cells exposed to sodium valproate using microarray combined with the connectivity map database. *J Biomed Biotechnol* 2012;**2012**(4)654291.

22. Hieronymus H, Lamb J, Ross KN, Peng XP, Clement C, Rodina A, et al. Gene expression signature-based chemical genomic prediction identifies a novel class of HSP90 pathway modulators. *Cancer Cell* 2006;**10**(4):321–30.

23. D'Arcy P, Brnjic S, Olofsson MH, Fryknäs M, Lindsten K, De Cesare M, et al. Inhibition of proteasome deubiquitinating activity as a new cancer therapy. *Nat Med* 2011;**17**(12):1636–40.

24. Liu J, Lee J, Salazar Hernandez MA, Mazitschek R, Ozcan U. Treatment of obesity with celastrol. *Cell* 2015;**161**(5):999–1011.

25. Lee KH, Lo HL, Tang WC, Hsiao HH, Yang PM. A gene expression signature-based approach reveals the mechanisms of action of the Chinese herbal medicine berberine. *Sci Rep* 2014;**4**:6394.

26. Tillhon M, Guamán Ortiz LM, Lombardi P, Scovassi AI. Berberine: new perspectives for old remedies. *Biochem Pharmacol* 2012;**84**(10):1260–7.

27. Chow MS, Huang Y. Utilizing Chinese medicine to improve cancer therapy-fiction or reality? *Curr Drug Discov Technol* 2010;**7**(1):1.

28. Zhou W, Song XG, Chen C, Wang SM, Liang SW. Study on action mechanism and material base of compound Danshen dripping pills in treatment of carotid atherosclerosis based on techniques of gene expression profile and molecular fingerprint. *China J Chin Mater Med* 2015;**40**(16):3308–12.

29. Yu S, Guo Z, Guan Y, YY L, Hao P, Li Y, et al. Combining ZHENG theory and high-throughput expression data to predict new effects of Chinese herbal formulae. *Evid Based Complement Alternat Med* 2012;**2012**(8). 986427.

30. Wen Z, Wang Z, Wang S, Ravula R, Yang L, Xu J, et al. Discovery of molecular mechanisms of traditional Chinese medicinal formula Si-Wu-Tang using gene expression microarray and connectivity map. *PLoS One* 2011;**6**(3). e18278.

31. Liu QS, Chen XY, Zhuang SJ. Research progress of gene expression profiles based on the application of it in traditional Chinese medicine network pharmacology. *Lishizhen Med Mater Med Res* 2014;**25** (2):502–4.

32. Wang Y, Gao X, Zhang B, Cheng Y. Building methodology for discovering and developing Chinese medicine based on network biology. *China J Chin Mater Med* 2011;**36**(2):228–31.

33. Chen C, Grennan K, Badner J, Zhang D, Gershon E, Jin L, et al. Removing batch effects in analysis of expression microarray data: an evaluation of six batch adjustment methods. *PLoS One* 2011;**6**(2). e17238.

34. Wang K, Sun J, Zhou S, Wan C, Qin S, Li C, et al. Prediction of drug-target interactions for drug repositioning only based on genomic expression similarity. *PLoS Comput Biol* 2013;**9**(11). e1003315.

35. Li Y, Hao P, Zheng S, Tu K, Fan H, Zhu R, et al. Gene expression module-based chemical function similarity search. *Nucleic Acids Res* 2008;**36**(20). e137.

Case Study on Shexiang Baoxin Pill

CHAPTER 7

The Study of the Material Basis of the Shexiang Baoxin Pill

Peng Jiang*, Runui Liu[†], Weidong Zhang[†]
*Shanghai Hutchison Pharmaceutical Limited Company, Shanghai, PR China
[†]Second Military Medical University, Shanghai, PR China

Abstract

It is well known that each piece of traditional Chinese medicine (TCM) contains many different chemical constituents, which are responsible for therapeutic effects in complex matrices. The Shexiang Baoxin Pill is a TCM for the treatment of myocardial ischemia with a long history. To identify the main material basis of the Shexiang Baoxin Pill, the LC-MS and GC-MS method were both used to analyze the components. In the end, 96 compounds were identified, illuminating the material basis of the Shexiang Baoxin Pill.

Keywords: Shexiang Baoxin Pill, Material basis, LC-MS, GC-MS.

The traditional method of identifying the single compounds in complex systems of TCM uses chromatography technology to obtain pure compounds; the pure compounds were then identified by nuclear magnetic resonance and mass spectrometry. The traditional method needs complex separation processes and a long time. It is hard to exhibit the diversity of chemical composition and the whole characteristic of TCM. In recent years, some technologies of chromatography coupled with mass spectrometry, such as gas chromatography coupled with mass spectrometry and liquid chromatography coupled with mass spectrometry, were applied in the compositional analysis of TCM. These modern technologies can quickly identify the composition of TCM.

The Shexiang Baoxin Pill originated from the Suhexiang Pill, which was recorded in the famous book of the Song Dynasty called "Prescriptions People's Welfare Pharmacy." The Shexiang Baoxin Pill took 8 years to develop by the Shanghai Zhongshan Hospital, the Shanghai Huashan Hospital, the Shanghai Institute of Cardiovascular Disease, the Shanghai First TCM factory, and a number of scientific research, medical, and production units. The Pill has the effects of opening an orifice mildly with aromatics, supplementing Qi, and reinforcing the heart. The Shexiang Baoxin Pill is a representative formula of the "warm and fragrant" prescription. It not only has the characteristics of relieving angina pectoris but also is the first TCM prescription for promoting therapeutic angiogenesis.

The chemical composition of the Shexiang Baoxin Pill is very complicated, having both volatile small molecules and large nonvolatile components such as cholic acid, ginsenoside, and bufanolide dienes. Therefore it is a very difficult task to quickly and

Systems Biology and Its Application in TCM Formulas Research
https://doi.org/10.1016/B978-0-12-812744-5.00007-2

accurately identify the general chemical substances in the whole formula. In this chapter, we use GC–MS and LC–MS methods to qualitatively analyze the main chemical components of the Shexiang Baoxin Pill in a fast and accurate way.

7.1. IDENTIFICATION OF NONVOLATILE CONSTITUENTS IN THE TCM-FORMULA SHEXIANG BAOXIN PILL BY LC COUPLED WITH DAD-ESI-MS-MS

7.1.1 Experimental

7.1.1.1 Materials and Chemicals

LC-grade acetonitrile and formic acid were purchased from Merck (Darmstadt, Germany). Ultrapure water from a Milli-Q50 SP Reagent Water System (Millipore Corporation, MA, USA) was used for the preparation of samples and the mobile phase. Other reagents were of analytical grade. The reference standards of cinnamic acid, cinnamaldehyde, bilirubin, benzyl benzoate, ursodeoxycholic acid, chenodeoxycholic acid, hyodeoxycholic acid, cholic acid, and 10 triterpene saponins including ginsenoside Rb_1, Rb_2, Rb_3, Rc, Rd., Re, Rf, Rg_1, Rg_3, and notoginsenoside R_1 were purchased from the National Institute for the Control of Pharmaceutical and Biological Products (Beijing, PR China). Seven standard compounds of bufadienolides including ψ-bufarenogin, gamabufotalin, arenobufagin, bufalin, resibufagin, resibufogenin, and cinobufagin, were isolated in our laboratory (purity >99.0%); their chemical structure was identified by spectral analysis and previous data. SBP (batch number 080508) and its raw materials including moschus, radix rhizoma ginseng, calculus bovis, cortex cinnamomi, styrax, venenum bufonis, and borneolum syntheticum were kindly offered by the Shanghai Hutchison Pharmaceuticals Company (Shanghai, China). The voucher specimens were deposited in our laboratory.

7.1.1.2 Preparation of Samples

SBP was ground into a fine powder and 500 mg were accurately weighed with a 6.5 mL mixed solvent (methanol:dichlormethane:water = 4:2:0.5, v/v) added. The sample was ultrasonically extracted for 20 min, then centrifuged and filtered through a syringe filter (0.45 μm). Aliquots (10 μL) were subjected to LC analysis. All the dry crude materials were ground into a fine powder. Moschus, radix rhizoma ginseng, cortex cinnamomi, and venenum bufonis (5 g) were ultrasonically extracted respectively in 10% methanol 20 mL for 30 min, and then extracted by 95% methanol 20 mL for 30 min. The operations were repeated twice, and the total extracts were combined. Each crude material solvent was removed at 50°C under vacuum by the Buchi rotavapor B-490. The residues were then dissolved in 25 mL methanol. Calculus bovis (5 g) was ultrasonically extracted with a mixed solvent (dichlormethane:methanol = 4:2, v/v) 20 mL for 30 min. This operation was also repeated twice. After the decompression drying process, the residue was

Table 7.1 Chemical structures of compounds identified in the extract of SBP

Type	Substituent groups	Name
	$R_1=CH_3$, $R_2=H$, $R_3=H$, $R_4=H$, $R_5=H$, $R_6=H$	Bufalin
	$R_1=CH_3$, $R_2=H$, $R_3=OH$, $R_4=H$, $R_5=H$, $R_6=H$	Gamabufotalin
	$R_1=CH_3$, $R_2=H$, $R_3=H$, $R_4=H$, $R_5=H$, $R_6=OH$	1β-Hydroxylbufalin
	$R_1=CH_3$, $R_2=H$, $R_3=OH$, $R_4==O$, $R_5=H$, $R_6=H$	Arenobufagin
	$R_1=CH_3$, $R_2=H$, $R_3==O$, $R_4=\alpha$-OH, $R_5=H$, $R_6=H$	ψ-Bufarenogin
	$R_1=CH_3$, $R_2=H$, $R_3==O$, $R_4=\beta$-OH, $R_5=H$, $R_6=H$	Bufarenogin
	$R_1=CHO$, $R_2=OH$, $R_3=H$, $R_4=H$, $R_5=H$, $R_6=H$	Hellebrigenin
	$R_1=CH_3$, $R_2=H$, $R_3=H$, $R_4=H$, $R_5=OAc$, $R_6=H$	Bufotalin
	$R_1=CH_3$, $R_2=OH$, $R_3=H$, $R_4=OH$	Desacetylcinobufotalin
	$R_1=CHO$, $R_2=OH$, $R_3=H$, $R_4=H$	Bufotalinin
	$R_1=CHO$, $R_2=OH$, $R_3=H$, $R_4=OAc$	19-Cinobufotalin
	$R_1=CH_3$, $R_2=H$, $R_3=H$, $R_4=OH$	Desacetylcinobufagin
	$R_1=CHO$, $R_2=H$, $R_3=H$, $R_4=H$	Resibufagin
	$R_1=CH_3$, $R_2=OH$, $R_3=H$, $R_4=H$	Marinobufagin
	$R_1=CH_3$, $R_2=OH$, $R_3=H$, $R_4=OAc$	Cinobufotalin
	$R_1=CH_3$, $R_2=H$, $R_3=H$, $R_4=OAc$	Cinobufagin
	$R_1=CH_3$, $R_2=H$, $R_3=H$, $R_4=H$	Resibufogenin
	$R_1=glc(2-1)glc$, $R_2=glc(6-1)glc(3-1)xyl$	Ginsenoside Ra_3
	$R_1=glc(2-1)glc$, $R_2=glc(6-1)arap(4-1)xyl$	Ginsenoside Ra_1
	$R_1=glc(2-1)glc$, $R_2=glc(6-1)araf(4-1)xyl$	Ginsenoside Ra_2
	$R_1=glc(2-1)glc(2-1)xyl$, $R_2=glc(6-1)xyl$	Ginsenoside Fc
	$R_1=glc(2-1)glc$, $R_2=glc(6-1)glc$	Ginsenoside Rb_1
	$R_1=glc(2-1)glc$, $R_2=glc(6-1)araf$	Ginsenoside Rc
	$R_1=glc(2-1)glc$, $R_2=glc(6-1)arap$	Ginsenoside Rb_2

Continued

Table 7.1 Chemical structures of compounds identified in the extract of SBP—cont'd

Type	Substituent groups	Name
	R_1=glc(2-1)glc, R_2=glc(6-1)xyl	Ginsenoside Rb_3
	R_1=glc(2-1)glc, R_2=glc	Ginsenoside Rd
	R_1=glc(2-1)glc, R_2=H	Ginsenoside Rg_3
	R_1=glc(2-1)glc(2-1)xyl, R_2=glc(6-1)glc	Notoginsenoside Fa
	R_1=glc(2-1)glc-Ac, R_2=glc(6-1)glc	Quinquenoside R_1
	R_1=glc(2-1)glc-Ac, R_2=glc(6-1) arap	Ginsenoside Rs_1
	R_1=glc(2-1)glc-Ac, R_2=glc(6-1) araf	Ginsenoside Rs_2
	R_1=glc(2-1)xyl, R_2=glc	Notoginsenoside R_1
	R_1=glc, R_2=glc	Ginsenoside Rg_1
	R_1=glc(2-1)rha, R_2=glc	Ginsenoside Re
	R_1=glc(2-1)glc, R_2=H	Ginsenoside Rf
	R_1=glc(2-1)xyl, R_2=H	Notoginsenoside R_2
	R_1=glc(2-1)rha, R_2=H	Ginsenoside Rg_2
	R_1=glucuronic acid-glc(2-1), R_2=glc	Ginsenoside Ro
	R_1=OH, R_2=H, R_3=α-OH	Cholic acid
	R_1=OH, R_2=H, R_3=H	Deoxycholic acid
	R_1=H, R_2=H, R_3=β-OH	Ursodeoxycholic acid
	R_1=H, R_2=H, R_3=α-OH	Chensodeoxycholic acid
	R_1=H, R_2=OH, R_3=H	Hyodeoxycholic acid
		Bilirubin

dissolved in a 25 mL mixed solvent (dichlormethane:methanol=4:2, v/v). A total of 0.2 g Styrax and borneolum syntheticum were dissolved in 25 mL methanol directly. All the samples were filtered through a 0.45-μm film before LC analysis.

7.1.1.3 LC-DAD-MS System

Liquid chromatographic analysis was carried out using an Agilent 1100 series LC system (Agilent Technologies, Palo Alto, MA, USA) equipped with a quaternary pump with an online degasser, autosampler, column oven, and diode array detector (DAD). Separation was performed on a Symmetry C18 column (5 µm, 4.6 mm × 250 mm, waters). The column temperature was kept constantly at 25°C, and the mobile phase flow rate was 0.8 mL min^{-1}. The mobile phase consisted of 0.5 vol.% aqueous formic acid (A) and (B) acetonitrile using a gradient elution of 20 vol.% B at 0–7 min, 20–30 vol.% B at 7–25 min, 30 vol.% B at 25–35 min, 30–35 vol.% B at 35–60 min, 35 vol.% B at 60–65 min, 35–70 vol.% B at 65–75 min, 70–100 vol.% B at 75–80 min, and 100 vol.%-B at 80–95 min. The DAD detector recorded UV spectra in the range from 190 to 500 nm and the monitored wavelengths were set at 203, 280, and 446 nm. The injection volume was 10 µL.

An Agilent LC-MSD Trap XCT mass spectrometer equipped with an ESI interface and an ion trap mass analyzer was used for carrying out the MS and MS$^{(2)}$ analysis. By solvent splitting, 0.2 mL min^{-1} portions of the column effluent were delivered into the ion source of the mass spectrometer. The conditions were as follows: drying gas (nitrogen) flow rate 10 L min^{-1}, temperature 350°C, pressure of nebulizer gas 30 psi, HV voltage 3.5 kV, target mass 600 amu, compound stability 100%, threshold 50,000 (ESI^{+}) and 10,000 (ESI^{-}), and scan range 100–1500 amu. An amplitude voltage of 1.0 V was typically used for fragmentation in the ion trap auto MS$^{(2)}$ experiments. Positive and negative mode data were acquired by using Agilent Chemstation Software. All the structure of identified compounds are shown in Table 7.1.

7.1.2 Results and Discussion

7.1.2.1 LC-DAD Analysis of SBP

The selection of LC conditions was guided by the requirement for obtaining chromatograms with better resolution of adjacent peaks. A linear gradient elution of CH_3CN and H_2O–HCOOH was found to be the optimal mobile phase in both LC and MS analyses. CH_3CN remarkably improved the separation of the major constituents in SBP as compared to CH_3OH. Studies showed that 0.5% formic acid added into the mobile phase (water) remarkably improved the symmetries of chromatographic peaks, especially for the bufadienolides. Otherwise the peaks were rather broad with poor separation.

By careful analysis of the chromatograms at different wavelengths in the range from 190 to 500 nm, it was found that the chromatograms at 203, 280, and 446 nm could well represent the profile of the constituents. Under the current LC condition, 39 peaks from SBP were detected. The peaks were characterized by the retention times and UV spectra as well as by comparing the chromatogram of SBP with those of single herb extracts. The representative LC-DAD chromatograms of the extract of SBP and single crude drugs are presented in Fig. 7.1. As revealed in Fig. 7.1A–C, the main constituents in SBP were well separated on the reversed-phase column with gradient elution. By comparing the chromatograms of SBP with those of its crude herbs' extracts (Fig. 7.1D–I), the major constituents in SBP were well assigned to the crude plants. As the solution of borneolum syntheticum showed no signal in DAD, its chromatography was not shown.

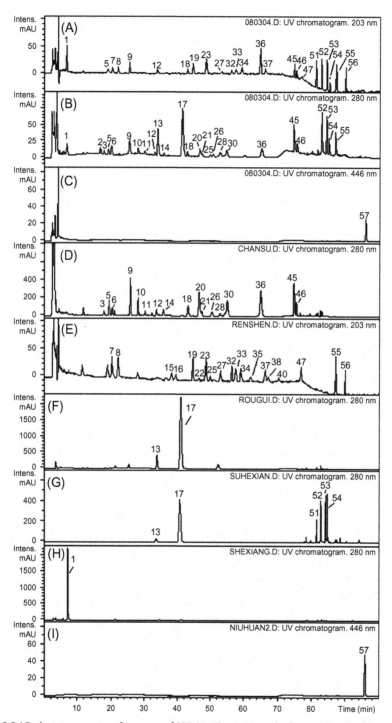

Fig. 7.1 LC-DAD chromatograms of extracts of SBP (A–C), venenum bufonis (D), radix rhizome ginseng (E), cortex cinnamom (F), styrax (G), moschus (H), and calculus bovis (I). All peak numbers as in Table 7.2.

According to the characteristic UV profile of some major constituents such as triterpene saponins giving end absorption at 203 nm, bufadienolides giving maximum UV absorption wavelengths at 300 nm, and phenylallyl compounds giving at 220 and 280 nm, the framework type of compounds could be rapidly identified based on their UV profiles.

7.1.2.2 ESI-MS$^{(2)}$ Analysis of Authentic Compounds

In order to obtain MS fragmentation patterns of constituents in SBP, MS$^{(2)}$ spectra of 11 reference compounds, that is, ursodeoxycholic acid, chenodeoxycholic acid, cholic acid, ginsenoside Rb$_1$, Rd., Re, notoginsenoside R$_1$, gamabufotalin, resibufogenin, bufalin, and cinobufagin, were first analyzed by direct infusion. MS and MS$^{(2)}$ data were obtained by CID. Their fragmentation patterns were summarized; it was very helpful for the constituents' structure identification in SBP, which had the similar framework.

In the full-scan mass spectra, most of the authentic compounds exhibited $[M+H]^+$ ions in the positive mode or their quasimolecular $[M-H]^-$ in the negative mode.

The characteristic fragmentation of four bufadienolides was studied in the positive ion mode. A neutral loss of 96 Da, resulting from elimination of the a-pyrone ring at the C-17 position, was common in the MS$^{(2)}$ spectra of bufadienolides in their MS$^{(2)}$ spectra. Because of substitutions of polyhydroxy and the a-pyrone ring in bufadienolides, most of the produced fragmentation ions also included $[M+H-H_2O]^+$, $[M+H-2H_2O]^+$, $[M+H-2H_2O-CO]^+$, $[M+H-3H_2O]^+$, and $[M+H-3H_2O-CO]^+$.

The characteristic fragmentation of four triterpene saponins and three bile acids was studied in the negative ion mode. Most triterpene saponins yielded prominent $[M-H]^-$ and $[M-H+HCOO]^-$ ions in the first order mass spectra. Their MS$^{(2)}$ spectra exhibited a fragmentation pattern corresponding to the loss of the glycosidic units. The fragmentation ions of $[M-H-2H_2O]^-$ and $[M-H-H_2O-HCOO]^-$ were characteristic ions of bile acids in the MS-MS spectra of the negative mode.

7.1.2.3 LC-DAD-MS-MS Analysis of SBP

Fig. 7.2 shows the total ion chromatogram of SBP in both positive ion mode (Fig. 7.2A) and negative ion mode (Fig. 7.2B). As we can see, it was difficult to screen and identify the components in the TIC chromatograms due to the poor signal-to-noise ratio in mass data. To reduce the noise of MS data, LC-MSD Trap Software version 5.2 (Agilent) was used. Fig. 7.2C and D shows the total ion chromatograms after reducing noise.

A total of 57 peaks were detected by using the LC-DAD-MS$^{(2)}$, among which 39 major peaks were detected by DAD; 30 of them had the corresponding peaks in the MS chromatogram, and 18 other peaks with low UV absorption were also detected in the MS chromatogram. Forty-seven of the 57 peaks were identified, and 21 peaks were unambiguously identified by comparing RT, UV spectra, and m/z value with the authentic compounds. Another 26 peaks were identified on the basis of the UV spectra,

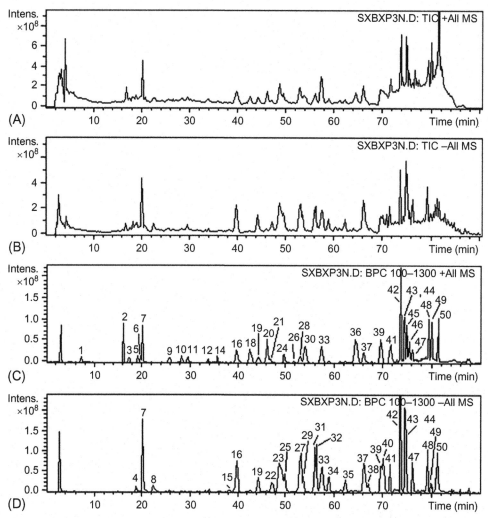

Fig. 7.2 Total ion current (TIC) chromatograms of SBP in positive ion mode MS spectra and negative ion mode MS spectra (A and B), base peak chromatograsms of SBP in positive ion mode MS spectra, and negative ion mode MS spectra (C and D). The peak numbers as in Table 7.2.

MS and $MS^{(2)}$ spectra with fragmentation patterns of the aforementioned, and the literature data.[1-7] All the detailed data are shown in Table 7.2.

Among these identified 47 compounds, there were 20 triterpene saponins from radix rhizoma ginseng, 18 bufadienolides from venenum bufonis, five bile acids from calculus bovis, two phenylallyl compounds from cortex cinnamomi and styrax, and two other compounds. All the identified compounds are the main components in these medicinal materials.

Table 7.2 Characterization of compounds in extract of SBP by HPLC-DAD-MS-MS

Peak no.	t (min)	Compound	λ_{max} (nm)	MS+ (m/z)	MS− (m/z)	Plant material	Fragments ions (m/z)
1	7.1	Unknown	265	359; 585			342; 278
2	16.7	Unknown	250, 300	679; 701			661; 435
3	17.4	ψ-Bufarenogin*	250, 300	417[M+H]+ 855 [2M+Na]+		1	399[M+H−H₂O]+; 363[M+H−3H₂O]+; 335[M+H−3H₂O−CO]+; 307[M+H−3H₂O−2CO]+
4	19.0	Notoginsenoside R₁*	—		932[M−H]−; 977[M−H+HCOO]−	2	799[M−H−Xyl]−; 769 [M−H−Glc]−; 637 [M−H−Glc−Xyl]−; 475 [Agl]−
5	19.2	Gamabufotalin*	250, 300	403[M+H]+ 827 [2M+Na]+		1	385[M+H−H₂O]+; 367[M+H−2H₂O]+; 349[M+H−3H₂O]+; 253[M+H−3H₂O−α-pyr]+
6	19.9	Bufarenogin	250, 300	417[M+H]+		1	399[M+H−H₂O]+; 371[M+H−H₂O−CO]+; 363[M+H−3H₂O]+; 353[M+H−2H₂O−CO]+; 335[M+H−3H₂O−CO]+
7	20.3	Ginsenoside Re*	—		946[M−H]−; 991[M−H+HCOO]−	2	799[M−H−Rha]−; 783 [M−H−Glc]−; 637 [M−H−Glc−Rha]−; 475 [Agl]−
8	22.2	Ginsenoside Rg₁*	—		800[M−H]−; 845[M−H+HCOO]−	2	637[M−H−Glc]−; 475[Agl]−
9	25.8	Arenobufagin*	260, 305	417[M+H]+ 855 [2M+Na]+		1	399[M+H−H₂O]+; 371[M+H−H₂O−CO]+; 353[M+H−2H₂O−CO]+; 335[M+H−2H₂OCO]+; 335[M+H−3H₂O−CO]+

Continued

Table 7.2 Characterization of compounds in extract of SBP by HPLC-DAD-MS-MS—cont'd

Peak no.	t (min)	Compound	λ_{max} (nm)	MS+ (m/z)	MS− (m/z)	Plant material	Fragments ions (m/z)
10	28.3	Hellebrigenin	250,300	417[M+H]+ 855 [2M+Na]+		1	363[M+H−3H$_2$O]+; 353[M+H−2H$_2$O−CO]+; 335[M+H−3H$_2$O−CO]+
11	29.7	Desacetylcinobufotalin	250, 300	417[M+H]+		1	399[M+H−H$_2$O]+; 381[M+H−2H$_2$O]+; 363[M+H−3H$_2$O]+; 335[M+H−3H$_2$O−CO]+
12	33.5	Bufotalinin	250,290	415[M+H]+		1	397[M+H−H$_2$O]+; 379[M+H−2H$_2$O]+; 351[M+H−2H$_2$O−CO]+; 361[M+H−3H$_2$O]+; 333[M+H−3H$_2$O−CO]+
13	33.8	Cinnamic acid*	216, 285				
14	35.8	19-oxo-Cinobufotalin	250, 300	473[M+H]+		1	395[M+H−H$_2$O−HOAC]+;377[M+H−2H$_2$O−HOAC]+; 349[M+H−2H$_2$O−HOAC−CO]+
15	38.2	Gnsenoside Ra$_3$/notoginsenoside Fa	—		1240 [M−H]−	2	1107[M−H−Xyl]−; 1077 [M−H−Glc]−; 945 [M−H−Xyl−Glc]−; 783 [M−H−Xyl−2Glc]−; 621 [M−H−Xyl−3Glc]−
16	39.7	Ginsenoside Rf*	—		800[M−H]− 845[M−H+HCOO]−	2	637[M−H−Glc]−; 475[Agl]−
17	41.1	Cinnamaldehyde*	225, 285				
18	42.7	1β-Hydroxylbufalin	295	403[M+H]+ 827 [2M+Na]+		1	385[M+H−H$_2$O]+;367[M+H−2H$_2$O]+;349[M+H−3H$_2$O]+; 339[M+H−3H$_2$O−CO]+; 253[M+H−3H$_2$O−α-pyr]+

No.	t_R	Compound	UV	Positive	Negative		Fragments
19	44.2	Notoginsenoside R_2	—		$770[M-H]^-$; $815[M-H+HCOO]^-$	2	$637[M-H-Xyl]^-$; $475[Agl]^-$
20	46.3	Bufotalin	255, 310	$445[M+H]^+$; $911[2M+Na]^+$		1	$409[M+H-2H_2O]^+$; $367[M+H-2H_2O-HOAC]^+$; $349[M+H-2H_2O-HOAC]^+$
21	46.8	Desacetylcinobufagin	255, 305	$401[M+H]^+$		1	$383[M+H-H_2O]^+$; $365[M+H-2H_2O]^+$; $347[M+H-3H_2O]^+$; $337[M+H-2H_2O-CO]^+$; $319[M+H-3H_2O-CO]^+$
22	47.3	Ginsenoside Ra_1/Ra_2/Fc	—		$1210[M-H]^-$	2	$1077[M-H-Xyl]^-$; $1047[M-H-Glc]^-$; $945[M-H-2Xyl/(Xyl-Ara)]^-$; $783[M-H-2Xyl'Glc/(Xyl-Ara-Glc)]^-$
23	48.9	Ginsenoside Rb_1*	—		$1108[M-H]^-$; $1153[M-H+HCOO]^-$	2	$945[M-H-Glc]^-$; $783[M-H-2Glc]^-$; $621[M-H-3Glc]^-$; $459[Agl]^-$
24	49.2	Resibufagin*	250, 300	$399[M+H]^+$; $421[M+Na]^+$		1	$381[M+H-H_2O]^+$; $353[M+H-H_2O-CO]^+$; $335[M+H-2H_2O-CO]^+$; $307[M+H-2H_2O-2CO]^+$; $257[M+H-CO-\alpha-pyr]^+$
25	49.7	Ginsenoside Rg_2	—		$784[M-H]^-$; $829[M-H+HCOO]^-$	2	$637[M-H-Rha]^-$; $621[M-H-Glc]^-$; $475[Agl]^-$
26	51.6	19-oxo-Cinobufagin	255, 300	$457[M+H]^+$		1	$421[M+H-2H_2O]^+$; $379[M+H-H_2O-HOAC]^+$; $361[M+H-2H_2O-HOAC]^+$; $333[M+H-2H_2O-HOAC-CO]^+$

Continued

Table 7.2 Characterization of compounds in extract of SBP by HPLC-DAD-MS-MS—cont'd

Peak no.	t (min)	Compound	λ_{max} (nm)	MS+ (m/z)	MS− (m/z)	Plant material	Fragments ions (m/z)
27	53.0	Ginsenoside Rc*	—		1078 [M−H]−	2	945[M−H−Araf]−; 783[M−H−Araf−Glc]−; 621[M−H−Araf−2Glc]−; 459[Agl]−
28	53.2	Marinobufagin	250, 300	401[M+H]+		1	383[M+H−H2O]+; 365[M+H−2H2O]+; 347[M+H−3H2O]+; 337[M+H−2H2O−CO]+; 319[M+H−3H2O−CO]+; 269[M+H−2H2O−α-pyr]+
29	53.7	Ginsenoside Ra1/Ra2/Fc	—		1210 [M−H]−	2	1077[M−H−Xyl]−; 1047[M−H−Glc]−; 945[M−H−2Xyl/(Xyl−Ara)]−; 783[M−H−2Xyl−Glc/(Xyl−Ara−Glc)]−
30	54.2	Cinobufotalin	250, 300	459[M+H]+ 939 [2M+Na]+		1	417[M+H−CH2CO]+; 381[M+H−2H2O−CH2CO−CH2CO]+; 363[M+H'-3H2O'-CH2CO]+
31	55.7	Ginsenoside Ra1/Ra2/Fc	—		1210 [M−H]−	2	1077[M−H−Xyl]−; 1047[M−H−Glc]−; 945[M−H−2Xyl/(Xyl−Ara)]−; 783[M−H−2Xyl−Glc/(Xyl−Ara−Glc)]−
32	56.2	Ginsenoside Ro	—		955[M−H]−	2	793[M−H−Glc]−; 613[M−H−2Glc−H2O]−; 455[Agl]−

No.	t_R	Compound					
33	57.6	Ginsenoside Rb_2	—		1078 [M−H]⁻ 1114 [M−H+2 H₂O]⁻	2	945[M−H−Arap]⁻;783 [M−H−Arap−Glc]⁻;621 [M−H−Arap−2Glc]⁻;459 [Ag]⁻
34	59.0	Ginsenoside Rb_3*	—		1078 [M−H]⁻ 1114 [M−H +2H₂O]⁻	2	945[M−H−Xyl]⁻;783 [M−H−Xyl−Glc]⁻;621 [M−H−Xyl−2Glc]⁻;459 [Ag]⁻
35	62.2	Quinquenoside R_1	—		1150 [M−H]⁻	2	1107[M−CH₃CO]⁻;987 [M−H−Glc]⁻;945 [M−GlcAc]⁻;927 [M−H−GlcAc−H₂O]⁻;783 [M−H−GlcAc−Glc]⁻
36	64.4	Bufalin*	255, 300	387[M +H]⁺ 795 [2M +Na]⁺		1	369[M+H+H₂O]⁺;351[M +H−2H₂O]⁺;333[M +H−3H₂O]⁺;305[M +H−3H₂O−CO]⁺;255[M +H−2H₂O−α-pyr]⁺
37	66.0	Ginsenoside Rd*	—		946[M−H]⁻ 991[M−H +HCOO]⁻	2	783[M−H−Glc]⁻;621 [M−H−2Glc]⁻;459[Ag]⁻
38	66.8	Ginsenoside Rs_1/Rs_2	—		1120 [M−H]⁻	2	1077[M−H−CH₂CO]⁻;1059 [M−H−H₂O−CH₂CO]⁻; 945[M−H−Arap (Araf)−CH₂CO]⁻;927 [M−H−Arap (Araf)−H₂O−CH₂CO]⁻; 459[Ag]⁻
39	69.5	Unknown	—	462; 480	514; 1030		
40	70.5	Ginsenoside Rs_1/Rs_2	—		1120 [M−H]⁻	2	1077[M−H−CH₂CO]⁻;1059 [M−H−H₂O−CH₂CO]⁻; 945[M−H−Arap (Araf)−CH₂CO]⁻;927 [M−H−Arap (Araf)−H₂O−CH₂CO]⁻; 459[Ag]⁻

Continued

Table 7.2 Characterization of compounds in extract of SBP by HPLC-DAD-MS-MS—cont'd

Peak no.	t (min)	Compound	λ_{max} (nm)	MS$^+$ (m/z)	MS$^-$ (m/z)	Plant material	Fragments ions (m/z)
41	71.5	Unknown	—	355;373	453; 815		
42	73.6	Cholic acid*	—		407[M−H]$^-$; 815; [2M−H]$^-$	3	371[M−H−2H$_2$O]$^-$; 353 [M−H−3H$_2$O]$^-$; 344 [M−H−H$_2$O−HCOO]$^-$; 326
43	74.5	Ursodeoxycholic acid*	—		391[M−H]$^-$; 783; [2M−H]$^-$	3	373[M−H−H$_2$O]$^-$; 355 [M−H−2H$_2$O]$^-$; 328 [M−H−H$_2$O−HCOO]$^-$
44	74.5	Hyodeoxycholic acid*	—		391[M−H]$^-$; 783; [2M−H]$^-$	3	373[M−H−H$_2$O]$^-$; 355 [M−H−2H$_2$O]$^-$; 328 [M−H−H$_2$O−HCOO]$^-$
45	74.8	Cinobufagin*	250, 300	443[M+H]$^+$		1	401[M+H−CH$_2$CO]$^+$; 383[M+H−HOAC]$^+$; 365[M+H−HOAC−H$_2$O]$^+$; 347[M+H−HOAC−2H$_2$O]$^+$
46	75.1	Resibufogenin*	250, 300	385[M+H]$^+$		1	367[M+H−H$_2$O]$^+$;349[M+H−2H$_2$O]$^+$; 321[M+H−2H$_2$O−CO]$^+$; 253[M+H−2H$_2$O−α−pyr]$^+$
47	76.7	Ginsenoside Rg$_3$*			784[M−H]$^-$; 829[M−H+HCOO]$^-$	2	621[M−H−Glc]$^-$; 459[Agl]$^-$
48	79.2	Chenodeoxycholic acid*	—		391[M−H]$^-$; 783; [2M−H]$^-$	3	373[M−H−H$_2$O]$^-$; 355 [M−H−2H$_2$O]$^-$; 328 [M−H−H$_2$O−HCOO]$^-$
49	79.8	Deoxycholic acid	—		391[M−H]$^-$; 783; [2M−H]$^-$	3	373[M−H−H$_2$O]$^-$; 355 [M−H−2H$_2$O]$^-$; 328 [M−H−H$_2$O−HCOO]$^-$

50	81.2	Unknown	–			
51	81.6	Benzyl benzoate*	240, 270			
52	82.7	Unknown	280			
53	84.0	Unknown	280			
54	85.5	Unknown	225			
55	87.0	Unknown	–			2
56	90.3	Unknown	–			2
57	95.9	Bilirubin*	446	520; 758	765; 812	3

*Structure confirmed by comparison with reference standards.

For example, peak 32 showed the same fragmentation pathway of triterpene saponins in the $MS^{(2)}$ spectrum as mentioned above and was suspected as a triterpene saponin. It was also confirmed by its UV spectrum. In the MS spectrum, peak 32 showed a base peak at m/z 955 and exhibited m/z 793 $[M-H-Glu]^-$, m/z 613 $[M-H-2Glu-O]^-$, and m/z 455 $[Agl]^-$ ions in the $MS^{(2)}$ spectra. The m/z 455 ion resulting from successive losses of all linked glucosidic bonds is a characterized fragmentation of the oleanolic acid-type ginsenoside. By comparison with the literature data, this compound was tentatively identified as the known compound ginsenoside Ro.

Peaks 3, 6, 9, 10, and 11 all showed m/z 417 $[M+H]^+$ and 855 $[2M+Na]^+$ ions in their MS spectra and gave the same fragmentation pathway of bufadienolides as mentioned above in their $MS^{(2)}$ spectra. Their UV spectra were also similar and gave the maximum absorption at 250 and 300 nm. These five components were then assumed to be bufadienolides-type compounds. By comparison with reference standards, peaks 3 and 9 were identified as ψ-bufarenogin and arenobufagin. The $MS^{(2)}$ spectra of peak 6 gave the base peak at m/z 399 $[M+H-H_2O]^+$, while peak 10 showed the base peak at m/z 335 $[M+H-3H_2O-CO]^+$ and peak 11 showed the base peak at m/z 363 $[M+H-3H_2O]^+$. As the different base peak in their MS-MS spectra, peaks 6, 10, and 11 were identified as bufarenogin, hellebrigenin, and desacetylcinobufotalin. The result was also confirmed by comparison with the literature data.

Peaks 43, 44, 48, and 49 derived from calculus bovis showed a low UV signal in DAD. All their MS spectra showed ions at m/z 391 $[M-H]^-$ and m/z 783 $[2M-H]^-$. By comparison with the reference standards, peaks 43, 44, and 48 were identified as ursodeoxycholic acid, hyodeoxycholic acid, and chenodeoxycholic acid. As peak 49 showed fragmentation ions at m/z 373 $[M-H-H_2O]^-$, m/z 355 $[M-H-2H_2O]^-$, m/z 346 $[M-H-HCOO]^-$, and m/z 328 $[M-H-H_2O-HCOO]^-$ in the $MS^{(2)}$ spectrum, which exhibited the same fragmentation pathway as other three bile acids, it was deduced that peak 49 was a bile acid-type compound. By comparison with the literature data, peak 49 was tentatively identified as deoxycholic acid.

By comparing LC-UV and LC-MS chromatograms of SBP with those of crude herbs, most peaks in the chromatogram of SBP were assigned to the corresponding crude herb (shown in Table 7.2). Several peaks, such as 2, 39, and 41, could not be assigned to any crude plant. One of the most likely reasons is that they were the intermediates of manufacture or sample preparation.

7.1.3 Conclusion

In this study, a reliable and simple analytical method by LC-DAD-ESI-$MS^{(2)}$ for rapid identification of multiple components in the extract of SBP was established. Based on retention time, UV spectra, and MS information, 47 components including triterpene saponins, bufadienolides, bile acids, phenylallyl compounds, and some other components in the complex system were successfully separated and identified by LC-DAD-ESI-MS[2]. The results of this study would be helpful in discovering the biologically active compounds in SBP while facilitating improvement in the quality control standard of this multiherbal formula.

7.2. THE STUDY ON VOLATILE COMPONENTS IN THE SHEXIANG BAOXIN PILL

7.2.1 Instrumentation and Materials

7.2.1.1 Instrumentation

Thermo GC DSQ II Gas Chromatograph, Xcalibur version software Chromatography workstation, KS5200H Ultrasonic cleaning (Shanghai Kudos Ultrasonic instrument Co., Ltd.), BP211D electronic balance (Sartorius, Germany), Milli-Q50 SP Pure Water System (Millipore, USA).

7.2.1.2 Reagents

Hexane, ethyl ether, acetone, chloroform were all of analytical grade and purchased from Chinese Medicine Group Chemical Reagent Co., Ltd. Water was prepared using a Milli-Q purification system.

7.2.1.3 Chemicals

The Shexiang Baoxin Pill (No. 080105) was kindly donated by the Shanghai Hutchison Pharmaceuticals (Shanghai, China). Muscone, Cinnamic acid, Cinnamic aldehyde, Borneol, Isoborneol, and benzyl benzoate were purchased from the National Institute for Food and Drug Control (Beijing, China).

7.2.2 Method and Results

7.2.2.1 Preparation of the Standard Solution

Each standard substance was accurately weighed, then dissolved in ether and diluted to appropriate concentration, respectively. All solutions were stored in the refrigerator at 4° C before analysis.

7.2.2.2 Preparation of Sample Solution

A 500 mg sample of powdered SBP (No. 080105) was extracted with 5 mL ether by ultrasonic for 20 min, followed by centrifugation. This extraction was repeated two times. The extracts were then combined and filtered through a membrane (0.45 μm). The subsequent filtrate was dried for 24 h by anhydrous sodium sulfate and stored in the refrigerator at 4°C as the sample solution until analysis.

7.2.2.3 Chromatographic Conditions

Chromatographic separation was carried out on a Thermo TR-5 ms column. Xcalibur version software was used for the data analysis. The carrier gas was helium and gas flow was set to 1.0 mL/min. The inlet temperature was 220°C, and source temperature was set to 250°C. The injection volume was 1 µL. Table 7.3 shows the temperature programmed and analysis time was 59 min. The GC–MS chromatography is shown in Fig. 7.3.

7.2.2.4 Identification of SBP

A total of 49 compounds were identified by comparing with the NIST05 database. Retention time, structure, and names of these compounds were shown in Table 7.4.

7.2.3 Conclusions

A total of 47 compounds were identified in 57 peaks by HPLC-DAD-MS/MS analysis of SBP, mainly ginsenosides, bufadienolides, and cholic acid. The chemical information of nonvolatile components in SBP was basically defined and the fragmentation regularities of mass spectra of ginsenosides, bufadienolides, and cholic acid were also summarized, which provided a good basis for the analysis of nonvolatile chemical constituents in

Table 7.3 Temperature programmed

Heating rate (/min °C)	Temperature (°C)	Residence time (min)
60		0
20	85	21
20	150	5
5	165	0
20	200	6
3	225	2
4	245	2

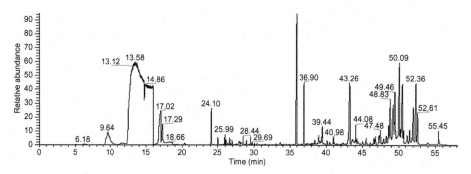

Fig. 7.3 Total ion chromatograms of GC-MS.

Table 7.4 GC-MS identified compounds

Retention time (min)	Compound	Structure
6.15	Benzyl alcohol	
9.27	Bicyclo[2,2,1]heptan-2-ol, 1,5,5–trimethyl	
9.74	Fenchol, *exo*–	
11.46	(–)-Alcanfor	
12.87	Borneol	
14.19	Isoborneol	
15.80	Methanol, oxo-benzoate	
16.18	*p*-Menth-8-en-3-ol, [1R,3R,4S]-[–]-	
20.38	Hexanoic acid, ethylester	
24.10	Cinnamaldehyde	

Continued

Table 7.4 GC-MS identified compounds—cont'd

Retention time (min)	Compound	Structure
25.01	Cinnamyl alcohol	
25.99	Hydrocinnamaldehyde	
26.12	Benzenepropyl aceate	
26.60	Isopatchoulane	
26.95	Caryophyllene	
28.03	Cinnamic acid	
28.46	Cinnamic acid, ethylester	
28.92	α-Amorphene	
29.50	Cadina-1(10),4-diene	
29.66	Cadina-1,3,5-triene	

29.95	Copaene	
30.42	Cinnamaldehyde, o-methexy-	
31.56	9-Isopropenyl-4,8a-dimethyl-1,2,3,5,6,7,8,8a-octahydro-naphthalen-2-ol	
33.06	Cubenol	
33.62	1β-Cadin-en-10-ol	
35.9	Benzylbenzoate	
36.9	Cycolpentadecanone, 3-methyl-	
38.43	5β-Androstane	
38.99	Hexadecanoic acid	
39.46	Palmitic acid, ethylester	
40.8	18-Norabietane	
43.22	18-Norabietane	

Continued

Table 7.4 GC-MS identified compounds—cont'd

Retention time (min)	Compound	Structure
43.26	Quinazolin-4(3H)-one, 1,2-dihydro-2-(3-cyclohexenyl)-3-(2-methylphenyl)	
44.07	Ethyl(9E,12E)-9,12-octadecadienoate	
45.53	Cinnamic acid, phenethylester	
46.80	Methylpimar-7-en-18-oate	
47.20	Podocarp-8-en-15-oic acid, (3α-ethy)-13-methyl-, methylester	
47.47	3-Hydroxy-13-methylpodocarp-7-ene-13-carbaldehyde	
48.0	Podocarpan-15-oic acid, 13β-isopropyl-, methylester	
48.28	Methylpimar-7-en-18-oate	
48.62	Cyclohexane,3,3,5,5-tetramethyl-1-(3,3,5,5-tetramethylcyclohexyldene)	
48.83	Podocarp-8en-15-oic acid, 13-isopropyl-, methylester	

49.20	α-Methylstyrene	
49.46	Podocarpa-8,11,13-trien-15-oic acid, 13-isopropyl-, methylester	
50.50	Podocarpa-8,11,13-trien-16-ol, 13-isopropyl	
51.49	Podocarpan-15-oic acid, 13α-ethyl-13-methyl-, methylester	
52.0	Methyl17-oxoabieta-9(11),8(14),12-trien-18-oate	
52.36	1-[5.5.8a-Trimethyl-2-methylenedecahydro-1-haphthalenyl]-3-methyl-3-pentanol	
52.60	Cinnamylcinnamate	

the serum after administration. In addition, a total of 49 compounds were identified by GC–MS analysis of SBP and basic understanding of the chemical information of volatile compounds in SBP as well as the analysis of the volatile chemical components in the serum after administration has a good foundation. The HPLC–DAD–MS/MS and GC–MS method provided reliable chromatographic conditions for the study of serum pharmacochemistry.

REFERENCES

1. Ye M, Guo DA. Analysis of bufadienolides in the Chinese drug ChanSu by high-performance liquid chromatography with atmospheric pressure chemical ionization tandem mass spectrometry. *Rapid Commun Mass Spectrom* 2005;**19**(13):1881–92.
2. Lai CM, Li SP, Yu H, Wan JB, Kan KW, Wang YT. A rapid HPLC–ESI–MS/MS for qualitative and quantitative analysis of saponins in "XUESETONG" injection. *J Pharm Biomed Anal* 2006;**40**(3):669–78.
3. Shu YL, Meng C, Liu ZQ, Feng RS, Wen JM. Structural analysis of saponins from medicinal herbs using electrospray ionization tandem mass spectrometry. *J Am Soc Mass Spectrom* 2004;**15**(2):133–41.
4. Zhang P, Zheng C, Liu YS, Wang D, Liu N, Yoshikawa M. Quality evaluation of traditional Chinese drug toad venom from different origins through a simultaneous determination of bufogenins and indole alkaloids by HPLC. *Chem Pharm Bull* 2005;**53**(12):1582–6.
5. Huang JW. Study on chemical components of essential oils in *Cinnamomum cassia* presl from different growth years by GC-MS. *Chin J Pharm Anal* 2005;**25**(3):288–91.
6. Zhang HF, Hu P, Luo GA, Liang QL, Wang YL, Yang SK, et al. Screening and identification of multi-component in Qingkailing injection using combination of liquid chromatography/time-of-flight mass spectrometry and liquid chromatography-ion trap mass spectrometry. *Anal Chim Acta* 2006;**577**(2):197–200.
7. Yao FY, Qiu Q, Cui ZJ, Su DM. Chemical components of essential oils from *Liquidambar orientalis* mill. *Chin J Pharm Anal* 2005;**25**(7):859–62.

CHAPTER 8

Study on the Serum Pharmacochemistry of the Shexiang Baoxin Pill

Peng Jiang*, Runui Liu†, Weidong Zhang†
*Shanghai Hutchison Pharmaceutical Limited Company, Shanghai, PR China
†Second Military Medical University, Shanghai, PR China

Abstract

This study was focused on the bioactive components of the Shexiang Baoxin pill. The serum pharmacology method was used in this study. LC-MS and GC-MS tools were combined to identify the absorbed components of the Shexiang Baoxin pill in rats' blood. In the end, 30 components were identified in the rats' blood after administration of the Shexiang Baoxin pill, basically elucidating the bioactive components of the Shexiang Baoxin pill.

Keywords: Shexiang Baoxin pill, Serum pharmacology, LC-MS, GC-MS.

The conventional procedure for finding bioactive components is extraction and isolation of the components from traditional Chinese medicine (TCM) followed by pharmacology screening. This procedure is not only arduous and time consuming but also cannot clarify the characteristics of the synergistic action of multiple components of TCM.[1] To date, hundreds of compounds have been isolated and identified from the Shexiang Baoxin pill. To avoid any ambiguity of pharmacological evaluation for each compound, an integrative method for screening bioactive components should be established.

The concept of serum pharmacology, which was first mentioned by Homma et al.,[2,3] is a new method for screening the bioactive components from TCM, which contains complicated components. This strategy is based on the hypothesis that active compounds could be absorbed into blood after the administration of TCM, and only the absorbed components have a chance to show effects. In recent years, serum pharmacology, which is very straightforward and helpful in discovering real bioactive constituents in TCMs, has been widely used.[4–7]

In this study, we applied serum pharmacology to screen and analyze multiple effective components of the Shexiang Baoxin pill. An HPLC coupled with ESI and the ion-trap mass spectrometry method was adopted to simultaneously separate the effective components from interfering ingredients and determine their structures in rat plasma. From a comprehensive analysis of the chromatography of the Shexiang Baoxin pill, controlled plasma, and dosed plasma, 17 components from the Shexiang Baoxin pill extract and four metabolites were observed in rat plasma (structures of identified compounds shown in

Systems Biology and Its Application in TCM Formulas Research
https://doi.org/10.1016/B978-0-12-812744-5.00008-4

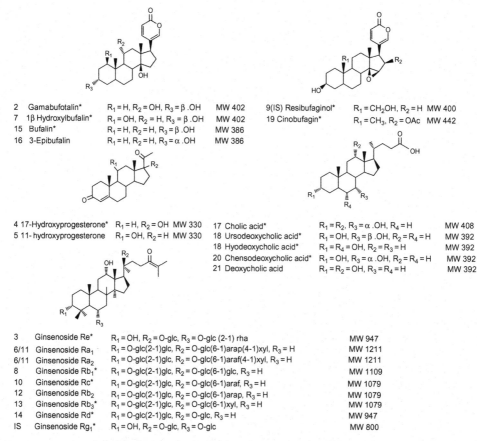

Fig. 8.1 Structures of identified compounds in rat plasma after oral administration of the Shexiang Baoxin pill. The asterisk refers to reference standards. IS means internal standards. The numbers of structures refer to Table 8.3.

Fig. 8.1). All the original form compounds from the Shexiang Baoxin pill and three of the metabolites were identified by comparing their retention times and MS and MS/MS spectra with the reported literature and reference standards. The method using HPLC-ESI-MS/MS technology coupled with serum pharmaceutical chemistry enhances the speed of screening the bioactive constituents in the Baoxin pill.

8.1. ANALYSIS OF THE NONVOLATILE CONSTITUENTS IN RAT PLASMA AFTER ORAL ADMINISTRATION OF THE BAOXIN PILL BY HPLC-ESI-MS/MS

8.1.1 Experimental

8.1.1.1 Chemicals and Reagents

HPLC-grade acetonitrile and formic acid were purchased from Merck (Merck, Darmstadt, Germany). Ultrapure water from a Milli-Q50 SP Reagent Water System (Millipore

Corporation, MA, USA) was used for the preparation of samples and the mobile phase. Other reagents were of analytical grade. The reference standards of ginsenoside Rb_1, Rb_3, Rc, Rd, Re, ursodeoxycholic acid, chenodeoxycholic acid, hyodeoxycholic acid, and deoxycholic acid were purchased from the National Institute for Food and Drug Control (Beijing, China). 17-Hydroxyprogesterone was purchased from Sigma Chemicals (St Louis, MO, USA). Five other standard bufadienolides, including gamabufotalin, 1β-hydroxylbufalin, resibufaginol, bufalin, and cinobufagin, were isolated in our laboratory (purity >99.0%) and their chemical structures were identified by several spectral analyses and previous data. The Shexiang Baoxin pill samples (batch number 080101) were kindly offered by the Shanghai Hutchison Pharmaceuticals Company.

8.1.1.2 Instrumentation and Conditions

An Agilent-1100 (Agilent Technologies, Palo Alto, CA, USA) HPLC system was coupled with an Agilent LC/MSD Trap XCT electrospray ion mass spectrometer equipped with a quaternary pump, vacuum degasser, autosampler, and column heater-cooler. Separation was performed on a Symmetry C_{18} column (5 μm, 4.6×250 mm, Waters) with the column temperature set at 30°C. The flow rate was $0.8 \, \text{mL min}^{-1}$. The mobile phase consisted of water containing (A) 0.5 vol% formic acid, and (B) acetonitrile. The following gradient program was used: 0–15 min, B 20–30 vol%; 15–20 min, B 30 vol%; 20–30 min, B 30–35 vol%; 30–50 min, B 35–40 vol%; 50–55 min, B 40 vol%; 55–85 min, B 40–90 vol%; and 85–90 min, B 90–100 vol%. The injection volume was 3 μL.

By solvent splitting, $0.2 \, \text{mL min}^{-1}$ portions of the column effluent were delivered into the ion source of the mass spectrometer. The MS conditions were as follows: drying gas (nitrogen) flow rate $10 \, \text{L min}^{-1}$, temperature 350°C, pressure of nebulizer gas 30 psi, HV voltage 3.5 kV, target mass 600 amu, compound stability 100%, threshold 50,000 (ESI^+), and 10,000 (ESI^-) and scan range 100–1500 amu. An amplitude voltage of 1.0 V was typically used for fragmentation in the ion trap auto MS^2 experiments. Positive and negative mode data were acquired using Agilent Chemstation software.

8.1.1.3 Animals, Drug Administration, and Blood Sampling

Ten male Sprague-Dawley (SD) rats (180–200 g body weight) were obtained from the Shanghai SLAC Lab Animal Co., Ltd. (Shanghai, China). The animals were acclimatized to the facilities for 5 days, and then fasted with free access to water for 12 h prior to the experiment. The Shexiang Baoxin pill was ground into fine powder and dissolved in a 0.5% carboxymethyl cellulose sodium salt (CMC-Na) aqueous solution. The prepared suspension was orally administered to six rats at a dose of 0.34 g Shexiang Baoxin pill/ 100 g body weight; a 0.5% CMC-Na aqueous solution was orally administered to four other rats used as control. Two hours after drug administration, the animals were anesthetized by intraperitoneal injection of 1% pentobarbital sodium (0.15 mL/100 g body weight). The blood was collected from the hepatic portal vein and then centrifuged at 3500 rpm for 10 min at 4°C. The supernatant obtained was frozen immediately and stored at −80°C, and thawed before analysis. All procedures were in accordance with the National Institute of Health's guidelines regarding the principles of animal care (2004).

8.1.1.4 Sample Preparation

A 0.5 g aliquot of the Shexiang Baoxin pill was dissolved in 5 mL of 50% methanol v/v and the mixture was extracted in an ultrasonic bath for 20 min,[8] followed by centrifugation for 10 min at 12,000 rpm. The supernatant was collected and filtered through a 0.45 μm membrane prior to HPLC-ESI-MS/MS analysis. The plasma sample (400 μL) was added into a 5 mL polypropylene test tube and 3 mL methanol was added using an Eppendorf repeater pipette. The mixture was vortexed by a vortex-mixer for 60 s and then centrifuged at 12,000 rpm for 10 min. Supernatant was pipetted into another clear tube and placed in a Speed Vacplus vacuum drier. The dried residue was dissolved in 200 μL of methanol and centrifuged, and then an aliquot of 3 μL of supernatant was injected into the analytical column. Each of the reference standard samples was accurately weighed, dissolved in methanol, and diluted to a series of proper concentration (50–5000 ng mL^{-1}). All the solutions were stored in the refrigerator at 4°C until analysis.

8.1.2 Results and Discussion

8.1.2.1 LC-ESI-MS/MS Analysis of Shexiang Baoxin Pill Extracts and Plasma Samples

Various sample preparation methods, including deproteinating by adding methanol, liquid–liquid extraction with ethyl acetate, and solid-phase extraction with various sorbents such as Waters Sep-pak Vac or Oasis HLB cartridge were tested to select an efficient cleanup of the plasma sample for obtaining a better recovery of the target compounds. The extraction recoveries were determined by comparing peak areas obtained from plasma samples with those found by direct injection of a standard solution of the same concentration. The solution of ginsenoside Re, bufalin, and chenodeoxycholic acid at three different concentrations (30, 300, and 900 ng mL^{-1}) ($n=6$) was used for analysis. The results showed that the method of deproteinating by adding methanol could ensure better extraction efficiency of all target compounds. By using this method, the mean extraction efficiency ($n=6$) of ginsenoside Re, bufalin, and chenodeoxycholic acid was 85.3%, 87.9%, and 81.0%, respectively. Finally, deproteinating by adding methanol was chosen because it not only ensured better extraction efficiency of all target compounds but also caused less interference from the coeluted endogenous matrixes.

Reference compounds, including ginsenoside Re, Rd, bufalin, cinobufagin, resibufaginol, deoxycholic acid, and chenodeoxycholic acid, were analyzed in order to optimize the MS conditions. The trials showed that saponins and bile acids can give better chromatograms in negative mode than in positive mode while bufadienolides showed better chromatograms in positive mode. To get high responses from all

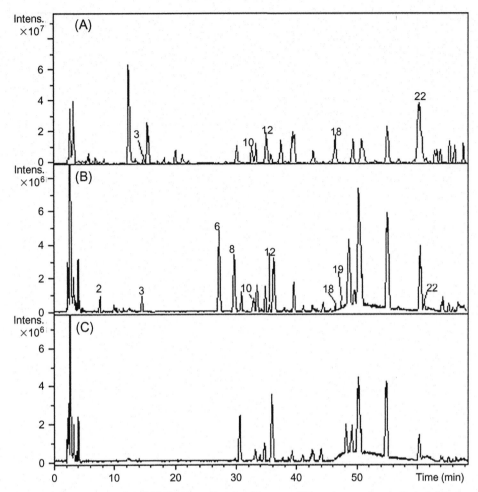

Fig. 8.2 Ion chromatography of (A) Shexiang Baoxin pill extract, (B) rat plasma after oral administration of the Shexiang Baoxin pill, (C) controlled rat plasma in positive ode. Peak 1, not identified; peak 2, gamabufotalin; peak 4, 7-hydroxyprogesterone; peak 5, 11-hydroxyprogesterone; peak 7, 1β-hydroxylbufalin; peak 9, resibufaginol; peak 15, bufalin; peak 16, 3-epi-bufalin; peak 19, cinobufagin.

compounds in MS spectra, the analysis was carried out in both positive and negative mode (Figs. 8.2 and 8.3).

The HPLC-ESI-MS/MS chromatography of plasma samples of the Shexiang Baoxin pill, collected at different times postdose, was measured. More peaks and higher responses were detected in the HPLC-ESI-MS/MS chromatography at 2 h postdose. Therefore, LC-ESI-MS/MS chromatography postdose at 2 h was used for comparison with the chromatography of the Shexiang Baoxin pill to study the multiple absorbed bioactive components and metabolites in rat plasma.

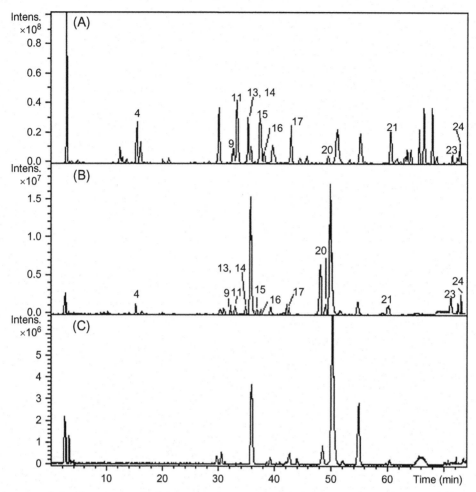

Fig. 8.3 Ion chromatography of (A) Shexiang Baoxin pill extract, (B) rat plasma after oral administration of Shexiang Baoxin pill, (C) controlled rat plasma in negative mode. Peak 3, ginsenoside Re; peak 6, ginsenoside Ra_1 or ginsenoside Ra_2; peak 8, ginsenoside Rb_1; peak 10, ginsenoside Rc; peak 11, ginsenoside Ra_1 or ginsenoside Ra_2; peak 12, ginsenoside Rb_2; peak 13, ginsenoside Rb_3; peak 14, ginsenoside Rd; peak 17, cholic acid; peak 18, hydroxycholic acid or ursodeoxycholic acid; peak 20, chenodeoxycholic acid; peak 21, deoxycholic acid.

8.1.2.2 Method Validation

As ginsenoside Re and bufalin showed a relatively lower peak area than other components in negative ion mode and positive ion mode chromatograms of postdose at 2 h respectively, the calibration curves, LLOQ (lower limit of quantification), and intra- and interday precisions of these two compounds were examined to validate the analysis method. Ginsenoside Re and bufalin were at first characterized by MS and MS/MS spectrum to ascertain their precursor ions and to select product ions for use in SRM mode. As ginsenoside Re and bufalin gave abundant ions in negative mode and positive mode respectively, ginsenoside Rg_1 was chosen as an internal standard for ginsenoside Re and resibufaginol was chosen as an internal standard for bufalin. The SRM transitions were chosen to be m/z 946→783 for ginsenoside Re and m/z 800→637 for Rg_1 in negative mode, m/z 387→351 for bufalin and m/z 401→383 for resibufaginol in positive mode.

Calibration curves ranging from 10 to 1000 ng mL^{-1} of ginsenoside Re and bufalin were run on three successive days. Calibration curves were constructed from the peak area ratios of each analyte to IS versus plasma concentrations using a $1/x^2$ weighted linear least squares regression model. The LLOQ is defined as the lowest concentration of standard that can be measured with an acceptable accuracy and precision ($\leq$20% for both parameters; data shown in Table 8.1).

Six replicates at three levels of ginsenoside and bufalin were included in each run to determine the intraday and interday precision of the assay. The accuracy was determined as the percentage difference between the mean detected concentrations and the nominal concentrations (data shown in Table 8.2). The results showed that the developed method was accurate and sensitive for analysis of the components in rat plasma.

Table 8.1 The linearity, lower limit of quantification of the assay for ginsenoside Re and bufalin

Compound	Linear range (ng mL^{-1})	Regressive equation	R^2	Lower limit of quantification (ng)
Ginsenoside Re	10–1000	$y=0.6250x+0.0237$	0.9980	4.0
Bufalin	10–1000	$y=0.2378x+0.3000$	0.9982	3.0

Table 8.2 Precision and accuracy of ginsenoside Re and bufalin from rat plasma extracts ($n=3$ days and six replicates per day)

Analyte	Added C (ng mL^{-1})	Found C (ng mL^{-1})	Intraday RSD (%)	Interday RSD (%)	Relative error (%)
Ginsenoside Re	30	31.32	7.21	7.04	4.40
	300	325.61	4.60	6.44	8.50
	900	936.27	4.32	5.72	4.03
Bufalin	20	19.24	10.34	12.31	−3.80
	200	205.61	8.13	10.50	2.81
	800	812.97	3.40	5.71	1.62

8.1.2.3 Identification of Prototype Components in Rat Plasma

By comparing the MS chromatograms of rat plasma after oral administration of the Shexiang Baoxin pill with controlled rat plasma in both positive mode and negative mode, 21 peaks were observed in dosed rat plasma but not in controlled rat plasma. Among the 21 peaks, 17 peaks were also found in the MS spectra of Shexiang Baoxin pill extract in both positive mode and negative mode, which indicated that these components were absorbed into rat plasma in the prototype. By comparing the retention times and MS and MS/MS data with literature data or reference standards,[8–10] these 17 compounds, including eight ginsenosides (peak 3, 6, 8, 10, 11, 12, 13, and 14), four bile acids (peak 17, 18, 20, and 21), and five bufadienolides (peak 2, 7, 9, 15, and 19) were all identified (data shown in Table 8.3).

In the MS spectra of the negative mode, all target peaks gave a base peak at $[M-H]^-$. The fragmention ions of peaks 3, 6, 8, 10, 11, 12, 13, and 14 exhibited a fragmentation pattern corresponding to the loss of the glycosidic units and showed aglycone ions at m/z 459 or 475 corresponding to protopanaxadiol aglycon moiety or protopanaxatriol aglycon moiety, respectively. This means that these components are ginsenosides. For example, peaks 10, 12, and 13 all showed a base peak at m/z 1078 both in their MS spectrum of dosed plasma samples and Shexiang Baoxin pill extract. In their MS/MS spectra, m/z 945, 783, 621, and 459 were observed, exhibiting a fragmentation pattern corresponding to the loss of the glycosidic units. The fragmentation ion at m/z 459 corresponding to the protopanaxadiol aglycon moiety is a characteristic ion to identify the structures of these components. In comparison with the literature data,[10] ginsenoside Rc, Rb$_2$, and Rb$_3$ correspond to these three peaks. By comparison with the reference standards, peaks 10 and 13 were identified as ginsenoside Rc and Rb$_3$. Peak 12 was identified as ginsenoside Rb$_2$ by comparison with literature data.[10] Peak 3 showed a base peak at m/z 946 $[M-H]^-$ and 991 $[M-H+HCOO]^-$ in the MS spectra and m/z 799 $[M-H-Rha]^-$, 783 $[M-H-Glc]^-$, 637 $[M-H-Glc-Xyl]^-$, and 475 $[Agl]^-$ in MS/MS spectra, which exhibited the same fragmentation pathway as ginsenosides. The fragmentation ion at m/z 459 indicated that the aglycon of this compound is protopanaxatriol. By comparing with reference standards, peak 3 was identified as ginsenoside Re.

Except for eight ginsenosides in negative mode, the other four components (peaks 17, 18, 20, and 21), which showed fragmention ions corresponding to the loss of the hydroxyl group and the carboxyl group and gave the characterized fragmentation ion at m/z 327, exhibited the same fragmentation pathways as bile acids. For example, peaks 18, 20, and 21 showed the abundant ion at m/z 391 $[M-H]^-$ and 783 $[2M-H]^-$ in their MS spectra. Their molecular weight could be confirmed to be 392. Fragmentation ions at m/z 373 $[M-H-H_2O]^-$, 355 $[M-H-2H_2O]^-$ and 327 $[M-H-H_2O-HCOO]^-$ were exhibited in their MS/MS spectra.

As the fragmentation pattern was similar to bile acids and ion m/z 327 was the characteristic ion of bile acids, these three isomers were tentatively identified as bile acid-type

Table 8.3 MS and MS/MS data (*m/z*, percentage of relative abundance) of the absorbed compounds and metabolites in rat plasma after oral administration of the Shexiang Baoxin pill

Peak	Name	Origin	RT (min)	MW	MS (pos.) (*m/z*)	MS (neg.) (*m/z*)	MS/MS (pos.) (*m/z*)	MS/MS (neg.) (*m/z*)
1	Not identified		7.8	201	202[M+H]$^+$ 425[2M+Na]$^+$		183 (80); 159 (70); 131 (100)	
2	Gamabufotalin[a]	Venenum Bufonis	14.7	402	403[M+H]$^+$ 425[M+Na]$^+$		385 (10) [M+H−H$_2$O]$^+$; 367 (40) [M+H−2H$_2$O]$^+$; 349 (100) [M+H−3H$_2$O]$^+$; 253 (30) [M+H−3H$_2$O−α-pyr[b]]$^+$	
3	Ginsenoside Re[a]	Panax Ginseng	15.3	947		946[M−H]$^-$ 991[M−H+HCOO]$^-$		799 (40) [M−H−Rha]$^-$; 783 (100) [M−H−Glc]$^-$; 637 (50) [M−H−Glc−Xyl]$^-$; 475 (20) [Agl[c]]$^-$
4	17-Hydroxypro-gesterone[a]		27.1	330	353[M+Na]$^+$ 683[2M+Na]$^+$		313 (35) [M+H−H$_2$O]$^+$; 271 (20) [M+H−H$_2$O−CH$_3$CO]$^+$; 163 (100) [M+H−C$_{13}$H$_{20}$O$_2$]$^+$; 125 (45) [M+H−C10H$_{16}$O$_2$]$^+$	
5	11-Hydroxypro-gesterone		29.4	330	353[M+Na]$^+$ 683[2M+Na]$^+$		313 (30) [M+H−H$_2$O]$^+$; 271 (23) [M+H−H$_2$O−CH$_3$CO]$^+$; 163 (100) [M+H−C$_{13}$H$_{20}$O$_2$]$^+$; 125 (42) [M+H−C$_{10}$H$_{16}$O$_2$]$^+$	
6	Ginsenoside Ra$_1$/Ra$_2$	Panax Ginseng	32.1	1211		1210[M−H]$^-$		1077 (100) [M−H−Xyl]$^-$; 1047 (5) [M−H−Glc]$^-$; 945 (20) [M−H−2Xyl]$^-$; 783 (15) (Xyl−Ara)$^-$

Continued

Table 8.3 MS and MS/MS data (m/z, percentage of relative abundance) of the absorbed compounds and metabolites in rat plasma after oral administration of the Shexiang Baoxin pill—cont'd

Peak	Name	Origin	RT (min)	MW	MS (pos.) (m/z)	MS (neg.) (m/z)	MS/MS (pos.) (m/z)	MS/MS (neg.) (m/z)
7	1β-Hydroxylbufalin[a]	Venenum Bufonis	32.5	402	403[M+H]$^+$ 425[M+Na]$^+$ 827[2M+Na]$^+$		385 (25) [M+H−H$_2$O]$^+$; 367 (75) [M+H−2H$_2$O]$^+$; 349 (100) [M+H−3H$_2$O]$^+$; 339 (20) [M+H−2H$_2$O−CO]$^+$; 253 (30) [M+H−3H$_2$O−α-pyr]$^+$	[M−H−2Xyl−Glc/(Xyl−Ara−Glc)]$^-$; 621 (5) [M−H−2Xyl−2Glc/(Xyl−Ara−2Glc)]; 459 (1) [Agl]$^-$
8	Ginsenoside Rb$_1$[a]	Panax Ginseng	33.1	1109		1108[M−H]$^-$		945 (100) [M−H−Glc]$^-$; 783 (40) [M−H−2Glc]$^-$; 621 (10) [M−H−3Glc]$^-$; 459 (2) [Agl]$^-$
9	Resibufaginol[a]	Resibufaginola Venenum Bufonis	34.6	400	401[M+H]$^+$ 423[M+Na]$^+$		383 (100) [M+H−H$_2$O]$^+$; 365 (50) [M+H−2H$_2$O]$^+$; 347 (50) [M+H−3H$_2$O]$^+$; 319 (20) [M+H−3H$_2$O−CO]$^+$; 251 (15) [M+H−3H$_2$O−α-pyr]$^+$	
10	Ginsenoside Rc[a]	Panax Ginseng	34.9	1079		1078[M−H]$^-$		945 (100) [M−H−Araf]$^-$; 783 (30) [M−H−Araf−Glc]$^-$; 621 (5) [M−H−Araf−2Glc]$^-$; 459 (1) [Agl]$^-$
11	Ginsenoside Ra$_1$/Ra$_2$	Panax Ginseng	34.9	1211		1210[M−H]$^-$		1077 (100) [M−H−Xyl]$^-$; 1047 (5) [M−H−Glc]$^-$; 945 (20) [M−H−2Xyl/(Xyl−Ara)]$^-$;

No.	Compound	Source	RT	MW	ESI+ ions	ESI− ions	Fragment ions (m/z, rel. int.)
							783 (15) [M−H−2Xyl−Glc/(Xyl−Ara−Glc)]−; 621 (5) [M−H−2Xyl−2Glc/(Xyl−Ara−2Glc)]−; 459 (1) [AgI]−
12	Ginsenoside Rb2	Panax Ginseng	37.1	1079		1078[M−H]−	945 (100) [M−H−Arap]−; 783 (45)[M−H−Araf−Glc]−; 621 (5) [M−H−Arap−2Glc]− (1) [AgI]−
13	Ginsenoside Rb3[a]	Panax Ginseng	37.8	1079		1078[M−H]−	945 (100) [M−H−Xyl]−; 783 (50) [M−H−Xyl−Glc]−; 621 (5) [M−H−Xyl−2Glc]−; 459 (1) [AgI]−
14	Ginsenoside Rd[a]	Panax Ginseng	42.3	947		946[M−H]−; 991[M−H+HCOO]−	783 (100) [M−H−Glc]−; 621 (10) [M−H−2Glc]−; 459 (2) [AgI]−
15	Bufalin[a]	Venenum Bufonis	46.1	386	387[M+H]+; 409[M+Na]+		369 (20) [M+H−H2O]+; 351 (100) [M+H−2H2O]+; 333 (25) [M+H−3H2O]+; 305 (15) [M+H−3H2O−CO]+; 255 (35) [M+H−2H2O−α-pyr]+
16	3-*epi*-Bufalin		47.5	386	387[M+H]+; 409[M+Na]+		369 (25) [M+H−H2O]+; 351 (100) [M+H−2H2O]+; 333 (20) [M+H−3H2O]+; 305 (15) [M+H−3H2O−CO]+; 255 (35) [M+H−2H2O−α-pyr]+

Continued

Table 8.3 MS and MS/MS data (m/z, percentage of relative abundance) of the absorbed compounds and metabolites in rat plasma after oral administration of the Shexiang Baoxin pill—cont'd

Peak	Name	Origin	RT (min)	MW	MS (pos.) (m/z)	MS (neg.) (m/z)	MS/MS (pos.) (m/z)	MS/MS (neg.) (m/z)
17	Cholic acid	Calculus Bovis	49.2	408		$407[M-H]^-$ $452[M-H+HCOO]^-$		371 (20) $[M-H-2H_2O]^-$; 353 (30) $[M-H-3H_2O]^-$; 343 (100) $[M-H-H_2O-HCOO]^-$; 327 (25) $[M-H-2H_2O-HCOO]^-$
18	Hyodeoxycholica/ursodeoxycholic acid[a]	Calculus Bovis	60.3	392		$391[M-H]^-$ 783 $[2M-H]^-$		373 (100) $[M-H-H_2O]^-$; 355 (10) $[M-H-2H_2O]^-$; 327 (10) $[M-H-H_2O-HCOO]^-$
19	Cinobufagin[a]	Venenum Bufonis	60.7	442	$443[M+H]^+$ $465[M+Na]^+$		401 (13) $[M+H-CH_2CO]^+$; 383 (20) $[M+H-HOAC]^+$; 365 (100) $[M+H-HOAC-H_2O]^+$; 347 (40) $[M+H-HOAC-2H_2O]^+$	
20	Chenodeoxycholic acid[a]	Calculus Bovis	71.2	392		$391[M-H]^-$ 783 $[2M-H]^-$		373 (100) $[M-H-H_2O]^-$; 355 (5) $[M-H-2H_2O]^-$; 327 (1) $[M-H-H_2O-HCOO]^-$
21	Deoxycholic acid[a]	Calculus Bovis	72.5	392		$391[M-H]^-$ 783 $[2M-H]^-$		373 (10) $[M-H-H_2O]^-$; 355 (50) $[M-H-2H_2O]^-$; 345 (100) $[M-H-HCOO]^-$; 327 (40) $[M-H-H_2O-HCOO]^-$

[a] Structure confirmed by comparison with reference standards.
[b] α-pyr refers to α-pyrone ring.
[c] Agl refers to aglycone.

compounds. By comparison with standard compounds, peaks 18, 20, and 21 were identified as hyodeoxycholic acid or ursodeoxycholic acid, chenodeoxycholic acid, and deoxycholic acid respectively. Peak 17, giving abundant peaks at m/z 407 $[M-H]^-$ and 452 $[M-H+HCOO]^-$ in MS spectra, eluted at 49.2 min. Its molecular weight was 18 Da higher than the other identified bile acids, and was confirmed to be 408. In the MS/MS spectra, peak 17 showed a similar fragmentation pathway to other bile acids, which indicated that peak 17 was also a bile acid-type compound and had one more hydroxyl group substituent than the other three identified bile acids. By comparison of literature data, peak 17 was identified as cholic acid.

In the MS spectra of positive mode, $[M+H]^-$ or $[M+Na]^-$ was observed as the base peak of peaks 2, 7, 9, 15, and 19. In MS/MS spectra, their produced fragmentation ions usually included $[M+H-H_2O]^-$, $[M+H-2H_2O]^-$, $[M+H-3H_2O-CO]^-$, and $[M+H-3H_2O-\alpha\text{-pyr}]^-$. Their characteristic fragmentation pathways were similar to those of bufadienolides. These five peaks were tentatively identified as bufadienolide-type compounds. Peaks 2, 7, 9, 15, and 19 were respectively identified as gamabufotalin, 1β-hydroxylbufalin, resibufaginol, bufalin, and cinobufagin by comparison with reference standards.

8.1.2.4 Identification of Metabolites in Rat Plasma

As the 17 peaks identified as the prototype, the other four of 21 peaks were tentatively identified as metabolites. By scrutinizing their MS and MS/MS spectrum, three of them were tentatively identified, and the other one was still in progress.

Both peaks 4 and 5 at 27.1 and 29.4 min gave the base peaks at m/z 353 $[M+Na]^+$ and 683 $[2M+Na]^+$ in positive mode. Therefore, m/z 330 was considered as their molecular weight. Their MS/MS spectra were also very similar, and both gave fragmentation ions at m/z 313, 271, and 163 in positive mode. The losses of 18 and 42 Da could be assigned as a hydroxyl substitute and an acetyl group in their structures. By comparing their retention times and MS and MS/MS data with those of the literature,[11] peak 5 was identified as 11-hydroxyprogesterone. Peak 4 was identified as 17-hydroxyprogesterone by comparison with reference standards. The MS and MS/MS spectra and fragmentation pathways of 17-hydroxyprogesterone in positive mode are shown in Fig. 8.4.

The component, eluted at 47.5 min (peak 16) in dosed plasma, showed the same MS and MS/MS fragmentation as that of bufalin. It was considered as an isomer of bufalin. By comparison with the literature data, it was identified as 3-epi-bufalin.[9,12,13] The identification of peak 1, which gave a base peak at 202 $[M+H]^+$ and 405 $[2M+Na]^+$ in positive mode in MS spectra, and showed fragmentation ions such as m/z 183, 159, and 131 in MS/MS spectra, is still in progress.

Finally, 17 components from the Shexinag Baoxin pill, including gamabufotalin, ginsenoside Re, ginsenoside Ra$_1$, ginsenoside Ra$_2$, 1β-hydroxylbufalin, ginsenoside Rb$_1$, resibufaginol, ginsenoside Rc, ginsenoside Rb$_2$, ginsenoside Rb$_3$, ginsenoside Rd, bufalin, cholic

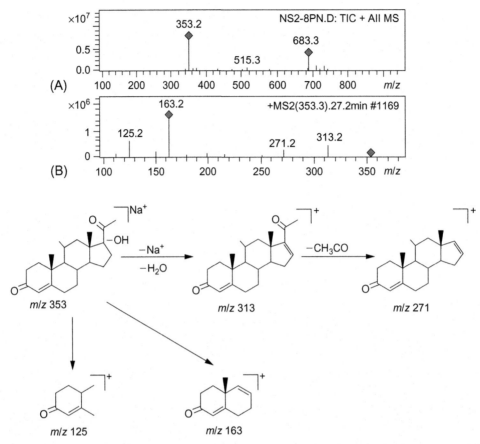

Fig. 8.4 MS (A) and MS/MS (B) spectra of 17-hydroxyprogesterone and its fragmentation pathway in positive mode.

acid, hyodeoxycholic/ursodeoxycholic acid, cinobufagin, chenodeoxycholic acid, and deoxycholic acid, were identified in dosed rat plasma in prototype. Four metabolites, including 3-epi-bufalin, which is a metabolite of bufalin; 11-hydroxyprogesterone and 17-hydroxyprogesterone, which may be endogenous components in plasma; and one peak, which is still being identified, were also observed in dosed rat plasma.

8.1.3 Conclusion

An identification method of the effective constituents in TCM was developed by analyzing the constituents of the Shexiang Baoxin pill in rat plasma using HPLC-ESI-MS/MS. In this study, 21 components including 17 components from the Shexiang Baoxin pill and four metabolites were simultaneously observed, which enhanced the speed and targeting of bioactive constituent analysis.

The proposed method was simple, reliable, and sensitive, which revealed that it was appropriate for rapid screening and compound identification of absorbed and metabolic components of the Shexiang Baoxin pill. This study developed an integrated method for screening the bioactive constituents in plasma after oral administration of Chinese herbal medicine.

8.2. ANALYSIS OF THE VOLATILE CONSTITUENTS IN RAT PLASMA AFTER ORAL ADMINISTRATION OF THE SHEXIANG BAOXIN PILL BY GC-MS

8.2.1 Instrument and Reagent

8.2.1.1 Mass Spectrometer

Thermo GC DSQ 1I gas chromatograph; Xcalibur chromatography workstation; KS5200H ultrasonic cleaners (Shanghai kudos ultrasonic instruments Co., Ltd.); BP211D type electronic balance (Germany Sartorius); Anke TGL-16-C type centrifuge; Vortex QL-901 type vortex.

8.2.1.2 Reagent

The Shexiang Baoxin Pill preparation (batch number 080105) was provided by Shanghai Hutchison Pharmaceutical Co., Ltd. The reference standard of musk ketone (batch number M0128), cinnamic acid (batch number ASB-00003655-025), cinnamaldehyde (batch number YY90307), borneol (batch number M0297), and isoborneol (batch number 111512) were bought from the National Institute for Food and Drug Control, and benzyl ester was bought from Shanghai Sunny Biotech Co., Ltd. Five kinds of reference substance were bought from the National Institute for Food and Drug Control, and benzyl ester was bought from Shanghai Sunny Biotech Co., Ltd. Pentobarbital sodium and sodium heparin were purchased from the Sinopharm Chemical Reagent Co., Ltd. Hexane, ether, acetone, and chloroform were analytically pure, purchased from the Sinopharm Chemical Reagent Co., Ltd.

8.2.1.3 Animal

SPF male SD rats (200 ± 20 g) were purchased from the Slac Laboratory Animal Co., Ltd. with animal license SCXK (Shanghai) 2003-0003, before the experiment fasting was 12 h (free water).

8.2.1.4 Shexiang Baoxin Pill Analysis and Sample Preparation

Precision said set of Shexiang Baoxin pill sample 500 mg, porphyrized and joined ether suspension in 10 µL volumetric flask and ultrasonic extraction 20 min, cool to room temperature, ether for volume loss, let stand for supernatant liquid, with the method of extracting twice, filtrate merged, 12,000 r/min centrifuge for 10 min. Take the supernatant (including 0.45 µm microporous membrane filter), inject 1 µL sample GC-MS analysis.

Precisely weigh each reference substance respectively, add ether to 10 mL volumetric flask and 4°C refrigerator cold storage, for GC-MS analysis.

Precision weighing the Shexiang Baoxin pill sample amount, then porphyrize and add 0.5% sodium carboxymethyl cellulose suspension liquid (concentration: 0.34 g/mL) to conical flask. 20 SD male rats were randomly divided into a control group and a drug group, each group of 10, solvent control group rats given 0.5% sodium carboxymethyl cellulose solution to fill. To medicine group rats was given the Shexiang Baoxin pill suspension liquid filling (doses: 3.4 g/kg). After 30 min, intraperitoneal injection of all rats 1% of pentobarbital sodium solution (dose: 0.15 mL/kg) anesthesia. Hepatic portal venous blood make 5 mL, put in besmear of heparin sodium EP tube, 4°C, 3000 r/min, the centrifugal 10 min, take the supernatant, −80°C refrigerator freezer, set aside.

8.2.1.5 Separate Condition

Thermo TR-5 ms column; Xcalibur workstation; the carrier gas was He; flow rate 1.0 mL min^{-1}; the inlet temperature was set at 220°C; ion source temperature was 250°C; the injection volume was 1 μL; gradient warming procedure following with Chapter 7; the total analysis time was 59 min.

8.2.1.6 Mass Condition

EI source, electronic energy was 70 eV, scan rate was 5 scan/s, emission current was 100 μA, scanning period was 3642 amu/s, ion source temperature was 250°C, and scanning mass range was 10–650 U. Xcalibur chromatography workstation was used for data analysis.

8.2.2 Results and Discussion

250 μL serum was added into 5 mL EP tube, 1 mL ether was then added, shaking for 1 min in vortex and centrifugal 12,000 r/min for 10 min. Repeat two times and upper liquid was then obtained and combined. Residue was added 50 μL ether after drying, shaking for 1 min in vortex and centrifugal. The upper liquid 1 μL was injected into GC-MS.

Comparing the mass spectra of the control group and the administrated SBP group, it could identify the different peaks. With the help of the online database of GC-MS, the different peaks could be identified. The result was shown in Table 8.4.

8.2.3 Conclusion

This study was based on the gas chromatography coupled with mass technology to analyze the violate components in rat serum after administration of the SBP. In the end, ten components, including six prototype components and four metabolites, were identified. These components may be playing an important role in the medical treatment of coronary heart disease.

Table 8.4 The identified components in rat serum after administration SBP using GC-MS

Retention time (min)	Name	Structure
12.6	Borneol	
13.5	Isoborneol	
24.2	Cinnamaldehyde	
25.7	Bicycle[2,2,1]heptan-2-ol, 2-allyl-1,7,7-trimethyl	
26.6	2,6,10-Trimethyltetradecane	
26.9	2-Butyl-5-methyl-3-[2-methylprop-2-enyl] cyclohexanone	
27.7	6-Methyloctodecane	
8.2	Cinnamic acid	
35.8	Benzyl benzoate	
36.8	Muscone	

REFERENCES

1. Qi L, Li P, Li SL, Sheng LH, Li RY, Song Y, et al. Screening and identification of permeable components in a combined prescription of Danggui Buxue decoction using a liposome equilibrium dialysis system followed by HPLC and LC–MS. *J Sep Sci* 2006;**29**:2211–20.
2. Homma M, Oka K, Yamada T, Niitsuma T, Ihto H, Takahashi N. A strategy for discovering biologically active compounds with high probability in traditional Chinese herb remedies: an application of Saiboku-to in bronchial asthma. *Anal Biochem* 1992;**202**:179–87.
3. Homma M, Oka K, Taniguchi C, Niitsuma T, Hayashi T. Systematic analysis of post-administrative Saiboku-To urine by liquid chromatography to determine pharmacokinetics of traditional chinese medicine. *Biomed Chromatogr* 1997;**11**:125–31.
4. Wang P, Liang YZ, Zhou N, Chen BM, Yi LZ, Yan Y, et al. Screening and analysis of the multiple absorbed bioactive components and metabolites of Dangguibuxue decoction by the metabolic fingerprinting tecnique and liquid chromatography/diode-array detection mass spectrometry. *Rapid Commun Mass Spectrom* 2007;**21**:99–106.
5. Xu F, Zhang Y, Xiao SY, XW L, Yang DH, Yang XD, et al. Absorption and metabolism of astragali radix decoction: in silico, in vitro, and a case study in vivo. *Drug Metab Dispos* 2006;**34**:913–24.
6. Wang XJ, Sun WJ, Sun H, Lv HT, ZM W, Wang P, et al. Analysis of the cnstituents in the rat plasma after oral administration of Yin Chen Hao Tang by UPLC/Q-TOF-MS/MS. *J Pharm Biomed Anal* 2008;**46**:477–90.
7. Pan JY, Cheng YY. Identification and analysis of absorbed and metabolic components in rat plasma after oral administration of 'Shuangdan' granule by HPLC-DAD-ESI-MS/MS. *J Pharm Biomed Anal* 2006;**42**:565–72.
8. Yan S, Zhang WD, Liu RH, Zhan YC. Chemical fingerprinting of Shexiang Baoxin pill and simultaneous determination of its major constituents by HPLC with evaporative light scattering detection and electrospray mass spectrmetric detection. *Chem Pharm Bull* 2006;**54**:1058–62.
9. Ye M, Guo DA. Analysis of bufadienolides in the chinese drug chansu by high-performance liquid chromatography with atmospheric pressure chemical ionization tandem mass spectrometry. *Rapid Commun Mass Spectrom* 2005;**19**:1881–92.
10. Lai CM, Li SP, Yu H, Wan JB, Kan KW, Wang YT. A rapid HPLC-ESI-MS/MS for qualitative and quantitative ananlysis of saponins in 'XUESETONG' injection. *J Pharm Biomed Anal* 2006;**40**:669–78.
11. Karl V, Price E, Gertrud S, Peter AS, Kelvin C, Laszlo T, et al. Steroid metabolism as a mechanism of escape from progesteronemediated growth inhibition in trichophyton mentagrophytes. *J Biol Chem* 1989;**264**:11186–92.
12. Ma XC, Cui J, Zheng J, Guo DA. Microbial trasformation of three bufadienolides by *Penicillium aurantigriseum* and its application for metabolite identification in rat. *J Mol Catal B Enzym* 2007;**48**:42–50.
13. Kazutake S, Yoshimichi M, Tadashi N. Characterization of in vitro metabolites of toad venom using high-performance liquid chromatography and liquid chromatography–mass spectrometry. *Biomed Chromatogr* 2006;**20**:1321–7.

CHAPTER 9

The Quality Study of the Shexiang Baoxin Pill

Peng Jiang*, Runui Liu†, Junjie Zhou*, Changsen Zhan*, Weidong Zhang†
*Shanghai Hutchison Pharmaceutical Limited Company, Shanghai, PR China
†Second Military Medical University, Shanghai, PR China

Abstract

The Shexiang Baoxin Pill (SBP) comprises seven medicinal materials or extracts thereof, including Moschus, Radix Ginseng, Calculus Bovis, Cortex Cinnamomi, Styrax, Venenum Bufonis, and Borneolum Syntheticum. These medicinal materials are often from different origins, sources, cultural manner, harvest times, and pretreatment processes. Quality control of SBP products is very critical to ensure their efficacy and safety. In this study, chemical fingerprinting and multicomponent determinations were both used to control the quality of SBP and also used in medicinal materials such as Calculus Bovis.

Keywords: Chemical fingerprint, Simultaneous determination, Shexiang Baoxin Pill, Quality control.

As mentioned above, the Shexiang Baoxin Pill (SBP) comprises seven medicinal materials or extracts including *Moschus*, *Radix Ginseng*, *Calculus Bovis*, *Cortex Cinnamomi*, *Styrax*, *Venenum Bufonis*, and *Borneolum Syntheticum*. These medicinal materials are often from different origins, sources, cultural manners, harvest times, and pretreatment and manufacturing processes, and accordingly will result in significant variances in the quality of SBP, even when produced by the same manufacturer. As a result, the quality control of SBP products is very critical to ensure their efficacy and safety. So far, chemical fingerprinting has been internationally accepted as an efficient tool for the integral quality control of traditional Chinese medicine (TCM).[1-3] Hence, developing the fingerprints of seven medicinal materials of SBP is urgently needed so as to ensure the efficacy, safety, and batch-to-batch uniformity.

There are four main kinds of components in SBP: ginsenosides, steroids, cardogenanes, and volatiles. So HPLC coupled with ELSD and GC coupled with flame ionization detection (FID) should be used as a quality-control technique. On the other side, we gave an example of the quality control method for *Calculus Bovis* in SBP to guarantee the quality of the medicinal material of SBP.

Systems Biology and Its Application in TCM Formulas Research
https://doi.org/10.1016/B978-0-12-812744-5.00009-6

9.1. THE QUALITY STUDY OF BOVIS CALCULUS IN THE SBP

9.1.1 Experimental

9.1.1.1 Reagents and Materials

Authentic standards, including cholic acid (CA), deoxycholic acid (DCA), ursodeoxycholic acid (UDA), chenodeoxycholic acid (CDA), hyodeoxycholic acid (HCA), and bilirubin, were purchased from the National Institute for the Control of Pharmaceutical and Biological Products (Beijing, PR China). Acetonitrile, methanol, and formic acid were of HPLC grade (Merck, Darmstadt, Germany). Ultrapure water was prepared from the Millipore water purification system (Millipore, Milford, MA, USA). Other reagents were of analytical grade.

Twenty-one batches of Calculus Bovis samples were purchased from local drug stores. Of those, six were natural (marked as samples 1–6), five were artificial (marked as samples 7–11), and others were in vitro cultured (marked as samples 12–21). Natural and artificial samples were from various districts in China, including Hebei, Anhui, Gansu, Guangxi, Shanxi, Shandong, and Shanghai; in vitro cultured Calculus Bovis samples were produced from the Wuhan Jianmin Dapeng Pharmceutical Co., Ltd. (Wuhan, PR China). Voucher specimens were deposited at the Herbarium of School of Pharmacy, Second Military Medical University, Shanghai, PR China.

9.1.1.2 Chromatographic System

Chromatographic analysis was performed on a Shimadzu LC2010A liquid chromatograph system (Shimadzu Co., Japan) consisting of a quaternary pump, a column oven, an autosampler, an ultraviolet (UV) detector, and a Sedex 75 ELSD detector (Sedere Co., France). Analytical data was acquired on a CLASS-VP workstation.

9.1.1.3 Analytical Conditions

A C18 RP-ODS column (4.6 mm × 250 mm, 5 μm, Agilent, USA) and a C18 guard column (4.6 mm × 7.5 mm, 5 μm, Merck, USA) were used. The mobile phases were composed of methanol/water/formic acid (70/30/0.3, v/v, A) and acetonitrile (B). The gradient was as follows: 0 min, 100% A, 0% B; 30–45 min, 0% A, 100% B. Elution was performed at a solvent flow rate of 0.8 mL/min. The column compartment was kept at the temperature of 25°C, and the sample injection volume was 10 μL. The drift tube temperature of ELSD was 40°C, and the gas pressure was set at 3.5 bar.

9.1.1.4 Sample Preparation

Six standards, including CA, DCA, UDA, CDA, HCA, and bilirubin, were accurately weighted, and were dissolved with acetonitrile in a 5 mL volumetric flask (to dissolve bilirubin, 1 mL dimethyl sulfoxide was added) and then diluted to the appropriate concentration. A mixed stock solution of standards containing CA 5.432 mg/mL, DCA 1.322 mg/mL, UDA 1.098 mg/mL, CDA 0.436 mg/mL, HCA 0.498 mg/mL, and bilirubin 0.424 mg/mL, was finally prepared. The stock solutions were further diluted to make working solutions.

Twenty-one batches of Calculus Bovis samples were ground into fine powder and 30 mg of each was accurately weighted, and with 3.5 mL mixed solvent (chloroform: methanol:formic acid = 4:2:1, v/v) added, the samples were ultrasonically extracted (15 min × 2), then centrifuged and filtered. All solutions were stored in the refrigerator at 4°C, and filtered through a syringe filter (0.45 μm) before HPLC analysis.

9.1.1.5 Calibration Curves

The calibration curves were constructed by analyzing at least five different concentrations of standard solutions. For the components by UV detection, their regression equations were calculated in the form of $Y = A*X + B$, where Y and X were peak area and sample amount respectively, while by ELSD detection, their regression equations could be described as $Y = aX^b$, so the calibration curves should be obtained in double logarithmic coordinates.[4]

9.1.2 Results and Discussion

9.1.2.1 Chromatographic Analysis

In this study, a mixed solvent of methanol, formic acid, and chloroform was thus used, and both bile acids and bilirubin can be acquired in acceptable yields. By the method of standard addition to a sample, the extraction recovery of UDA, HCA, CA, CDA, DCA, and Bilirubin, respectively, was calculated as 87.2%, 91.5%, 94.3%, 82.7%, 81.6%, and 70.7%.

Under the proposed condition, HPLC/UV/ELSD chromatograms of various Calculus Bovis were acquired. Just as Fig. 9.1 shows, in ELSD chromatograms, the peaks of bile acids are eluted within 15 min, and at a time of 37 min, the peak of bilirubin appears but is rather weak; while in the UV chromatogram, no peaks of bile acids can be seen, only that of bilirubin. Peaks of these components are observed by their retention times in comparison with those of reference standards, and also by the method of standard addition to the sample.

9.1.2.2 Validation

The linearity study was carried out by preparing the calibration curves described above. Aliquots of standard solutions ranging from 0.106 to 3.580 μg/mL were analyzed to obtain LOD values. Table 9.1. shows the regression data and LODs of the components determined, and each has a regression coefficient over 0.995.

The intraday and interday precisions were determined by analyzing calibration samples during a single day and on three different days, respectively. To confirm the repeatability, five different working solutions prepared from the same sample were analyzed.

The accuracy tests were carried out by spiking known contents of standard samples into a Calculus Bovis sample and comparing the determined amount of these standards with the amount originally added. The relative standard deviation (RSD) was taken as a measure of precision, repeatability, and accuracy. Table 9.2 lists the validation results of the precision, stability, and accuracy tests. It shows that most bile acids have RSDs less

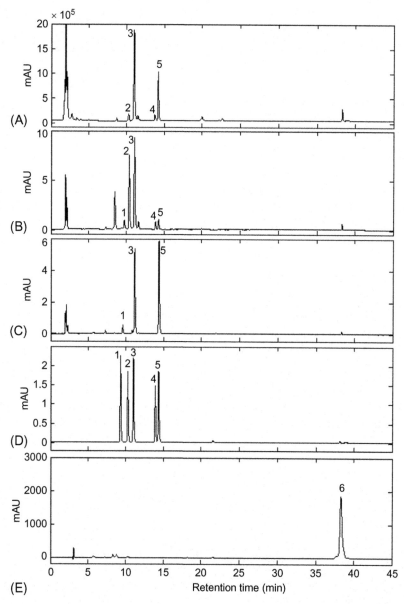

Fig. 9.1 HPLC/UV/ELSD chromatograms of various Calculus Bovis and reference chemicals. 1. ursodexsycholic acid; 2. hyodeoxycholic acid; 3. cholic acid; 4. chensodeoxycholic acid; 5. deoxycholic acid; and 6. bilirubin. (A–C) Representative profiles of natural, artificial, and in vitro cultured Calculus Bovis; (D and E) HPLC/ELSD.

Table 9.1 Linear regression data and LODs of the compounds to be qualified.

Compound	Linear function[a]	Regression coefficient (r^2)	Linear range (µg/mL)	LOD (µg/mL)
UDA	$y = 0.5126x + 3.7726$	0.9960	54.9–1098	2.745
HCA	$y = 0.5424x + 3.7853$	0.9953	24.9–498	1.245
CA	$y = 0.5557x + 3.8688$	0.9960	271.6–5432	3.580
CDA	$y = 0.4985x + 3.6239$	0.9984	21.8–436	1.090
DCA	$y = 0.6899x + 4.8845$	0.9980	66.1–1322	3.305
Bilirubin	$A = 0.9317B + 6.4982$	0.9985	0.170–42.4	0.106

[a]y and x, respectively, denote the logarithmic value of content and peak area, while A and B directly denote the content and peak area.

Table 9.2 Precision, repeatability, and accuracy data of the proposed method

		Precision							
		Intraday ($n = 5$)		Interday ($n = 3$)		Repeatability ($n = 5$)		Accuracy ($n = 5$)	
Peak no.	Compounds	Mean (µg/mL)	RSD (%)	Mean (µg/mL)	RSD (%)	Mean (µg/mL)	RSD (%)	Mean (µg/mL)	RSD (%)
1	UDA	113.4	2.59	101.8	2.47	112.5	3.05	97.16	2.68
2	HCA	257.1	4.28	347.1	4.36	355.7	0.84	93.76	1.82
3	CA	390.0	0.70	327.7	5.09	357.7	3.73	101.8	1.26
4	CDA	118.2	5.75	88.43	3.28	101.5	3.10	104.3	4.53
5	DCA	147.8	2.98	152.0	4.90	159.4	0.59	95.82	3.84
6	Bilirubin	86.1	5.94	77.11	7.60	85.65	5.22	84.57	5.92

than 5% while validation tests on bilirubin achieve a higher RSD (but no more than 8%). It is reported that bilirubin would be stable in 4 h.[5] Therefore, if the analysis is not delayed too long, the method is still acceptable.

9.1.2.3 Sample Analysis

Using the proposed method, 21 Calculus Bovis samples were analyzed. Table 9.3 lists the analysis data, from which we find that there are great variations for the content of each investigated constituent in Calculus Bovis and its substitutes; it indicates that the developmental condition is closely related to the quality of Calculus Bovis. Among three kinds of Calculus Bovis samples, in vitro cultured ones have the most abundant amounts of CA, DCA, and bilirubin but contain no HCA and CDA, which could be employed as the most important characteristic to identify or discriminate cultured Calculus Bovis. Although it is usually accepted that natural Calculus Bovis has the best therapeutic effects in clinic, the contents of bioactive components are not the highest, and some integrants (e.g., UCA and HCA) are even much lower than those of its substitutes.

In this study, total bile acids and bilirubin were compared to evaluate the quality variance of different samples. Fig. 9.2 shows the average contents of total bile acids and

Table 9.3 Quantitative analysis data of various Calculus Bovis samples (µg/mL)

Sample no.	Source	Lot no.	UDA	HCA	CA	CDA	DCA	Bilirubin
Natural								
1	Hebei	050705			0.907	0.130	0.420	0.002
2	Hebei	050706	0.015	0.064	0.186	0.160	0.046	0.308
3	Hebei	050720		0.023	0.103	0.069	0.034	0.206
4	Gansu	050415		0.242	0.414	0.021		0.001
5	Guangxi	050804	0.018	0.021	0.126	0.118	0.017	0.149
6	Shanxi	050512			0.501	0.092	0.270	0.056
Artificial								
7	Anhui	050507	0.386	1.240	1.383	0.486	0.022	0.027
8	Shandong	060301	0.061	1.241	1.308	0.151	0.023	0.009
9	Shanxi	051004	0.267	1.202	1.097	0.199	0.215	0.005
10	Shanghai	050606	0.244	1.072	1.178	0.237	0.291	0.003
11	Zhejiang	050810	0.226	1.001	1.234	0.228	0.227	0.003
In vitro cultured								
12	Wuhan	060501	0.110		1.393		1.208	0.113
13	Wuhan	060502	0.106		1.385		1.201	0.114
14	Wuhan	060503	0.101		1.293		1.148	0.122
15	Wuhan	060504	0.114		1.363		1.171	0.102
16	Wuhan	060505	0.102		1.096		1.578	0.108
17	Wuhan	060506	0.091		1.060		1.545	0.112
18	Wuhan	060507	0.102		1.077		1.536	0.108
19	Wuhan	060508	0.093		1.075		1.507	0.109
20	Wuhan	060509	0.047		1.074		1.470	0.114
21	Wuhan	060510	0.005		1.118		1.528	0.095

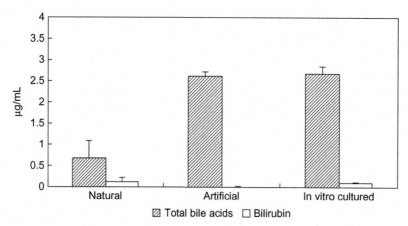

Fig. 9.2 Contents of total bile acids and bilirubin in three kinds of Calculus Bovis.

bilirubin and their standard deviations. It shows that natural Calculus Bovis contains bilirubin the most, but the content of total bile acids is rather low; in artificial samples, less bilirubin is contained. in vitro cultured samples have almost equivalent bilirubin as natural products but the content of total bile acids is much higher, even though HCA and CDA are absent. Artificial Calculus Bovis contains total bioactive constituents no less than natural products and have the best batch-to-batch uniformity, sufficient to be used as substitutes of natural Calculus Bovis.

9.1.3 Conclusions

The proposed method allows simultaneous determination of bile acids and bilirubin. The method has been applied to comparatively study the variations of bile acids and bilirubin in natural, artificial, and in vitro cultured Calculus Bovis samples. The results demonstrate the variations in three kinds of samples. Natural Calculus Bovis is often considered to have the best therapeutic effects, but the major bioactive components thereof are actually lower and the batch-to-batch uniformity is poor. Artificial Calculus Bovis contains total bioactive constituents no less than natural products and has the best batch-to-batch uniformity, sufficient to be used as substitutes of natural Calculus Bovis.

9.2. THE QUALITY STANDARD OF THE SBP

9.2.1 The Quality Standard of Nonvolatile Components in the SBP

9.2.1.1 Experimental

Reagents and Materials

Authentic standards were purchased from the National Institute for the Control of Pharmaceutical and Biological Products (Beijing, PR China). Acetonitrile and formic acid were of HPLC grade (Merck, Darmstadt, Germany). Ultrapure water was prepared from the Millipore water purification system (Millipore, Milford, MA, USA). Other reagents were of analytical grade.

Chromatographic System

HPLC/ELSD analysis was performed on a Shimadzu LC 2010A liquid chromatograph system (Shimadzu Co., Japan) consisting of a quaternary pump, a column oven, an autosampler, and a Sedex 75 ELSD detector (Sedere Co., France) coupled with a CLASS-VP workstation.

Analytical Conditions

A C18 RP-ODS column (4.6 mm × 250 mm, 5 μm, Agilent, USA) and a C18 guard column (4.6 mm × 7.5 mm, 5 μm, Merck, USA) were used. The mobile phases were composed of water/formic acid (100/0.5, A) and acetonitrile (B). The gradient was as follows:

0 min, 80% A, 20% B; 27 min, 42% A, 58% B; 37–60 min, 0% A, 100% B. Elution was performed at a solvent flow rate of 0.8 mL/min. The column compartment was kept at a temperature of 25°C, and the sample injection volume was 10 mL. The drift tube temperature of ELSD was 40°C, and the gas pressure was set at 3.5 bar.

Sample Preparation

Nine batches of SBP samples were kindly offered by the Shanghai Hutchison Pharmaceuticals Co. (Shanghai, China), three of which were produced in the year 2004 (marked as samples 1–3) and the others were produced in 2005 (marked as samples 4–9). Samples were ground into fine powder and 2.00 g of each was accurately weighted. A total of 50 mL 50% ethanol (v/v) was added; the samples were ultrasonically extracted (15 min ×2) under the same conditions, then centrifuged and filtered. All solutions were stored in the refrigerator at 4°C, and filtered through a syringe filter (0.45 μm) before HPLC analysis.

9.2.1.2 Results and Discussion

Chemical Fingerprint of SBP

Using the proposed method, HPLC/ELSD chromatograms of the extracts of SBP were acquired, in which there were mainly 26 peaks eluted (shown in Fig. 9.3) in total. Reduplicate analysis showed that the 26 peaks represented the common major constituents of different SBPs with consistent retention values (RSDs of retention times lower than 1%, and those of most peak areas lower than 8%).

In this work, HPLC/ELSD chromatograms of its medicinal materials were also studied, and by comparing those chromatograms to that of SBP, it suggested that the HPLC/ELSD chromatogram represented the characteristic chemical information of most of the nonvolatile constituents in SBP. However, some volatile constituents from Moschus, Calculus Bovis, Cortex Cinnamomi, and Borneolum Syntheticum were not detected.

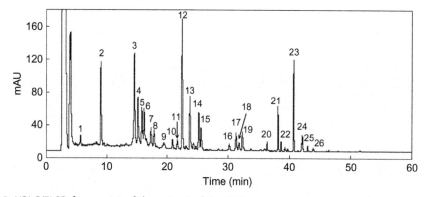

Fig. 9.3 HPLC/ELSD fingerprint of the extract of the SBP.

The obtained HPLC/ELSD chromatogram, therefore, can be applied as the chemical fingerprint of SBP for quality-control purposes.

Sample Analysis and Quality Evaluation

Using the proposed method, nine SBP samples were analyzed, including HPLC/ELSD fingerprint analysis and the quantitative determination of seven constituents. Table 9.4 lists the determination results of seven major constituents of these samples.

The approach of similarity measurement is commonly used in quality evaluation. Similarity measurement between the fingerprint of a test sample and that of a reference sample is often employed to quantitatively conduct quality evaluation. In this study, the Similarity Evaluation System for Chromatographic Fingerprint of TCM (Chinese Pharmacopoeia Committee, version 2004A) was used to achieve the similarity values as follows: 0.975, 0.920, 0.934, 0.979, 0.958, 0.983, 0.991, 0.974, and 0.984. All similarity values vary in the range of 0.92–0.99, and accordingly it concludes that there are no obvious differences among these products. From the above analysis, it concludes that the integral qualities of various SBP products are similar in general.

9.2.1.3 Conclusions

The proposed method allows obtaining chemical fingerprints of multiple constituents of TCM. The method has been applied to develop fingerprints of various SBP samples for quality-control purposes. The results demonstrate that the integral qualities of various SBP products are similar in general.

9.2.2 The Quality Standard of Volatile Components in the SBP

9.2.2.1 Experimental

Instruments

The GC/FID analysis was performed on an Agilent 6890N gas chromatograph system coupled with a flame ionization detector (Agilent Corporation, MA, USA). The chromatographic column was a CP8944 VF-5 capillary column (30 m × 0.25 mm, 0.25 μm).

Reagents and Materials

Eleven batches of SBP samples were kindly offered by the Shanghai Hutchison Pharmaceuticals Co. (Shanghai, China). Those batch numbers were: 000103, 001001, 010601, 020103, 020602, 030204, 030805, 040709, 040109, 050606, and 060109. A standard sample of cinnamaldehyde was purchased from the National Institute for the Control of Pharmaceutical and Biological Products (Beijing, China). Acetone was of a chromatographic grade (Merck, Darmstadt, Germany). Helium (99.999%) was used as a carrier gas, and H_2 (99.999%) and air were used for the FID detection (Chengkung Gas Industry Co., Shanghai, China).

Table 9.4 Quantitative analysis data of seven components in various SBP samples (μg/mL)

Components	Sample 1	Sample 2	Sample 3	Sample 4	Sample 5	Sample 6	Sample 7	Sample 8	Sample 9
Rb_1	31.45	34.06	29.57	33.19	30.62	29.65	24.83	30.01	25.81
CA	73.61	73.92	84.09	95.06	91.17	79.92	71.64	90.08	84.93
UDA	29.50	31.31	23.59	35.52	32.66	30.49	22.84	33.28	28.75
CIN	19.96	22.49	21.53	25.03	23.68	19.33	14.94	23.06	23.46
REC	8.14	8.41	9.37	10.64	9.42	10.23	8.86	9.55	10.50
CDA	8.14	8.90	9.63	10.48	9.08	7.51	6.33	9.55	9.24
DCA	16.39	16.90	17.41	19.25	17.29	18.96	17.22	17.18	16.55

GC Analysis

The GC/FID conditions were as follows: 1.5 mL/min carrier gas flow rate; 65°C initial oven temperature, ramped to 96°C at 6°C/min and held for 6 min, and to 190°C at 18°C/min, then to 225°C at 5°C/min and held for 10 min; injector temperature 220°C; heater temperature 250°C; flow rate of H_2, air, and makeup gas, respectively, set at 30, 400, and 25 mL/min; spite ratio 1:1; and the injection volume 1 μL.

Sample Preparation

A standard sample of cinnamaldehyde was accurately weighted, dissolved in acetone, and then diluted into the appropriate concentration. The stock solution was further diluted to make working standard solutions. Eleven batches of SBP samples were ground into a fine powder, and 2.00 g of each was accurately weighted. Next, 50 mL of acetone was added, the samples were ultrasonically extracted (15 min × 2), and then centrifuged and filtered. All samples were dried with anhydrous Na_2SO_4 over 12 h, then filtered and stored in the refrigerator at 4°C before analysis.

9.2.2.2 Results and Discussion
Chemical Fingerprinting Analysis

Using the proposed method, GC/FID chromatographic analyses were performed. Fig. 9.4 shows a representative gas chromatographic fingerprint. The fingerprint contains

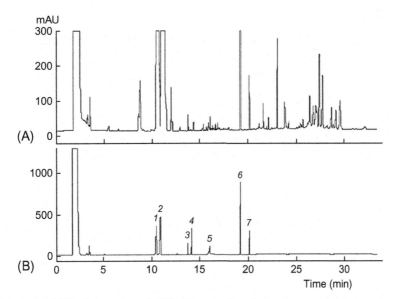

Fig. 9.4 Typical GC/FID fingerprint of SBP (A) and the chromatogram of seven standards (B): 1-isoborneol, 2-borneol, 3-cinnamaldehyde, 4-isopropyl methylphenol, 5-cinnamic acid, 6-benzyl benzoate, and 7-mascone.

more than 30 peaks. Reduplicate analysis showed that these peaks represented the major common constituents of different SBP samples with consistent retention values (RSDs of retention times lower than 0.5% and those of most peak areas were no more than 8%). The sum of the relative peak areas is almost 92% of the total content. The similarities of chemical fingerprinting of 11 SBPs were all above 0.95, which demonstrated that the batch stability of SBP was perfect.

Validation

The intraday and interday precisions were determined by analyzing calibration samples during a single day and on four different days, respectively. To confirm the repeatability, five different solutions prepared from the same sample were analyzed. The stability test was performed with sample solutions over a period of 2, 4, 8, 12, and 24 h.

RSD was calculated as a measure of the precision, repeatability, and accuracy. Most RSDs are less than 5%, which indicates that the method is precise and repeatable; the sample is stable when analyzed within 24 h. The proposed method is acceptable.

9.2.2.3 Conclusions

In this study, the chemical fingerprint of the SBP extract was established, and the fingerprint involved over 30 chromatographic peaks. The results indicate that the batch stability of SBP was perfect.

REFERENCES

1. Luo GA, Wang YM. Classification and development of TCM fingerprint. *Chin J New Drugs* 2002;**11**(1):46–51.
2. Yan SK, Xin WF, Luo GA, Wang YM, Cheng YY. An approach to develop two-dimensional fingerprint for the quality control of Qingkailing injection by high-performance liquid chromatography with diode array detection. *J Chromatogr A* 2005;**1090**(1–2):90.
3. Cheng YY, Chen MJ, Welsh WJ. Fractal fingerprinting of chromatographic profiles based on wavelet analysis and its application to characterize the quality grade of medicinal herbs. *J Chem Inf Comput Sci* 2003;**43**(6):1959–65.
4. Manoj MKB. Simultaneous separation and quantitation of four antiepileptic drugs—a study with potential for use in patient drug level monitoring. *J Pharm Biomed Anal* 2004;**34**(2):315–24.
5. Cao L, Sun Z, Cao L. Influence factors of content determination of bilirubin in artificial bezoar. *Chin J Public Health Eng* 2005;**4**(2):91–2.

CHAPTER 10

Pharmacokinetic Study of the Shexiang Baoxin Pill

Runui Liu, Weidong Zhang
Second Military Medical University, Shanghai, PR China

Abstract

Generally, there are hundreds and thousands of chemical compounds in one traditional Chinese medicine (TCM) formula. But only those that can be absorbed into the blood are the active ingredients of TCM, according to serum pharmacochemistry theory. Based on our previous serum pharmacochemistry study, 23 prototype components and seven metabolites from the Shexiang Baoxin Pill were detected in rat plasma, including eight gensinosides, five bufadienolides, four cholic acids, and six volatile compounds among those protype components. As the physicochemical characteristics of these plasma-absorbed compounds varied greatly, their in vivo pharmacokinetics (PKs) properties, such as the absorption speed, tissue distribution, and metabolism differences, were different from one another. In this chapter, the PK characteristics of gensinosides, bufadienolides, and four volatile compounds were studied to explain the in vivo process of these main active compounds of the Shexiang Baoxin Pill as an important guarantee for safe clinical use.

Keywords: Pharmacokinetics, TCM formula, Bufadienolide, Ginsenoside, Volatile components, The Shexiang Baoxin Pill.

10.1. PHARMACOKINETIC STUDY OF FIVE GINSENOSIDES FOLLOWING SINGLE AND MULTIPLE ORAL ADMINISTRATIONS OF THE SHEXIANG BAOXIN PILLS TO RATS

As a famous traditional Chinese medicine (TCM) formula, the *Shexiang Baoxin Pill* (SBP) has been widely used for treating coronary heart disease (CHD) in China for 35 years. SBP is composed of seven medicinal materials: *Moschus, Panax Ginseng, Calculus Bovis, Cortex cinnamomi, Styrax, Venenum Bufonis,* and *Borneolum Syntheticum,* which contain thousands of components such as ginsenosides, bufadienolides, cholic acids, and volatile constituents. Among the complex compounds of the SBP, ginsenosides from *Radix Ginseng* are the main type of therapeutic effects of the SBP, which have many bioactivities such as the treatment of myocardial ischemia, arrhythmia, and atherosclerosis; protecting neurons and endothelial cells; antithrombosis; and promoting angiogenesis.[1–4] A previous plasma pharmacochemistry study of the SBP also demonstrated that ginsenosides can be absorbed into the blood and have pharmacological actions (see Chapter 8).

Ginsenoside Rg1 (GRg1), ginsenoside Re (GRe), ginsenoside Rb3 (GRb3), ginsenoside Rc (GRc), and ginsenoside Rb1 (GRb1) are major ginsenosides in SBP. GRg1

Systems Biology and Its Application in TCM Formulas Research
https://doi.org/10.1016/B978-0-12-812744-5.00010-2

and GRe are ppt-type ginsenosides while GRb3, GRc, and GRb1 are ppd-type ginseno-sides. The information about pharmacokinetic (PK) properties of ginsenosides of the SBP is limited. Moreover, the PK behaviors after multiple-dose oral administration of the SBP had not been reported yet. Therefore, the accurate and comprehensive PK study of five ginsenosides in the SBP, including single-dosing and multiple-dosing PK, is essential for the safe clinical use of the SBP.

For the PK evaluation of five ginsenosides, development of a sensitive and reliable analytical method to simultaneous quantify GRg1, GRe, GRb3, GRc, and GRb1 in biological fluids is the key prerequisite. Because ginsenosides have poor ultraviolet (UV) radiation, the liquid chromatography-mass spectrometry (LC-MS) and liquid chromatography-tandem mass spectrometry (LC-MS/MS) methods are widely used for determining ginsenosides. Earlier publications have described various methods based on mass spectrometry.[4–7] However, these methods have some disadvantages such as insufficient sensitivity and a long analysis time.

Therefore, this study was aimed at developing a rapid, sensitive, and new LC-MS/MS method for simultaneous determination of GRg1, GRe, GRb3, GRc, and GRb1 and investigating the PK character of the five ginsenosides after single and multiple oral administrations of the SBP in rats. In addition, whether the PK behaviors of the five gin-senosides in the SBP were linear or nonlinear was also assessed.

10.1.1 Experimental

10.1.1.1 Chemicals and Reagents

GRg1, GRe, GRb3, GRc, GRb1, and digoxin (internal standard, IS) (purity >98%) were purchased from Shanghai Sunny Biotech Co., Ltd. Their chemical structures are shown in Fig. 10.1. The SBP (batch NO.: 120716) was kindly supplied by the Shanghai Hutchison Pharmaceuticals Company.

LC-MS grade acetonitrile was obtained from Merck. HPLC grade methanol was pro-vided by J&K Scientific Ltd. HPLC grade formic acid was purchased from Sigma-

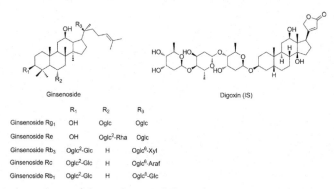

	R$_1$	R$_2$	R$_3$
Ginsenoside Rg$_1$	OH	Oglc	Oglc
Ginsenoside Re	OH	Oglc^2-Rha	Oglc
Ginsenoside Rb$_3$	Oglc^2-Glc	H	Oglc^6-Xyl
Ginsenoside Rc	Oglc^2-Glc	H	Oglc^6-Araf
Ginsenoside Rb$_1$	Oglc^2-Glc	H	Oglc^6-Glc

Fig. 10.1 Chemical structures of the analytes and IS.

Aldrich. All other reagents were of analytical grade. Purified water used throughout the study was prepared by a Milli-Q50 SP Reagent Water System.

10.1.1.2 Animals

Male Sprague-Dawley rats (180–220 g) were obtained from the Laboratory Animal Center of the Chinese Academy of Sciences. The animal protocols were approved by the Ethical Committees and the Institutional Animal Care and Uses Committee of the Second Military Medical University. The animal experiments were performed in accordance with the guide for the Care National Institutes of Health. Rats were kept in an environmentally controlled room (temperature: $22 \pm 2°C$, humidity: $50 \pm 10\%$, 12 h dark-light cycle) for 5 d before the experiments.

10.1.1.3 Preparation of the SBP Extract and the Determination of Five Ginsenosides in the Extract

To calculate the administration dosage, the contents of GRg1, GRe, GRb3, GRc, and GRb1 in the SBP were determined using the LC-MS/MS method described in the paper. The SBP was powdered and sieved through a NO. 40 mesh sieve to get a homogeneous size. The powder (10 mg), weighed accurately, was dissolved by methanol in a 10 mL volumetric flask and ultrasonically extracted for 30 min, then cooled at room temperature. The lost volume was compensated by adding the same solvent. The extracted solution was centrifuged at $14,000 \times g$ for 10 min. The supernatant was filtered through a 0.22-μm membrane filter to obtain samples. Finally, an aliquot of 5 μL of supernatant was injected into the LC-MS/MS system. The contents of GRg1, GRe, GRb3, GRc, and GRb1 in the SBP with three replicates were 3.88, 3.27, 4.38, 3.31, and 3.52 mg/g, respectively.

10.1.1.4 Preparation of Calibration Standards and Quality Control (QC) Samples

The primary stock standard solutions of five ginsenosides and digoxin were separately prepared by dissolving the required amount of reference standards in methanol at a concentration of 200 μg/mL. After serially diluting the mixture stock standard solution containing GRg1, GRe, GRb3, GRc, and GRb1 with methanol, working standard solutions of desired concentrations were provided. The IS working solution (1 μg/mL) was prepared by diluting the stock solution with methanol. All solutions were stored at about 4°C until use.

Calibration standard solutions were prepared by spiking these working solutions into drug-free rat plasma (1:19, V/V) to obtain final concentrations in the ranges of 2.5–1000 ng/mL for GRg1, 2.5–2000 ng/mL for GRe, 4.0–4000 ng/mL for GRb3 and GRc, and 4.0–8000 ng/mL for GRb1. Quality control (QC) samples were also obtained in the same fashion at concentrations of 5, 50, and 500 ng/mL for GRg1; 10, 100, and 1000 ng/mL for GRe; 20, 200, and 2000 ng/mL for GRb3 and GRc; and 40, 400, and 4000 ng/mL for GRb1, which represented low, medium, and high concentrations of QC samples, respectively. All spiked plasma samples were then treated according to the sample preparation procedure.

10.1.1.5 Instruments and LC-MS/MS Conditions

The Agilent 1200 rapid resolution liquid chromatography system consisted of a G1312B binary pump, a G1322A vacuum degasser, a G1316B thermostated column oven, and a G1329B autosampler. Mass spectra were performed using a triple-quadrupole tandem mass spectrometer equipped with electrospray ionization (ESI) of the Agilent 6410 system. The Masshunter software (version B.03.01) was used to control all parameters of LC and MS.

Chromatographic separation was achieved at 40°C using an ACQUITY HSS T3 column (100 × 2.1 mm I.D., 1.8 μm) in a run time of 8.0 min. Acetonitrile and 0.1% aqueous formic acid were used as the mobile phase at a flow rate of 0.3 mL/min. A gradient elution was applied with the initial mobile phase composed of 20% acetonitrile. The optimal gradient conditions were as follows: 0.0–1.0 min, 20–45% acetonitrile; 1.0–2.5 min, 45% acetonitrile; 2.5–4.0 min, 45%–20% acetonitrile; and 4.0–8.0 min, 20% acetonitrile. The injection volume was held constant at 5 μL. A divert valve was used to divert the eluent to waste from 0 to 1.0 min, and to MS from 1.0 to 8.0 min.

Quantification was operated in the negative ion mode using the multiple reaction monitoring (MRM) mode. High purity nitrogen served as both a nebulizing and drying gas. The parameters in the source were set as follows: capillary voltage 4000 V; source temperature 350°C; nebulizer gas pressure 40 psi; and drying gas flow rate 10 L/min. The optimized MRM parameters of ginsenosides and IS are given in Table 10.1.

10.1.1.6 Sample Preparation

Frozen plasma samples from rats were thawed to room temperature prior to preparation. A 100 μL aliquot of plasma was spiked with 1 mL n-butanol containing digoxin (IS) of 10 ng/mL. The mixture was vortexed for 10 min. The well-vortexed solutions were then centrifuged at 14,000 × g, 4°C for 10 min. The supernatant was transferred into a new centrifuge tube and evaporated to dryness under a centrifugal vacuum evaporator. Then, the residue was reconstituted in 100 μL methanol. After further centrifugation at 14,000 × g, 4°C for 10 min, 5 μL of the supernatant was injected into the LC-MS/MS system for analysis.

Table 10.1 MRM transitions and parameters for the detection of the ginsenosides and IS

Analyte	MRM transitions (m/z)	Fragmentor (V)	Collision energy (eV)	Dwell time (ms)
Ginsenoside Rg1	845.5 → 637.5	180	28	100
Ginsenoside Re	945.5 → 118.9	240	52	100
Ginsenoside Rb3	1077.6 → 148.9	200	56	100
Ginsenoside Rc	1077.6 → 148.9	200	56	100
Ginsenoside Rb1	1107.6 → 118.9	230	64	100
Digoxin (IS)	779.4 → 649.4	240	36	100

10.1.1.7 Method Validation

The method was fully validated according to the United States Food and Drug Administration (USFDA) guidelines for selectivity, linearity, lower limits of quantification (LLOQ), accuracy, precision, recovery, matrix effect, and stability (USFDA 2001).

The selectivity of the method was evaluated by the comparison of blank plasma from six individual rats to the corresponding spiked plasma sample at the LLOQ level to investigate the potential interferences at the LC peak region for analytes and IS. The signal-to-noise ratio (S/N) of the LLOQ samples was at least five times the response compared to the blank samples.

Each calibration curve was constructed using a weighted ($1/x^2$) linear least square regression model by plotting the peak area ratio (y) of analyte to IS versus the nominal concentration (x) of analyte. The LLOQ was defined as the lowest concentration on the calibration curve with S/N of at least 10 where precision and accuracy were less than or equal to 20% by five replicate analyses.

Intraday and interday precision and accuracy were estimated by analyzing QC samples at low, middle, and high concentrations with five replicates on the same day and on three consecutive days, respectively. Relative standard deviation (RSD) and relative error (RE) were used to express the precision and accuracy, respectively. The precision should not exceed 15% and the accuracy ranged from −15% to 15% of the nominal concentration.

The recovery of the five components was determined at three QC levels with three replicates by comparing the peak areas of plasma extracts spiked with analytes before extraction with those of the postextraction spiked samples at the same concentration. Matrix effects were investigated by comparing the peak areas of the analytes dissolved in the pretreated blank plasma with the corresponding concentrations prepared in the reconstitution solution with three replicates.

The stability of the analytes in rat plasma was assessed by analyzing five replicates of plasma samples at low, medium, and high QC levels under four different conditions. Short-term stability was evaluated after the exposure of the QC samples to room temperature for 4 h before processing and analysis. The freeze-thaw stability was tested after three repeated thawings at room temperature and freezing at about −20°C. The long-term stability was assessed after storage at −20°C for 30 days. The postpreparative stability was examined after the exposure of the processed samples at ambient temperature for 12 h.

10.1.1.8 PK Study

Experimental Design for Animals

Rats were fasted for 12 h with free access to water prior to and during the PK study. The SBP power was suspended in a 0.5% carboxymethyl cellulose sodium salt (CMC-Na) aqueous solution to obtain a concentration of 333 mg/mL. Rats were divided randomly into six groups ($n = 6$ in each group). Three groups of SD rats were given a single oral dose of the SBP at 4, 8, or 12 g/kg (via gavage). Serial blood samples (about 250 μL) were collected from the postorbital venous plexus veins in heparin pretreated polypropylene tubes at 0, 15, 30, 45 min, 1, 1.5, 2, 3, 4, 6, 8, 12, and 24 h after dosing.

Another three groups of rats for a multiple-dose study were orally given the SBP 4 g/kg once daily for 8, 15, or 22 consecutive days, respectively. On days 8, 15, and 22, blood samples (about 250 µL) were collected in the same way at 15, 30, 45 min, 1, 1.5, 2, 3, 4, 6, 8, 12, and 24 h after dosing. All blood samples were immediately centrifuged at 14,000 × g for 10 min at 4°C and stored frozen at about −70°C until analysis.

PK Calculation and Statistics

PK parameters including the area under the concentration-time curve from time zero to the last time point (AUC_{0-t}), the area under the concentration-time curve from time zero to infinity (AUC_{INF}), and the terminal elimination half-life ($T_{1/2}$) were determined by noncompartmental methods using WinNonlin 5.2 from Pharsight Corporation. The peak concentration (C_{max}) and time to reach peak concentration (T_{max}) were observed values directly. All results were expressed as mean ± SD.

A dose proportionality study on AUC_{0-t} was conducted by the regression of log-transformed data (power model). Statistics were performed using SPSS Statistics version 18. Differences were considered significant when P values were less than 0.05 ($P < 0.05$).

10.1.2 Results and Discussion

10.1.2.1 Method Development

MS parameters were optimized by infusing a standard analyte solution of 200 ng/mL into the mass spectrometer with ESI. It was discovered that the response observed in negative ion mode was higher than that in positive mode. In the precursor ion full-scan spectra, the most abundant ions were $[M+HCOO]^-$ m/z 845.5 for GRg1, $[M-H]^-$ m/z 945.5, 1077.6, 1077.6, 1107.6, and 779.4 for GRe, GRb3, GRc, GRb1, and IS, respectively. Fig. 10.2 shows the predominant product ions for the analytes and IS. The precursor→product ion transitions of m/z 845.5→637.5 for GRg1, m/z 945.5→118.9 for GRe, m/z 1077.6→148.9 for GRb3 and GRc, m/z 1107.6→118.9 for GRb1, and m/z 779.4→649.4 for IS were employed for quantitative analysis with the MRM mode. The fragmentor, collision energy, and dwell time were optimized to obtain maximal signal intensities.

Chromatographic conditions were optimized to obtain a high sensitivity and a short run time. Different columns, different mobile phase compositions, different column temperatures, and different flow rates of the mobile phase were tested. As a result, the ACQUITY HSS T3 column (100 × 2.1 mm I.D., 1.8 µm) was used in terms of response and peak shape. Acetonitrile water as the mobile phase was the most appropriate to give best sensitivity, efficiency, and peak shape. The addition of 0.1% formic acid was an important factor for enhancing the sensitivity and getting better peak shape. The column temperature was optimized at 40°C. The flow rate of 0.3 mL/min proved to be suitable. The employed gradient elution could provide satisfactory separations for all the analytes including isomers.

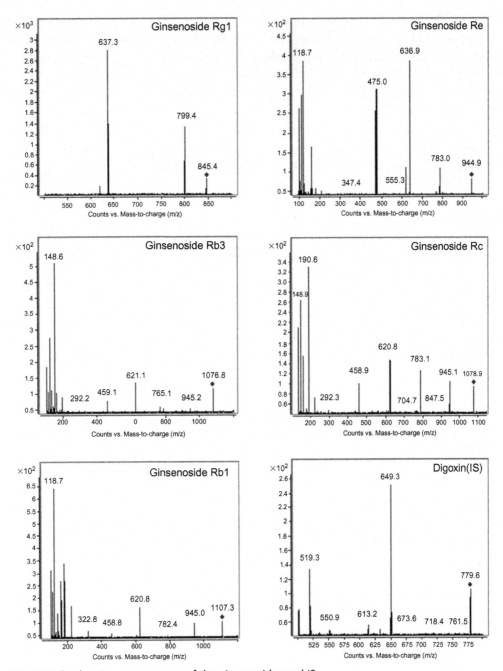

Fig. 10.2 Product ion mass spectra of the ginsenosides and IS.

Two different methods including protein precipitation (PPT) and liquid-liquid extraction (LLE) were investigated and compared for the sample preparation. The PPT with methanol or acetonitrile method was initially developed but the recoveries were low and could not eliminate the interferences from the sample matrix. LLE with different extraction solvents (ethyl acetate, diethyl ether, cyclohexane, tertbutyl methyl ether, *n*-butanol, or their different combinations) was explored. Finally, LLE using *n*-butanol was found to offer better recovery and fewer matrix effects for all the analytes.

In this study, digoxin has a similar basic structure, chromatographic behavior, and ionization efficiency to the ginsenosides. Moreover, digoxin could not be found in the plasma sample and is stable during the sample preparation. So, it was selected as the IS.

10.1.2.2 Method Validation
Fig. 10.3 shows the typical MRM chromatograms of the blank rat plasma, blank plasma spiked with the analytes at LLOQs and IS, and an in vivo plasma sample obtained at

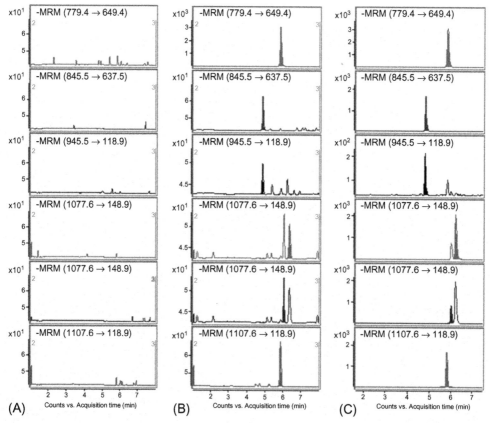

Fig. 10.3 Representative multiple reaction monitoring chromatograms of the ginsenosides and IS: (A) blank plasma sample; (B) blank plasma sample spiked with the ginsenosides at LLOQs and IS; and (C) plasma sample from a rat orally administered 4 g/kg at a time point of 30 min postdose.

Table 10.2 Regression data and LLOQs of the ginsenosides

Analyte	LLOQ (ng/mL)	Linear range (ng/mL)	Linear regression equation	r^2
Ginsenoside Rg1	2.5	2.5–1000	$y = 0.3422x + 0.0006$	0.9999
Ginsenoside Re	2.5	2.5–2000	$y = 0.0357x + 0.0007$	0.9998
Ginsenoside Rb3	4.0	4.0–4000	$y = 0.0992x + 0.0184$	0.9997
Ginsenoside Rc	4.0	4.0–4000	$y = 0.0549x + 0.0107$	0.9993
Ginsenoside Rb1	4.0	4.0–8000	$y = 0.0561x + 0.0142$	0.9997

30 min after a single oral administration of the SBP (4 g/kg). The retention time was about 5.83, 4.80, 4.77, 6.28, 6.02, and 5.81 min for digoxin (IS), GRg1, GRe, GRb3, GRc, and GRb1, respectively. No endogenous substances were observed to interfere with peaks of the analytes and IS, suggesting good selectivity of the developed method.

All the calibration curves exhibited good linearity at 2.5–1000 ng/mL for GRg1, 2.5–2000 ng/mL for GRe, 4.0–4000 ng/mL for GRb3 and GRc, and 4.0–8000 ng/mL for GRb1 (Table 10.2). The LLOQs of this assay were 2.5 ng/mL for GRg1 and GRe and 4.0 ng/mL for GRb3, GRc, and GRb1. These results proved more satisfactory in the analysis of PK behaviors of five ginsenosides in SBP.

The intraday and interday precision and accuracy values for five replicates of QC samples are summarized in Table 10.3. The mean accuracy of the analytes ranged from −4.49% to 9.33% (RE), and the intraday and interday precision were in the range of 1.39%–8.73% and 0.57%–8.18% (RSD), respectively. All the assay values met the requirements of FDA guidance, indicating that the established method was precise and accurate.

As shown in Table 10.4, the mean extraction recovery of the analytes was in the range of 85.69%–102.64% at different concentration levels, which indicated the recoveries of the five analytes were consistent, precise, and reproducible in various plasma samples. The matrix effect was examined to assess the possibility of ionization suppression or enhancement. The matrix effect ranged from 85.11% to 96.95% for all the analytes, indicating that the matrix effect contributing to the ionization suppression was not significant.

A summary of stability data in different storage conditions was presented in Table 10.5. The new method offered satisfactory stability with RSD in the range of 0.49%–12.54%. The results showed that the samples were stable during the routine analysis for the PK study.

10.1.2.3 PK Study

Single Dosing

The well-validated and new method was successfully applied to the PK study of the five ginsenosides after single and multiple oral administrations of the SBP. This is the first

Table 10.3 Precision and accuracy for the ginsenosides in rat plasma ($n = 15$, 5 replicates per day for 3 days)

Analyte	Nominal concentration (ng/mL)	Intraday			Interday		
		Concentration found (ng/mL) Mean ± SD	Precision (%, RSD)	Accuracy (%, RE)	Concentration found (ng/mL) Mean ± SD	Precision (%, RSD)	Accuracy (%, RE)
Ginsenoside Rg1	5	4.81 ± 0.42	8.73	−3.72	4.88 ± 0.15	3.13	−2.40
	50	48.65 ± 2.17	4.46	−2.71	48.28 ± 0.37	0.76	−3.44
	500	509.05 ± 7.08	1.39	1.81	490.34 ± 16.61	3.39	−1.93
Ginsenoside Re	10	9.74 ± 0.51	5.22	−2.65	10.36 ± 0.64	6.20	3.56
	100	96.54 ± 2.59	2.68	−3.46	95.52 ± 0.89	0.93	−4.49
	1000	1015.57 ± 29.66	2.92	1.56	1048.99 ± 34.02	3.24	4.90
Ginsenoside Rb3	20	19.85 ± 0.76	3.82	−0.74	19.90 ± 0.11	0.57	−0.53
	200	202.86 ± 5.44	2.68	1.43	206.03 ± 3.87	1.88	3.02
	2000	1966.69 ± 84.79	4.31	−1.67	1986.74 ± 25.96	1.31	−0.66
Ginsenoside Rc	20	20.02 ± 1.24	6.20	0.11	19.14 ± 1.57	8.18	−4.30
	200	205.75 ± 5.77	2.80	2.88	200.86 ± 4.28	2.13	0.43
	2000	2106.64 ± 170.28	8.08	5.33	2186.69 ± 80.45	3.68	9.33
Ginsenoside Rb1	40	40.56 ± 2.20	5.42	1.40	39.81 ± 0.81	2.03	−0.49
	400	412.78 ± 10.87	2.63	3.19	416.36 ± 6.62	1.59	4.09
	4000	4069.51 ± 172.78	4.25	1.74	3999.32 ± 61.27	1.53	−0.02

Table 10.4 Extraction recovery and matrix effect for the ginsenosides in rat plasma ($n = 3$)

Analyte	Nominal concentration (ng/mL)	Extraction recovery Mean ± SD	RSD (%)	Matrix effect Mean ± SD	RSD (%)
Ginsenoside Rg1	5	100.01 ± 3.78	3.78	95.86 ± 1.52	1.59
	50	88.28 ± 3.62	4.10	87.07 ± 1.25	1.44
	500	98.95 ± 0.27	0.27	85.7 ± 0.45	0.52
Ginsenoside Re	10	87.64 ± 4.61	5.26	87.06 ± 3.52	4.04
	100	97.05 ± 1.62	1.67	91.27 ± 2.65	2.91
	1000	97.06 ± 1.64	1.69	85.28 ± 1.01	1.18
Ginsenoside Rb3	20	95.93 ± 2.24	2.34	89.96 ± 2.85	3.17
	200	97.58 ± 1.87	1.92	94.98 ± 3.79	3.99
	2000	90.03 ± 1.20	1.33	95.98 ± 3.16	3.29
Ginsenoside Rc	20	102.64 ± 9.43	9.18	95.49 ± 10.13	10.61
	200	90.56 ± 1.03	1.14	85.11 ± 1.26	1.48
	2000	94.72 ± 0.85	0.90	95.18 ± 1.37	1.44
Ginsenoside Rb1	40	98.70 ± 5.37	5.44	92.00 ± 3.35	3.64
	400	85.69 ± 2.86	3.34	89.89 ± 2.49	2.77
	4000	86.83 ± 2.15	2.48	96.95 ± 0.55	0.57

systemic and comprehensive PK study of ginsenosides after single and multiple oral administrations of the SBP. The mean plasma concentration time profiles of GRg1, GRe, GRb3, GRc, and GRb1 after a single oral dose of 4, 8, or 12 g/kg are shown in Fig. 10.4 and the PK parameters are summarized in Tables 10.6A and 10.6B. After the SBP was orally administrated to rats, the five ginsenosides could be detected in rat plasma for up to 24 h postdose. Our method could be considered to be sufficiently sensitive. As shown in Fig. 10.4, double or triple plasma concentration peaks were observed in mean plasma concentration curves of GRe, GRc, and GRb1. The phenomenon might be attributed to the absorption at different rates in different intestinal segments. Except for GRc and GRb1 following a single oral dose of 12 g/kg, the maximal plasma concentrations of the ginsenosides occurred 0.25–1.08 h after single dosing, indicating they underwent rapid absorption, which might be explained by the effects of promoting absorption exerted by borneol in the SBP on ginsenosides (see Chapter 10.5). Although their total amounts present in the SBP were comparable, the AUC_{0-t} and C_{max} of the ppd-type ginsenosides Rb3, Rc, and Rb1 were significantly greater than those of the ppt-type ginsenosides Rg1 and Re. The $T_{1/2}$ values of all ginsenosides were long. Different excretion was the major factor. The ppd-type ginsenosides Rc and Rb1 were subject to slow extensive renal and biliary excretion, resulting in their long $T_{1/2}$ values and high systemic exposure levels, indicative of low bile/plasma distribution ratios of 0.2–0.4. Owing to the similar structures with GRc and GRb1, GRb3 has parallel excretion,

Table 10.5 Stability of the ginsenosides in rat plasma ($n = 5$)

Analyte	Nominal concentration (ng/mL)	Short-term stability (4 h at room temperature)		Freeze-thaw stability (3 cycles)		Autosampler stability (12 h room temperature)		Long-term stability (30 days at −20°C)	
		Concentration found (%) Mean ± SD	RSD (%)	Concentration found (%) Mean ± SD	RSD (%)	Concentration found (%) Mean ± SD	RSD (%)	Concentration found (%) Mean ± SD	RSD (%)
Ginsenoside Rg1	5	108.62 ± 6.34	5.84	89.43 ± 4.81	5.38	95.24 ± 11.87	12.47	94.58 ± 9.11	9.64
	50	99.61 ± 3.67	3.69	99.27 ± 2.15	2.17	98.29 ± 1.10	1.12	97.06 ± 0.48	0.49
	500	96.70 ± 1.54	1.60	90.30 ± 5.66	6.26	95.77 ± 3.94	4.12	92.71 ± 4.65	5.01
Ginsenoside Re	10	111.16 ± 10.11	9.10	88.60 ± 4.40	4.96	98.87 ± 8.07	8.16	95.51 ± 6.60	6.91
	100	96.05 ± 4.83	5.03	96.18 ± 2.90	3.02	99.33 ± 4.99	5.02	97.32 ± 4.02	4.13
	1000	99.21 ± 6.00	6.05	92.45 ± 5.72	6.18	95.23 ± 5.22	5.48	96.60 ± 4.34	4.49
Ginsenoside Rb3	20	106.94 ± 9.21	8.62	101.79 ± 10.04	9.86	110.42 ± 5.18	4.69	104.28 ± 7.82	7.50
	200	99.52 ± 1.53	1.54	92.56 ± 1.28	1.38	91.29 ± 1.29	1.42	91.05 ± 0.95	1.04
	2000	99.71 ± 4.14	4.15	94.32 ± 5.78	6.13	96.76 ± 9.38	9.70	95.41 ± 5.64	5.91
Ginsenoside Rc	20	112.19 ± 14.07	12.54	99.94 ± 4.45	4.45	95.13 ± 3.92	4.12	109.99 ± 11.02	10.02
	200	96.37 ± 3.74	3.88	95.73 ± 4.59	4.80	96.07 ± 1.66	1.73	95.74 ± 4.94	5.16
	2000	99.20 ± 5.17	5.21	93.60 ± 6.57	7.02	97.12 ± 9.85	10.14	95.12 ± 6.85	7.20
Ginsenoside Rb1	40	110.12 ± 10.05	9.13	107.36 ± 11.45	10.66	97.35 ± 10.35	10.64	104.86 ± 6.55	6.25
	400	96.10 ± 3.31	3.44	94.46 ± 4.59	4.86	91.98 ± 3.45	3.75	94.58 ± 2.59	2.73
	4000	100.15 ± 4.38	4.37	95.13 ± 5.16	5.42	98.98 ± 9.99	10.10	96.87 ± 6.27	6.47

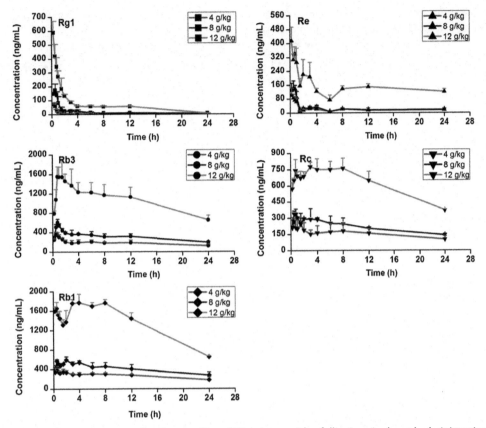

Fig. 10.4 Plasma concentration-time profiles of the ginsenosides following single oral administration of the SBP at 4, 8, or 12 g/kg to rats (mean $\pm$ SD, $n = 6$ in each group).

resulting in similar long $T_{1/2}$ values and high systemic exposure levels. The ppt-type ginsenosides were subject to rapid extensive biliary excretion through active transport, resulting in their high clearance and low systemic exposure levels, indicative of high bile/plasma distribution ratios of 22-1907.[8] However, their $T_{1/2}$ values were indeed long. This is worth thinking about. Considering that the administration route was oral, the $T_{1/2}$ reflected not only the elimination rate but also the absorption rate.[9] According to the literature,[10] GRg1 remains in the large intestine for a long time (6–24 h after administration). There is a possibility that the absorption rate of GRg1 and GRe in the large intestine was much higher than their elimination rate, resulting in long oral $T_{1/2}$. Thus, the significant variations ($P < 0.05$) of $T_{1/2}$ of the ppt-type compounds at different doses make no sense.

Fig. 10.5 presents the properties of a nondose-dependent exposure of ginsenosides. The exposure levels of all ginsenosides in AUC and C_{max} increased directly with the

Table 10.6A PK parameters of the ginsenosides Rg1 and Re following single oral administration of the SBP at 4, 8, or 12 g/kg to rats ($n = 6$ in each group)

Paramaters	Ginsenoside Rg1			Ginsenoside Re		
	4 g/kg Mean ± SD	8 g/kg Mean ± SD	12 g/kg Mean ± SD	4 g/kg Mean ± SD	8 g/kg Mean ± SD	12 g/kg Mean ± SD
T_{max} (h)	0.25 ± 0.00	0.50 ± 0.00	0.25 ± 0.00	0.38 ± 0.14	0.33 ± 0.14	0.50 ± 0.35
C_{max} (ng/ mL)	62.77 ± 11.38	173.85 ± 46.27	589.49 ± 82.56	106.45 ± 38.19	159.61 ± 30.01	428.25 ± 61.7
AUC_{0-t} (ng/mL h)	221.98 ± 22.69	310.94 ± 69.23	1413.63 ± 62.94	485.10 ± 64.13	512.30 ± 28.88	3466.13 ± 596.82
AUC_{INF} (ng/mL h)	347.55 ± 75.45	458.36 ± 61.21	1543.57 ± 50.91	616.64 ± 227.30	727.99 ± 58.48	15844.67 ± 3173.47
$T_{1/2}$ (h)	26.11 ± 8.14	8.97 ± 7.64	7.30 ± 2.13	36.34 ± 3.90	11.97 ± 6.62	59.74 ± 25.34

SBP dose from 4 to 12 g/kg but nonlinearly. In particular, when the single oral dose was 12 g/kg, the values of AUC and C_{max} increased sharply. The increases might be related to the saturation reached by active transporters. These might also be because of the increasing membrane permeability owing to the damaged intestinal membrane following a single large dose. However, the elucidation of the mechanism of the phenomenon requires further detailed study.

Mutiple Dosing

The PK parameters after multiple oral doses are listed in Tables 10.7A and 10.7B. The C_{max}/AUC-duration of administration profiles of the ginsenosides in the SBP is illustrated in Fig. 10.6. In the multiple-dose study, the plasma AUC_{0-t} and C_{max} of the five ginsenosides decreased from day 1 to day 8. The decreases of the plasma levels might be explained by some components of the SBP inducing some related transporters such as P-glycoprotein (P-gp), multidrug resistance-associated protein (MRP) after repeated oral dosing of SBP, or the adaptive acceleration of their metabolism mediated by the gut microflora in the stimulation of long-term administration. A previous study reported[8] that transporters played the major role in the overall elimination of ginsenosides. Moreover, the relative contributions of tissue deglycosylation and tissue oxidation to overall elimination appeared to be poor. However, compared with the minor tissue deglycosylation, the preabsorption deglycosylation of ginsenosides mediated by the gut microflora

Table 10.6B PK parameters of the ginsenosides Rb3, Rc, and Rb1 following single oral administration of the SBP at 4, 8, or 12 g/kg to rats ($n = 6$ in each group)

Paramaters	Ginsenoside Rb3			Ginsenoside Rc			Ginsenoside Rb1		
	4 g/kg Mean ± SD	8 g/kg Mean ± SD	12 g/kg Mean ± SD	4 g/kg Mean ± SD	8 g/kg Mean ± SD	12 g/kg Mean ± SD	4 g/kg Mean ± SD	8 g/kg Mean ± SD	12 g/kg Mean ± SD
T_{max} (h)	0.56 ± 0.13	0.92 ± 0.14	1.08 ± 0.38	1.00 ± 0.58	0.63 ± 0.18	3.25 ± 2.63	0.50 ± 0.00	1.08 ± 0.80	2.25 ± 1.47
C_{max} (ng/mL)	377.60 ± 35.08	615.61 ± 61.73	1612.67 ± 394.13	299.23 ± 106.28	359.69 ± 78.72	875.30 ± 125.69	506.73 ± 19.93	624.28 ± 74.41	2051.26 ± 685.56
AUC_{0-t} (ng/ mL h)	4284.56 ± 311.36	7258.45 ± 467.34	25172.82 ± 712.59	3644.65 ± 166.16	5111.12 ± 98.59	14545.17 ± 393.77	6990.19 ± 274.79	9655.90 ± 205.36	31331.58 ± 147.65
AUC_{INF} (ng/ mL h)	8917.68 ± 166.63	12851.52 ± 898.08	42389.39 ± 1377.98	6637.19 ± 810.66	9364.77 ± 172.40	22604.63 ± 724.39	12194.53 ± 386.37	19160.91 ± 434.36	41560.01 ± 222.94
$T_{1/2}$ (h)	27.34 ± 4.92	20.34 ± 3.17	17.60 ± 3.37	20.53 ± 1.86	20.81 ± 5.62	14.80 ± 1.96	19.19 ± 1.51	24.66 ± 10.34	10.89 ± 0.16

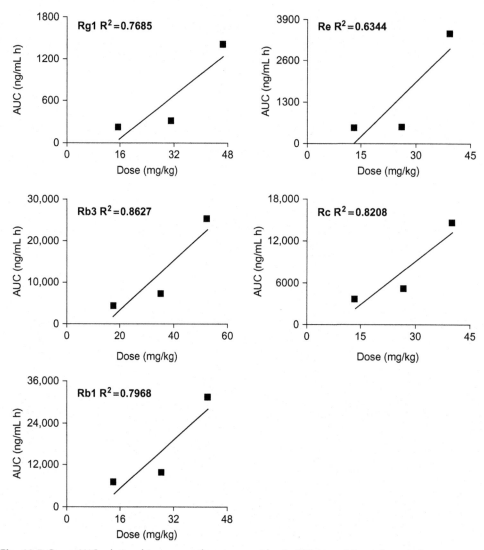

Fig. 10.5 Dose-AUC relationship among the ginsenosides in SBP ($n = 6$ in each group).

appeared to be relatively extensive. Thus, we made the above presumption. An earlier study[11] demonstrated that the levels of mdr1a and mdr1b (mdr1a and mdr1b could express P-gp) in small intestines of the rats treated orally with the SBP for six consecutive days increased significantly. These data provided evidence for our presumption. The longer T_{max} of the ppd-type ginsenosides on day 8 compared with those on day 1 might be also related to the above presumption. However, the differences of these ppd-type ginsenosides were not statistically significant ($P > 0.05$), while the AUC_{0-t} and C_{max} of GRe and the C_{max} of GRg1 decreased remarkably ($P < 0.05$) from day 1 to day 8

Table 10.7A PK parameters of the ginsenosides Rg1 and Re after 8, 15, and 22 days oral administration of the SBP (4 g/kg) to rats ($n = 6$ in each group)

Paramaters	Ginsenoside Rg1			Ginsenoside Re		
	8 days Mean $\pm$ SD	15 days Mean $\pm$ SD	22 days Mean $\pm$ SD	8 days Mean $\pm$ SD	15 days Mean $\pm$ SD	22 days Mean $\pm$ SD
T_{max} (h)	0.38 $\pm$ 0.25	0.55 $\pm$ 0.21	0.31 $\pm$ 0.13	0.42 $\pm$ 0.29	0.50 $\pm$ 0.20	0.44 $\pm$ 0.34
C_{max} (ng/ mL)	36.66 $\pm$ 3.78	36.90 $\pm$ 10.59	34.39 $\pm$ 14.66	34.74 $\pm$ 7.38	36.40 $\pm$ 6.61	33.38 $\pm$ 11.78
AUC_{0-t} (ng/mL h)	199.29 $\pm$ 18.02	186.03 $\pm$ 41.35	152.65 $\pm$ 25.57	158.18 $\pm$ 65.86	170.95 $\pm$ 11.46	158.77 $\pm$ 10.57
AUC_{INF} (ng/mL h)	318.75 $\pm$ 92.19	286.59 $\pm$ 62.11	240.21 $\pm$ 18.55	293.59 $\pm$ 137.97	244.70 $\pm$ 74.88	263.21 $\pm$ 174.62
$T_{1/2}$ (h)	35.88 $\pm$ 14.22	25.34 $\pm$ 11.22	18.90 $\pm$ 4.94	45.14 $\pm$ 2.56	12.44 $\pm$ 7.48	12.34 $\pm$ 7.33

for the ppt-type ginsenosides. The results might be attributed to slow excretion of the ppd-type ginsenosides. Then, the plasma AUC_{0-t} and C_{max} of the ppt-type ginsenosides had appeared to reach the steady state since day 8 while those of the ppd-type ginsenosides increased slightly ($P > 0.05$). The reason for these increases remains to be explored. Collectively, no significant differences ($P > 0.05$) were observed on AUC_{0-t} and C_{max} of these ppd-type ginsenosides between the single and multiple doses while compared with the single dose, the AUC_{0-t} and C_{max} of the ppt-type ginsenoside Re and the C_{max} of the ppt-type ginsenoside Rg1 decreased remarkably ($P < 0.05$) after multiple oral administration. All the ginsenosides were not accumulating after multiple doses. The values of $T_{1/2}$ of the ginsenosides were not significantly different ($P > 0.05$) between the single and multiple doses, indicating that no obvious accumulation was identified after multiple-dose administration.

10.1.3 Conclusions

A rapid, sensitive and new LC-MS/MS method for simultaneous determination of GRg1, GRe, GRb3, GRc, and GRb1 in rat plasma was developed and validated. It was successfully applied to investigate the systemic and comprehensive PK study of ginsenosides after single and multiple oral administration of the SBP. All the ginsenosides exhibited the nonlinear PK properties. No significant accumulation of the ginsenosides was observed after multiple oral administration of the SBP. Moreover, the ppd-type ginsenosides Rb3, Rc, and Rb1 have more favorable PK properties compared with the ppt-type ginsenosides Rg1 and Re. The results of the PK study provide a scientific basis for

Table 10.7B PK parameters of the ginsenosides Rb3, Rc, and Rb1 after 8, 15, and 22 days oral administration of the SBP (4 g/kg) to rats ($n = 6$ in each group)

Paramaters	Ginsenoside Rb3			Ginsenoside Rc			Ginsenoside Rb1		
	8 days Mean ± SD	15 days Mean ± SD	22 days Mean ± SD	8 days Mean ± SD	15 days Mean ± SD	22 days Mean ± SD	8 days Mean ± SD	15 days Mean ± SD	22 days Mean ± SD
T_{max} (h)	1.45 ± 0.45	0.88 ± 0.14	1.31 ± 0.24	1.70 ± 0.27	0.88 ± 0.14	0.81 ± 0.52	3.50 ± 1.09	2.38 ± 1.43	0.75 ± 0.45
C_{max} (ng/mL)	285.38 ± 46.78	281.25 ± 12.04	343.30 ± 75.12	226.58 ± 42.32	230.49 ± 19.26	253.55 ± 19.99	389.07 ± 56.04	428.75 ± 60.93	660.15 ± 49.90
AUC_{0-t} (ng/mL h)	3755.69 ± 699.49	3983.78 ± 737.58	4892.58 ± 164.74	3061.24 ± 138.84	3108.36 ± 646.28	3529.80 ± 241.89	6333.00 ± 208.19	6462.66 ± 175.57	9797.28 ± 955.87
AUC_{INF} (ng/mL h)	7538.24 ± 255.94	9154.06 ± 297.71	10325.46 ± 217.82	5060.73 ± 173.86	5177.33 ± 56.84	6827.89 ± 176.25	11533.21 ± 198.76	12294.46 ± 199.65	17420.28 ± 234.85
$T_{1/2}$ (h)	26.57 ± 7.49	28.95 ± 6.42	19.64 ± 4.16	17.50 ± 1.07	18.85 ± 4.61	19.53 ± 6.77	20.81 ± 5.16	21.28 ± 4.91	20.11 ± 1.44

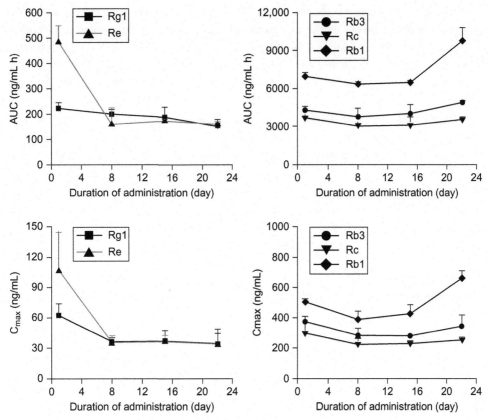

Fig. 10.6 C_{max}/AUC-duration of administration profiles of the ginsenosides in SBP (mean $\pm$ SD, $n = 6$ in each group).

exploring the efficacy and safety of the SBP and selecting suitable PK markers for the prescription.

10.2. PHARMACOKINETICS AND TISSUE DISTRIBUTION OF FIVE BUFADIENOLIDES FROM THE SBP IN MICE

It is well known that proper animal models are very important to obtain a good understanding of the PK properties of any drug. Differences between species concerning the metabolism of the drugs may contribute to the different PK properties in vivo after oral or injected administrations,[12] and the varied metabolites and their concentrations can potentially affect the in vivo bioactivities and toxicities. It had been reported that bufalin, cinobufagin, and resibufogenin were mainly metabolized by CYP3A4 in human liver microsomes.[13] However, the comparative metabolism of cinobufagin in liver microsomes from mouse, rat, dog, minipig, monkey, and human, significant species differences in cinobufagin metabolism were revealed.[14] In detail, deacetylation or epimerization are major metabolic pathways in the rat, while in the mouse, similarly to what occurs in humans, the major metabolites were found to be hydroxylate via CYP3A4. A similar phenomenon also arose in bufalin.[15] Accordingly, to select the mouse as the animal model may potentially more accurately reflect the information of the metabolism of bufadienolides in vivo.

In this chapter, five bufadienolides were simultaneous determined in plasma and tissues samples after oral administration of the SBP in mice. For the first time, the plasma PKs and tissue distribution of bufadienolides in the SBP were studed in mice, a more proper animal model than rat. A specific and sensitive LC–MS/MS method has been developed for the simultaneous determination of bufadienolides in mice plasma and tissue; it has been validated and successfully applied to the PK study of bufadienolides in mice plasma and tissue samples. The obtained results would be helpful for evaluating the clinical application of these components in SBP.

10.2.1 Experimental

10.2.1.1 Chemicals and Reagents

Resibufogenin (RBG), bufalin (BF), gamabufatalin (GBL), arenobufagin (ABG), bufotalin (BL), and internal standard (IS) tinidazole were purchased from the National Institute for Food and Drug Control. The purity of each reference standard was above 98.0% and their structures were shown in Fig. 10.7. Acetonitrile of LC-MS grade was obtained from Honeywell Burdick and Jackson Muskegon. Methanol and formic acid were of HPLC grade. Deionized water was purified with a Milli–Q50 SP Reagent Water System. Other reagents were of analytical grade. SBP samples were kindly offered by the Shanghai Hutchison Pharmaceuticals Company.

10.2.1.2 Animals

Male ICR mice (18–22 g) were purchased from the Shanghai SLAC Laboratory Animal Co. Ltd and acclimated in an environmentally controlled breeding room for 5 days prior to the experiments and housed in separate cages at a temperature of $23 \pm 2°C$ with a 12 h light/dark cycle and a relative humidity of 50%. All mice had free access to standard diet and water, and were fasting overnight before experiments. The study was approved by the Animal Ethics Committee of the Second Military Medical University.

10.2.1.3 Instruments and Conditions

Liquid Chromatography

Chromatographic analysis was performed on an Agilent 1200 Series high performance liquid chromatography (HPLC), which was equipped with a quaternary pump with online degasser, auto-sampler, and column oven. Chromatographic conditions including types of reversed-phase chromatographic columns, mobile phase compositions, choice of additives, column temperature, and the flow rate of the mobile phase were optimized to

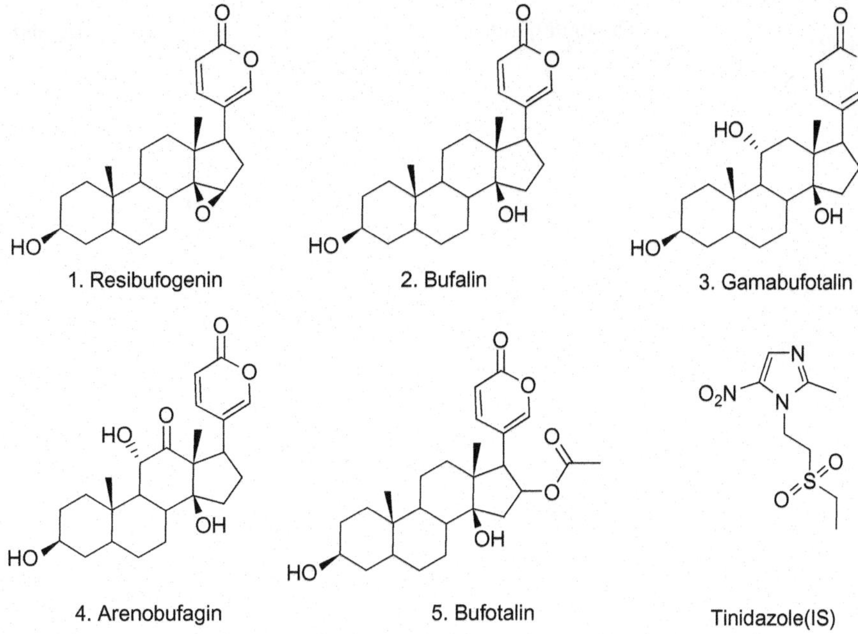

Fig. 10.7 Chemical structures of the analytes and IS.

achieve short retention time, symmetric peak shape, and satisfactory ionization. An Agilent Zorbax Eclipse Plus C_{18} column (3.0 × 100 mm I.D., 1.8μm) was employed and the column temperature was maintained at 30°C. The mobile phase consisted of A (0.1% formic acid in water) and B (acetonitrile) with the following gradient elution: 20%–50% B from 0 to 1 min, 50% B from 1 to 2.5 min, 50%–80% B from 2.5 to 4 min, 80% B from 4 to 6.5 min, 80%–20% B from 6.5 to 7 min, 20% B from 7 to 12 min with a 2 min equilibration time at a flow rate of 0.3 mL/min, and the sample injection volume was 5 μL.

Mass Spectrometric Conditions

Mass spectrometric detection was performed on an Agilent 6410 triple-quadrupole mass spectrometer equipped with an ESI source. Under the ESI condition chosen, the analytes and IS all exhibited higher sensitivity in the positive mode than in the negative mode. The MS/MS product ion spectra of the analytes and IS are shown in Fig. 10.8. Based on the optimization of mass spectrometry, the ESI source was set in positive ionization mode with the capillary voltage set at 3500 V. The dwell time was 100 ms, and the other parameters in the source were set as following: source temperature 350°C; desolvation gas flow 10 L/min; and nebulizer gas (N_2) pressure 40 psi. The mass spectrometer scanned in MRM mode, and the cone voltage and collision energy were optimized for each analyte and selected values were listed in Table 10.8.

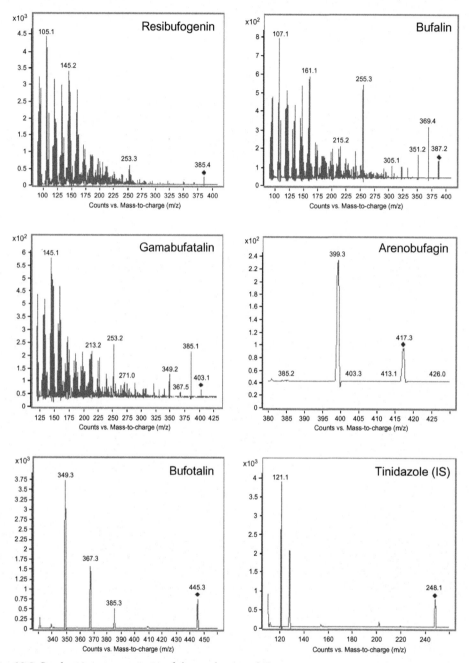

Fig. 10.8 Product ion mass spectra of the analytes and IS.

Table 10.8 MRM transitions and parameters for the detection of RBG, BF, GBL, ABG, BL, and IS

Analyte	MRM transitions (*m/z*)	Fragmentor (V)	Collisionenergy (eV)	Dwell time (ms)
Resibufogenin	385.4 → 105.1	140	36	100
Bufalin	387.2 → 107.1	150	30	100
Gamabufatalin	403.1 → 105.1	150	34	100
Arenobufagin	417.3 → 399.3	180	44	100
Bufatalin	445.3 → 349.3	150	22	100
Tinidazole (IS)	248.1 → 121.1	110	18	100

10.2.1.4 Determination of Five Bufadienolides in the SBP

The SBP was ground into fine powder. 10 mg was accurately weighed in a vial. A 10.0 mL mixed solution of methanol-water (1:1, V/V) was added and ultrasonically extracted for 20 min to prepare a uniform suspension, then centrifuged at 14,000 rpm for 10 min. The supernatant was filtered through a syringe filter (0.22 µm) and an aliquot of 5 µL of supernatant was subjected to LC-ESI-MS/MS analysis. The contents of BF, RBG, GBL, ABG, and BL were measured quantitatively using the same conditions described above, as 597.22, 454.86, 121.53, 250.00, and 157.89 µg/g, respectively.

10.2.1.5 Standard and Sample Preparation

Preparation of Calibration Standards and Quality Control Samples

Stock solutions of RBG, BF, GBL, ABG, BL, and IS were separately prepared by dissolving the compounds in methanol at a concentration of 200 µg/mL, and all solutions were stored at 4°C. Tissues (heart, liver, spleen, lung, kidney, and small intestine) were homogenized with physiological saline solution (2 mL/g). Calibration work solutions and QC samples were prepared by adding the diluted stock solutions into blank rat plasma and tissue homogenates (5/95, v/v).

Calibration standards of plasma samples working solutions with RBG, BF, GBL, ABG, and BL were prepared at final concentrations in the range of 2.50–5000, 5.00–10000, 2.50–1000, 2.00–2000, and 0.25–500 ng/mL, respectively. The final standard concentrations of tissue samples were in the range of 5.00–1000, 5.00–2000, 5.00–5000, 5.00–1000, and 0.20–200 ng/mL, respectively. And the I.S. solution was prepared at a final concentration of 10 ng/mL in methanol.

For validation of the method, QC plasma samples of RBG, BF, GBL, ABG, and BL were prepared separately at three concentrations of 25, 250, and 2500 ng/mL; 50, 500, and 5000 ng/mL; 5, 50, and 500 ng/mL; 10, 100, and 1000 ng/mL; and 2.5, 25, and 250 ng/mL, respectively. And three concentrations of 5, 50, and 500 ng/mL; 10, 100, and 1000 ng/mL; 5, 25, and 250 ng/mL; 5, 50, and 500 ng/mL; and 1, 10, and 100 ng/mL for tissue (liver) homogenatesm samples, respectively.

Samples Preparations

To eliminate interference from the sample matrix and achieve satisfactory recovery, several sample preparation methods including PPT with acetonitrile or methanol, LLE with ethyl acetate, and solid phase extraction (SPE) with Waters Oasis HLB cartridges were evaluated. Finally, we choose the method of LLE to prepare samples with comprehensive consideration. Plasma samples or tissue homogenates (100 µL) were treated with 1 mL ethyl acetate containing the IS tinidazole (10 ng/mL). The mixture was vortexed for 10 min and then centrifuged at 14,000 rpm for 10 min. The supernatant fluid was transferred into a 1.5 mL centrifuge tube and evaporated to dryness in a rotary evaporator at 37°C. The residue was reconstituted in 100 µL of the mobile phase, and then centrifuged at 14,000 rpm for 10 min at 4°C. The supernatants were transferred to a vial, and 5 µL was injected into the LC-ESI-MS/MS system for analysis.

10.2.1.6 Method Validation

The method was validated according to the USFDA bioanalytical method validation guidance (USFDA, 2001).

Specificity and Selectivity

The specificity and selectivity were investigated by comparing the chromatograms of blank plasma and tissue homogenates (liver was chosen as representative tissue) obtained from six mice with those of corresponding standard plasma and tissue homogenates samples spiked with analytes and IS (10 ng/mL), and the samples after an oral dose.

Linearity and LLOQ

The linearity of the method was evaluated by analysis of five calibration curves containing eight nonzero concentrations. The calibration curves were fitted by least square regression using $1 \times^{-2}$ as the weighting factor of the peak area ratio of each analyte to IS versus individual plasma and tissue homogenates concentrations. The lower limit of quantification (LLOQ) was determined at the lowest concentration to be detected taking into consideration a 1:10 baseline noise-calibration point ratio. It was repeated five times for confirmation with the precision and accuracy less than 20%.

Precision and Accuracy

The intraday precision and accuracy were assessed by determining the concentrations of QC samples of plasma and liver at three levels using six replicates during the same day. The concentration of each QC sample was obtained using calibration curves prepared that day. Three batches of QC samples were analyzed on three consecutive days to measure the interday precision and accuracy. Precision was expressed by RSD and accuracy was assessed by comparing the measured concentration to its nominal value, expressed as the RE.

Extraction Recovery Rates and Matrix Effects

Extraction recovery was calculated by comparing the responses of QC samples at three levels that were spiked with analytes prior to extraction with the response of those that were spiked with blank plasma and tissue homogenates. The matrix effect was assessed in a similar fashion. Analytes for all five compounds were added to the extract of precipitated blank plasma and tissue homogenates to achieve three concentration levels. These peak areas were compared with those obtained by adding the same concentration of analytes in acetonitrile, and it was considered negligible if values below $\pm 15\%$ were observed.

Stability

The stability was tested by analyzing QC samples at three concentration levels exposed to different conditions: at room temperature for 4 h before sample preparation (short-term stability), at room temperature for 12 h in autosampler after sample preparation (autosampler stability), after three freeze/thaw cycles from $-20°C$ to ambient temperature (freeze-thaw stability), and at $-20°C$ for 4 weeks (long-term stability). The obtained results were compared with the freshly prepared QC samples and the percentage concentration deviation was calculated to evaluate stability.

10.2.1.7 Pharmacokinetics and Tissue Distribution Study

Sixty male ICR mice (18 ± 2 g) were used in the PK study. All mice were orally administered with the SBP suspended in 0.5% carboxymethyl cellulose odium aqueous solution at 2.88 g/kg (equivalent to 1.31 mg/kg of RBG, 1.72 mg/kg of BF, 0.35 mg/kg of GBL, 0.57 mg/kg of ABG, and 0.36 mg/kg of BL). Then blood samples (250 μL) were drawn from the retro-orbital plexus of each mouse at 5, 15, 30 min, 1, 1.5, 2, 3, 4, 6, 8, 10, 12, and 24 h, and placed into heparinized microfuge tubes according to the specific schedule. All the collected blood samples were immediately centrifuged at 14,000 rpm for 10 min to obtain plasma, which were labeled and frozen at $-20°C$ until analysis.

For the tissue distribution study, six mice were assigned to each group representing 15, 30, 60, 180, and 360 min after oral administration. The tissues, including heart, liver, spleen, lung, and kidney, were excised immediately, thoroughly rinsed with ice-cold physiological saline solution to remove the blood or content, and then blotted dry with filter paper and stored at $-20°C$ until treatment.

10.2.1.8 Statistical Analysis

The PK parameters including the area under the blood concentration-time curve from time zero to the last measured concentration (AUC_{0-t}), the area under the plasma concentration-time curve extrapolated to infinity (AUC_{0-INF}), total body mean residence time (MRT), and elimination half-life ($T_{1/2}$) were calculated by noncompartmental methods using WinNonlin trial version 5.2 from Pharsight Corporation. The maximum plasma concentration (C_{max}) and the time to reach maximum concentration (T_{max}) were directly obtained from the experimental data.

10.2.2 Results and Discussion

10.2.2.1 Method Validation

Specificity and Selectivity

In MRM mode, a specific voltage at the optimum value was set to provide the best sensitivity and specificity for each analyte while the mass transition ion-pair was followed as m/z 385.4 → 105.1 for RBG, m/z 387.2 → 107.1 for BF, m/z 403.1 → 145.1 for GBL, m/z 417.3 → 399.3 for ABG, m/z 445.3 → 349.3 for BL, and m/z 248.1 → 121.1 for IS. The retention times for RBG, BF, GBL, ABG, BL, and IS were approximately 7.29, 6.17, 4.67, 5.22, 6.15, and 2.66 min, respectively. Typical chromatograms of blank plasma, blank plasma spiked with analytes, and the plasma sample at 45 min after oral administration of the SBP are shown in Fig. 10.9. No significant interferences from

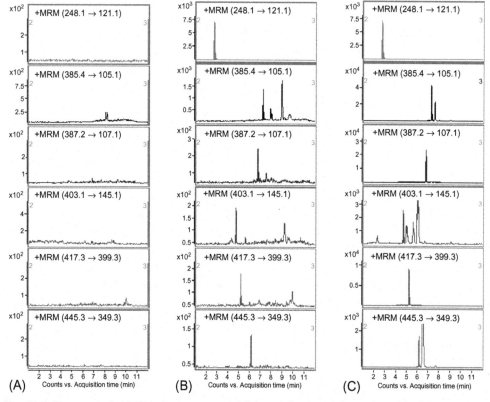

Fig. 10.9 Representative MRM chromatograms of the analytes and internal standards: (A) a blank plasma sample, (B) a blank plasma sample spiked with the analytes at LLOQs and IS, and (C) a plasma sample from a rat at 45 min after oral administration. Peak 1: tinidazole (IS), 2: resibufogenin, 3: bufalin, 4: gamabufotalin, 5: arenobufagin, and 6: bufotalin.

endogenous substances were observed at the retention times of the analytes and IS. Also, studies showed that there were no endogenous interferences in blank tissues.

Linearity and LLOQ

The standard curves correlation, coefficients, and linear ranges of plasma and tissue homogenates are listed in Table 10.9. The calibrations were linear over a certain range in all biosamples with a correlation coefficient (r) larger than 0.9950. The LLOQ of RBG, BF, GBL, ABG, and BL were 2.5, 2.0, 2.5, 2.0, and 0.1 ng/mL, respectively, for the plasma sample, and 5.0, 5.0, 5.0, 5.0, and 0.2 ng/mL in tissue homogenates, respectively.

Precision and Accuracy

Analytical accuracy and precision data were shown in Table 10.10. For all concentration quality control (QC) samples of plasma and tissue homogenates, the interday and intraday precision (RSD) of the method were determined to be <15%. For plasma, the intraday and interday accuracy (RE) were from −7.76% to 6.51% and −7.79% to 4.76%, respectively. For tissue homogenates, the intraday and interday accuracy (RE) were from −7.29% to 7.40 and −6.11% to 4.30, respectively. The results indicated an acceptable precision and accuracy of the present method.

Extraction Recovery Rates and Matrix Effects

The extraction recovery and matrix effects of each QC concentration were listed in Table 10.11. The result showed that the extraction recoveries were over 85% at different concentration levels in various biosamples. For the matrix effect, all the ratios were in the range of 88.71%–102.54% for plasma samples and 86.78%–96.87% for live samples, which indicated that no significant matrix effect was observed for the analytes.

Stability

The data of frozen-thaw stability, short-term temperature stability, long term stability, and postpreparative stability in different storage conditions were summarized in Table 10.12. The results were well within the acceptable limit, which suggested that the established method for sample extraction, storage, and intermittent analysis were validated and suitable for large-scale sample analysis.

10.2.2.2 Pharmacokinetic Studies

PKs aims to describe quantificationally the regularity of dynamic variation of a drug in vivo, which involves drug adsorption, distribution, metabolism, and excretion. In this study, the plasma concentrations of five bufadienolides were successfully determined by the established method. The plasma drug-time curves of five bufadienolides after oral administration of the SBP at 2.88 g/kg (RBG 1.31 mg/kg, BF 1.72 mg/kg, GBL

Table 10.9 Regression data and LLOQs of RBG, BF, GBL, ABG, and BL

Biosamples	Analytes	Standard curve	Correlation coefficient (R^2)	Linear range (ng/mL)	LLOQ (ng/mL)
Plasma	Resibufagin	$y = 0.0312x + 0.0593$	0.9998	2.50–5000	2.50
	Bufalin	$y = 0.0207x + 2.2099$	0.9967	5.00–10,000	2.00
	Gamabufotalin	$y = 0.0115x + 0.0683$	0.9996	2.50–1000	2.50
	Arenobufagin	$y = 0.0199x + 0.0629$	0.9999	2.00–2000	2.00
	Bufotalin	$y = 0.1146x + 0.1252$	0.9999	0.25–500	0.10
Heart	Resibufagin	$y = 0.0308x + 0.0719$	0.9988	5.00–1000	5.00
	Bufalin	$y = 0.0196x + 0.1463$	0.9989	5.00–2000	5.00
	Gamabufotalin	$y = 0.0086x - 0.0229$	0.9958	5.00–500	5.00
	Arenobufagin	$y = 0.0102x + 0.0925$	0.9984	5.00–1000	5.00
	Bufotalin	$y = 0.0725x + 0.0461$	0.9988	0.20–200	0.20
Liver	Resibufagin	$y = 0.0226x - 0.5210$	0.9950	5.00–1000	5.00
	Bufalin	$y = 0.0172x - 0.2173$	0.9997	5.00–2000	5.00
	Gamabufotalin	$y = 0.0073x - 0.0255$	0.9992	5.00–500	5.00
	Arenobufagin	$y = 0.0112x - 0.0331$	0.9996	5.00–1000	5.00
	Bufotalin	$y = 0.0698x - 0.0027$	0.9981	0.20–200	0.20
Spleen	Resibufagin	$y = 0.0303x - 0.1845$	0.9994	5.00–1000	5.00
	Bufalin	$y = 0.0193x - 0.0274$	0.9997	5.00–2000	5.00
	Gamabufotalin	$y = 0.0070x + 0.0172$	0.9998	5.00–500	5.00
	Arenobufagin	$y = 0.0106x - 0.0449$	0.9997	5.00–1000	5.00
	Bufotalin	$y = 0.0716x - 0.0508$	0.9995	0.20–200	0.20
Lung	Resibufagin	$y = 0.0296x - 0.0819$	0.9988	5.00–1000	5.00
	Bufalin	$y = 0.0191x - 0.0747$	0.9984	5.00–2000	5.00

Table 10.9 Regression data and LLOQs of RBG, BF, GBL, ABG, and BL—cont'd

Biosamples	Analytes	Standard curve	Correlation coefficient (R^2)	Linear range (ng/mL)	LLOQ (ng/mL)
	Gamabufotalin	$y = 0.0069x + 0.0338$	0.9993	5.00–500	5.00
	Arenobufagin	$y = 0.0097x - 0.0531$	0.9952	5.00–1000	5.00
	Bufotalin	$y = 0.0702x - 0.0522$	0.9976	0.20–200	0.20
Kidney	Resibufagin	$y = 0.0247x - 0.2723$	0.9982	5.00–1000	5.00
	Bufalin	$y = 0.0172x - 0.2376$	0.9989	5.00–2000	5.00
	Gamabufotalin	$y = 0.0070x - 0.0019$	0.9993	5.00–500	5.00
	Arenobufagin	$y = 0.0095x + 0.1104$	0.9995	5.00–1000	5.00
	Bufotalin	$y = 0.0673x - 0.0811$	0.9991	0.20–200	0.20
Small intestine	Resibufagin	$y = 0.0227x - 0.1193$	0.9999	5.00–1000	5.00
	Bufalin	$y = 0.0244x + 0.1205$	0.9994	5.00–2000	5.00
	Gamabufotalin	$y = 0.0081x - 0.0211$	0.9987	5.00–500	5.00
	Arenobufagin	$y = 0.0124x + 0.0566$	0.9999	5.00–1000	5.00
	Bufotalin	$y = 0.0865x - 0.0608$	0.9999	0.20–200	0.20

0.35 mg/kg, ABG 0.57 mg/kg, and BL 0.36 mg/kg) were presented in Fig. 10.10 and the main PK parameters were reported in Table 10.13.

Owing to the similar structures, RBG, BF, GBL, ABG, and BL have parallel PK parameters and concentration-time curves in vivo, being absorbed and eliminated with a similar rate. From the results, the time to reach the maximum plasma concentrations (T_{max}) was 0.14 h for RBG, 0.35 h for BF, 0.63 h for GBL, 0.31 h for ABG, and 0.11 h for BL, which demonstrated that these compounds were rapidly absorbed in mouse plasma by short T_{max} (less than 1 h). The C_{max} values and the mean AUC_{0-t} for RBG, BF, GBL, and ABG were 654.33 ng/mL and 452.12 ng/mL h, 1786.24 ng/mL and 1620.80 ng/mL h, 155.62 ng/mL and 235.27 ng/mL h, and 471.83 ng/mL and 368.97 ng/mL h, respectively. It showed that the four bufadienolides shared high plasma concentrations. Caco-2 cell culture studies of main components from the SBP

Table 10.10 Precision and accuracy for RBG, BF, GBL, ABG, and BL in mice plasma and liver homogenate (n = 15, 5 replicates per day for 3 days)

Biosamples	Analytes	Analyte concentration (ng/mL)	Intraday Concentration found (ng/mL) Mean	SD	RSD (%)	RE (%)	Interday Concentration found (ng/mL) Mean	SD	RSD (%)	RE (%)
Plasma	Resibufagin	25.00	25.66	0.95	3.69	2.64	26.18	0.48	1.85	4.73
		250.00	230.61	7.21	3.13	−7.76	230.48	4.30	1.87	−7.71
		2500.00	2553.93	119.16	4.67	2.16	2529.67	22.76	0.90	1.19
	Bufalin	50.00	49.66	3.45	6.94	−0.68	47.13	2.28	4.84	−5.73
		500.00	517.81	16.75	3.24	3.56	523.84	9.59	1.83	4.76
		5000.00	4638.68	96.45	2.08	−7.22	4620.83	35.68	0.77	−7.58
	Gamabufotalin	5.00	5.01	0.34	6.84	0.27	4.84	0.20	4.16	−3.23
		50.00	47.14	2.31	4.90	−5.73	47.35	0.52	1.09	−5.29
		500.00	467.70	9.82	2.10	−6.46	461.06	10.47	2.27	−7.79
	Arenobufagin	10.00	9.42	0.46	4.84	−5.84	9.53	0.12	1.22	−4.67
		100.00	97.39	1.82	1.87	−2.61	96.51	0.93	0.96	−3.49
		1000.00	1038.65	31.06	2.99	3.87	1008.17	30.65	3.04	0.82
	Bufotalin	2.50	2.34	0.05	2.14	−6.39	2.39	0.80	3.37	−4.51
		25.00	24.59	0.80	3.26	−1.62	23.91	0.68	2.83	−4.37
		250.00	266.26	4.67	1.75	6.51	255.71	11.52	4.50	2.28
Liver	Resibufagin	5.00	4.65	0.18	3.95	−6.97	4.71	0.12	2.65	−5.88
		50.00	46.90	2.15	4.59	−6.20	48.25	1.51	3.13	−3.50
		500.00	513.56	16.95	3.30	2.71	518.66	7.79	1.50	3.73
	Bufalin	10.00	9.92	0.51	5.10	−0.77	9.85	0.07	0.68	−1.54
		100.00	97.85	3.96	4.05	−2.15	97.40	1.16	1.19	−2.60
		1000.00	1048.81	69.35	6.61	4.88	1042.97	13.56	1.30	4.30
	Gamabufotalin	5.00	4.79	0.07	1.56	−4.13	4.83	0.05	1.14	−3.48
		25.00	23.48	1.73	7.38	−6.05	23.78	0.96	4.02	−4.86
		250.00	231.51	3.15	1.36	7.40	235.86	3.89	1.65	−5.66
	Arenobufagin	5.00	5.11	0.29	5.59	2.12	4.90	0.08	1.58	−2.02
		50.00	50.33	2.50	4.96	0.66	48.06	1.02	2.11	−3.88
		500.00	503.01	35.69	7.10	0.60	483.21	17.20	3.56	−3.36
	Bufotalin	1.00	0.93	0.04	4.53	−7.29	0.94	0.01	1.09	−6.11
		10.00	10.05	0.26	2.55	0.49	9.91	0.13	1.33	−0.93
		100.00	102.62	4.88	4.76	2.62	100.38	1.95	1.94	0.38

Table 10.11 Extraction recovery and matrix effect for RBG, BF, GBL, ABG, and BL in mice plasma and liver homogenate (n = 3)

Biosamples	Analytes	Analyte concentration (ng/mL)	Matrix effect			Extraction recovery		
			Mean	SD	RSD (%)	Mean	SD	RSD (%)
Plasma	Resibufagin	25.00	98.74	4.06	4.11	90.42	3.33	3.68
		250.00	88.71	2.39	2.70	91.89	4.81	5.24
		2500.00	89.07	7.68	8.62	94.17	1.16	1.23
	Bufalin	50.00	98.10	7.83	7.98	98.49	9.08	9.22
		500.00	94.58	5.63	5.96	93.56	4.36	4.66
		5000.00	98.25	5.91	6.01	90.35	5.04	5.58
	Gamabufotalin	5.00	102.54	7.33	7.15	93.45	5.76	6.16
		50.00	100.59	6.08	6.04	93.60	5.08	5.43
		500.00	102.21	8.04	7.86	93.40	5.66	6.06
	Arenobufagin	10.00	98.31	5.29	5.39	99.78	5.25	5.26
		100.00	90.04	7.10	7.89	92.85	5.99	6.45
		1000.00	99.02	7.52	7.59	97.10	3.69	3.80
	Bufotalin	2.50	96.95	2.87	2.96	96.69	3.73	3.86
		25.00	94.05	2.61	2.78	92.55	2.50	2.70
		250.00	99.49	7.30	7.34	92.12	4.88	5.29
Liver	Resibufagin	5.00	89.42	5.05	5.65	88.55	6.15	6.94
		50.00	89.38	10.58	11.85	90.77	10.08	11.10
		500.00	90.47	2.47	2.74	99.56	5.35	5.37
	Bufalin	10.00	86.84	5.47	6.29	86.55	9.83	11.35
		100.00	87.08	2.65	3.04	91.14	8.93	9.79
		1000.00	89.81	2.43	2.71	90.00	11.38	12.65
	Gamabufotalin	5.00	89.15	4.25	4.76	97.23	9.10	9.36
		25.00	88.50	7.46	8.43	99.23	10.97	11.05
		250.00	87.28	5.36	6.14	93.35	6.89	7.38
	Arenobufagin	5.00	96.87	5.91	6.10	87.69	2.44	2.78
		50.00	89.06	5.14	5.77	89.37	4.14	4.63
		500.00	87.21	6.47	7.42	90.95	4.83	5.31
	Bufotalin	1.00	87.06	2.43	2.79	95.15	9.10	9.56
		10.00	89.37	3.95	4.41	85.72	1.74	2.03
		100.00	86.78	2.32	2.68	92.98	6.34	6.82

Table 10.12 Stability of RBG, BF, GBL, ABG, and BL in mice plasma and liver homogenate ($n = 5$)

Biosamples	Analytes	Analyte concentration (ng/mL)	Short-term stability (4 h at room temperature) Concentration found (%) Mean	SD	RSD (%)	Long-term stability (4 weeks at −20°C) Concentration found (%) Mean	SD	RSD (%)	postpreparative stability (12 h at room temperature) Concentration found (%) Mean	SD	RSD (%)	Freeze-thaw stability (3 cycles) Concentration found (%) Mean	SD	RSD (%)
Plasma	Resibufagin	25.00	108.51	1.28	1.18	101.07	5.19	5.13	107.36	3.57	3.33	105.05	6.66	6.34
		250.00	102.05	5.71	5.59	102.06	5.93	5.81	104.11	3.38	3.25	102.39	6.71	6.56
		2500.00	102.18	4.95	4.84	97.20	7.06	7.26	93.91	5.71	6.08	96.50	6.47	6.71
	Bufalin	50.00	101.73	3.55	3.49	101.68	5.83	5.74	103.15	5.31	5.15	99.03	6.45	6.51
		500.00	106.25	7.83	7.37	101.53	6.17	6.08	101.95	5.48	5.38	103.73	5.52	5.32
		5000.00	101.22	2.09	2.06	98.74	6.55	6.64	97.85	2.35	2.41	99.05	4.99	5.03
	Gamabufotalin	5.00	93.29	3.05	3.27	92.75	5.80	6.26	92.60	5.02	5.42	94.97	4.46	4.69
		50.00	94.77	5.14	5.43	98.35	5.42	5.51	98.78	3.92	3.97	96.64	6.56	6.79
		500.00	96.93	4.50	4.64	96.27	7.61	7.91	96.71	2.10	2.17	92.61	1.63	1.76
	Arenobufagin	10.00	93.88	5.87	6.25	104.16	5.80	5.57	93.47	5.62	6.01	92.10	2.31	2.50
		100.00	94.65	4.28	4.53	99.24	6.68	6.73	92.17	5.52	5.99	93.93	4.70	5.00
		1000.00	93.59	5.87	6.27	95.97	2.36	2.46	92.69	3.16	3.41	94.57	8.21	8.68
	Bufotalin	2.50	92.17	3.52	3.82	98.19	3.04	3.10	93.70	4.92	5.25	94.03	7.14	7.60
		25.00	97.45	4.23	4.34	97.57	4.42	4.53	92.51	4.60	4.98	95.16	1.51	1.58
		250.00	93.33	6.22	6.67	100.24	4.70	3.10	95.32	3.98	4.17	92.46	4.57	4.94
Liver	Resibufagin	5.00	106.23	1.69	1.60	104.18	6.89	6.62	103.77	9.55	9.21	104.55	3.11	2.98
		50.00	107.88	7.87	7.30	101.85	7.49	7.35	102.36	6.42	6.28	97.14	6.53	6.72
		500.00	92.94	3.63	3.91	101.00	9.08	8.99	103.78	8.30	8.00	93.87	6.31	6.72
	Bufalin	10.00	96.46	7.03	7.29	99.02	6.02	6.08	98.70	9.30	9.43	93.18	8.67	9.30
		100.00	98.68	8.23	8.34	98.68	7.62	7.72	105.36	8.79	8.34	92.36	3.24	3.50
		1000.00	92.21	3.73	4.04	100.22	3.25	3.24	102.55	7.41	7.23	93.21	3.50	3.75
	Gamabufotalin	5.00	93.10	5.17	5.55	104.48	7.25	6.94	94.12	7.28	7.73	92.90	4.40	4.73
		25.00	91.25	2.28	2.50	108.11	9.05	8.37	91.50	8.28	9.05	92.29	1.84	1.99
		250.00	92.29	3.32	3.60	103.61	8.18	7.90	91.85	4.02	4.37	91.66	4.50	4.91

Arenobufagin	5.00	94.47	8.58	9.08	96.28	5.89	6.12	109.35	5.96	5.45	91.16	9.16	9.95
	50.00	92.24	7.22	7.83	93.25	8.04	8.62	102.20	5.97	5.97	92.26	8.73	9.46
	500.00	96.01	9.28	9.66	94.62	7.24	7.65	99.86	4.06	4.07	91.12	7.62	8.36
Bufotalin	1.00	92.19	3.80	4.12	96.95	9.34	9.64	94.42	9.15	9.70	97.61	8.20	8.40
	10.00	91.69	3.47	3.79	98.29	6.29	6.39	98.31	6.93	7.05	92.30	4.97	5.38
	100.00	92.48	3.69	3.99	97.06	5.35	5.51	103.75	9.11	8.78	92.24	4.77	5.17

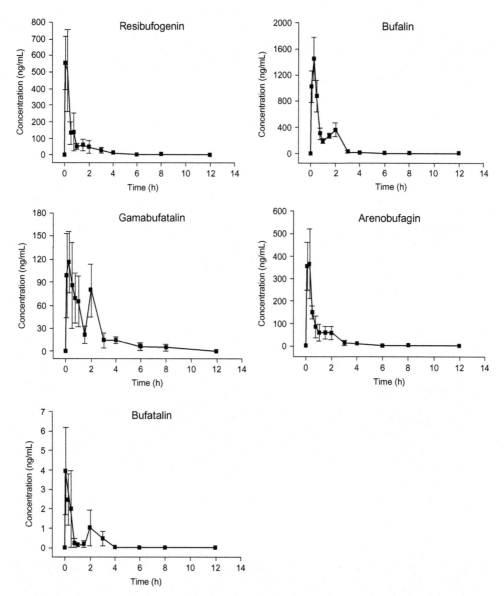

Fig. 10.10 Plasma concentration-time profiles of the analytes following a single oral administration of the SBP to mice (mean ± SD, $n = 6$).

in our laboratory revealed that bufalin (BF) had a high apparent infiltration rate, which may explain the rapid absorption of this kind of compound. The values of $T_{1/2}$ ranging from 0.99–2.47 h illustrated the four bufadienolides eliminated fast in mice. Previous PK studies in rats showed a similar phenomenon,[16–22] but the compounds are better absorbed in mice. By comparing the parameters of these four bufadienolides, bufatalin (BL)

Table 10.13 PK parameters of the five analytes following single oral administration of the SBP to mice ($n = 6$)

Paramaters	Resibufagin Mean	Resibufagin SD	Bufalin Mean	Bufalin SD	Gamabufotalin Mean	Gamabufotalin SD	Arenobufagin Mean	Arenobufagin SD	Bufotalin Mean	Bufotalin SD
Dose (mg/kg)	1.31	0.00	1.72	0.00	0.35	0.00	0.57	0.00	0.36	0.00
T_{max} (h)	0.14	0.09	0.35	0.24	0.63	0.81	0.31	0.23	0.11	0.07
C_{max} (ng/mL)	654.33	144.24	1786.24	521.40	155.62	33.16	471.83	57.32	4.40	1.86
AUC_{0-t} (ng/mL h)	452.12	217.64	1620.80	890.59	235.27	102.92	368.97	155.30	4.57	3.23
$AUC_{0-\infty}$ (ng/mL h)	473.82	209.23	1663.72	868.86	256.56	97.92	381.70	150.19	11.91	11.47
$T_{1/2}$ (h)	2.47	1.41	1.13	0.22	1.69	0.71	0.99	0.23	14.25	18.32
MRT (h)	2.05	0.71	1.38	0.51	2.62	0.79	1.28	0.44	26.01	33.80

represents a different specialty. The maximum mean plasma concentration (C_{max}) for BL was 4.40 ng/mL, much lower than the given dose (0.36 mg/kg), revealing that the compound had an extremely low oral bioavailability. Generally, oral bioavailability is affected by several factors including solubility, intestinal microorganisms, intestinal permeability, and first-pass extraction.[23] And complex interaction of components also occurred in the composite formula. Therefore, elucidation of the mechanism of the phenomenon needs further detailed studies.

As shown in Fig. 10.10, distinct double peaks were observed in both individual and mean plasma concentration-time curves of all these bufanolides. The phenomenon of multipeaks might be from the following reasons: (1) reabsorption of the intestinal tract because of the enterohepatic recirculation; (2) intertransformation among the compounds. Owing to the similar structures, some other bufadienolides might transform to these constituents; (3) variable gastric emptying[24] and distribution; or (4) double-site absorption involving the stomach and intestine.[25] For bufadienolides, these similar structure components such as bufalin, resibufagenin, and cinobufagin were metabolized by human SULTs to produce sulfonated metabolites in the phase II metabolism study (unpublished), which was provided by Dr. Ling Yang's team (Laboratory of Pharmaceutical Resource Discovery, Dalian Institute of Chemical Physics). These sulfonated metabolites may be hydrolyzed to obtain the archetypal compounds and then reabsorbed by the intestine. It was the potential reason for the phenomenon of double peaks of the bufadienolides, and this presumption needed to be verified by further experiments. As we knew, drug absorption is a very complex process that manifests itself through potential interaction with a host of physicochemical and physiological variables. So more detailed absorption studies are needed to elucidate the mechanism of the double-peak phenomenon in PKs.

10.2.2.3 Tissue Distribution Studies

The distribution of RBG, BF, GBL, ABG, and BL was investigated in mice following a single i.g. dose of SBP (2.88 g/kg) from tissues including the heart, liver, spleen, lung, kidney, and small intestines (Fig. 10.11). The results of the present study indicated that all the analytes underwent a rapid and wide distribution into tissues within the time course examined, with no long-term accumulation of the components in tissues.

Within 30 min of the SBP administration, the highest tissue concentration of RBG was detected in the small intestine (162.00 ng/g), followed by the lung (85.74 ng/g) and kidney (66.50 ng/g). And for BL, the highest tissue concentration was observed in the small intestine (392.54 ng/g), followed by the lung (226.35 ng/g) and kidney (183.75 ng/g). For GBL, the highest tissue concentration was observed in the small intestine (164.21 ng/g), followed by the liver (109.87 ng/g), and kidney (59.29 ng/g). For ABG, the highest tissue concentration was observed in the small intestine (324.57 ng/g), followed by the kidney (121.80 ng/g), and liver (86.70 ng/g). While for BL,

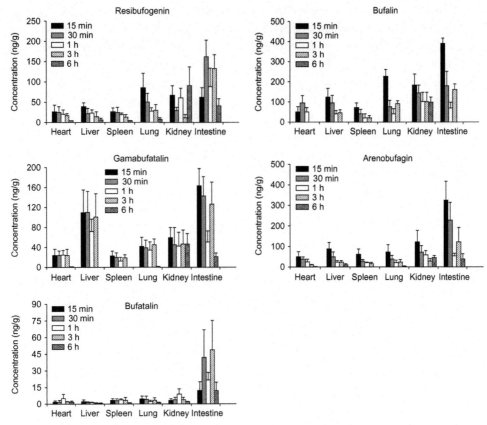

Fig. 10.11 Mean concentrations of the analytes in tissues at different time points after a single oral administration of the SBP to mice (mean ± SD, $n = 6$).

the highest tissue concentration was observed in the small intestine (42.14 ng/g), followed by the lung (4.73 ng/g), and kidney (3.21 ng/g).

From the results, we found that the maximum concentration of all the analytes was observed in the small intestine, which might mainly be attributed to the oral administration. Bufadienolides were mainly distributed in abundant blood-supply tissues such as the lung, kidney, and liver, which implied that the distribution of the components depended on the blood flow or perfusion rate of the organ. The relatively high distribution in the lung confirmed the reports that bufadienolides have an excitatory effect on respiration.[26] However, the concentration of bufadienolides was relatively low in the heart tissue, the target organ of the components. As members of the cardiac glycoside family, the bufadienolides mechanism of the positive inotropic effect has been well characterized. By combining with the phosphorylated intermediates of Na^+ K^+-ATPase, they inhibited the activity of the enzyme to increase the intracellular concentration of Na^+, thereby decreasing the driving force for the Na^+/Ca^{++} exchanger, leading to enhanced heart contractility.[27] It may explain the reason for the low concentration on the heart but the good curative affect on cardiovascular diseases. And different from the other four bufadienolides, GBL had relatively high accumulation in the liver, which may be caused by the PK interaction of other chemical constituents. Because the analytes are metabolized by the same enzyme, CYP3A4, the interactions and subsequent CYP3A4 inhibition may led to the reduced clearance or increased absorption of the affected drugs. A previous study also demonstrated that bufalin had a significant inhibition of CYP3A4 both in vitro and in vivo.[28] The metabolism base on CYP3A4 in liver of GBL may be inhibited by the other components, which was one of the conceivable reasons leading the high liver concentration of GBL.

10.2.3 Conclusion

To the best of our knowledge, this is the first report to evaluate the PKs and tissue distribution of bufadienolides in mice from the SBP, which can more accurately reflect dynamic variations of drugs in humans. A rapid, reliable, and sensitive HPLC-MS/MS method was validated for quantitative analysis of five bufadienolides in mice biological samples such as plasma and tissue samples. Following a single oral administration of the SBP, bufadienolides were rapidly distributed in mice plasma and tissues. The PK curve showed double peaks, which may due to the reabsorption of intestine. The major distribution tissues of bufadienolides in mice were the lung, kidney, and liver, and there was no long-term accumulation in the tissues. The achieved results of PKs and tissue distribution may be useful for the clinical application of the SBP, which also can provide reliable scientific data for ameliorating drug treatment regimens.

10.3. PHARMACOKINETIC STUDY OF FOUR VOLATILE COMPOUNDS IN THE SBP

In our former serum pharmaceutical chemistry study, six volatile compounds of SBP including isoborneol, borneol, muscone, cinnamaldehyde, cinnamic acid, and benzyl benzoate were detected by GC-MS.[29] Here, the simultaneous determination of isoborneol, borneol, muscone, and cinnamaldehyde and the PKs after oral administration of the SBP in rats were studied.

Solid-phase dynamic extraction (SPDE), a recently commercialized technique based on the same principle as solid-phase micro extraction (SPME), is a solvent-free technique containing extraction, enrichment, and desorption of the sample. Compared to the fragile fiber of SPME, SPDE has a significantly higher extraction speed and practical aspects of a stable steel needle.[30] SPDE efficiently enriches the sample after several extraction

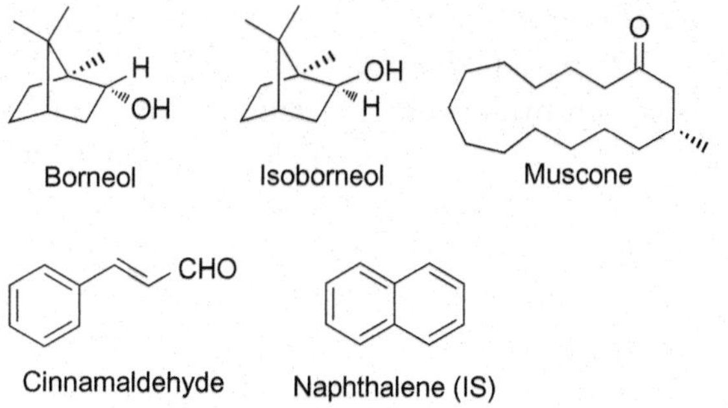

Fig. 10.12 Chemical structures of the analytes and IS.

cycles online, and then relatively improves the peak response of compounds. It has been extensively used in environmental,[31,32] pharmaceutical, and biomedical studies.[33–36] In the preliminary experiment, we found that the concentration of volatile compounds in plasma was too low to quantitate by the normal preparation method of a plasma sample, so we developed and validated a simple, rapid, and sensitive HS-SPDE-GC-MS/MS method to simultaneously determine isoborneol, borneol, muscone, and cinnamalde-hyde (Fig. 10.12) in rat plasma. To the best of our knowledge, this is the first report on simultaneous determination of the major volatile compounds in rat plasma after oral administration of the SBP. The method was successfully applied to PK studies of volatile compounds of the SBP, which would be very helpful for evaluating the clinical applica-tion of this formula in the further research. The SPDE-GC-MS/MS method, which contains simple plasma sample preparation, can be a quite promising tool for the analysis of the complex samples in vivo such as TCM.

10.3.1 Experimental

10.3.1.1 Chemicals and Reagents

Methanol from J&K Scientific Ltd was HPLC grade. Isoborneol, borneol, muscone, cin-namaldehyde, and naphthalene (purity ≥98%) were purchased from National Institute for the Control of Pharmaceutical and Biological Products. Ultrapure water was prepared by a Milli-Q50 SP Reagent Water System throughout the study. SBP samples (batch number 130401) were kindly offered by the Shanghai Hutchison Pharmaceuticals Company.

10.3.1.2 Instrumentation and Analytical Conditions

The analysis was performed by a GC-MS/MS system consisted of an Agilent 7890A gas chromatograph equipped with a 7000 tripie-quadrupole mass spectrometry detector. Data acquisition, processing, and evaluation were performed with Masshunter version

B.05.02 1032 software. The chromatographic column was a CP9205 VF-WAXms capillary column (30 m × 0.25 mm, 0.25 μm).

The conditions for gas chromatographic separation were as follows: 80°C initial oven temperature, ramped to 245°C at 25°C/min and held for 4 min, and the temperature at the injection port was 250°C. Helium was used as the carrier gas and set at the flow rate of 2.8 mL/min, and the injection was in the splitless mode. The temperatures of the transfer line, ion source, and quadrupoles were 250, 300, and 150°C, respectively. The multiplier voltage was 2056 V. The mass detector was operated in multiple-reaction monitoring (MRM) mode. The optimized mass transition ion pairs (m/z) and collision energy (CE) were described in Fig. 10.13. The scan time of all segments was 200 ms.

SPDE was performed with a CTC-Combi PAL autosampler supplied by Chromtech. The fiber was coated with a poly dimethylsiloxane (PDMS) phase (50 μm film thickness and 56 mm film length).

The 0.1 mL plasma sample spiked with 0.1 mL HCL (0.1 M, contain 500 ng/mL IS) was placed into a 10 mL vial. The samples were kept at 90°C for 5 min in the single-magnet mixer to equilibrium between the HS and the water phase. Then, the needle was inserted 20 mm into the sample vial through the septum into the vial at 200 μL/s for 40 times to extract the analytes. Then 1 mL of nitrogen gas was aspirated into the syringe at the gas station and was derived into the injector with a flow rate of 50 μL/s. The fiber was desorbed into the injector port of GC–MS at 250°C for 20 s. The parameters that affect the extraction rate such as incubation time, extraction temperature, the number of extraction cycles, desorption time, desorption volume, and pH have been optimized to obtain the highest extraction efficiency.

10.3.1.3 Assaying the Dosage of Oral Administration of Four Volatile Compounds

The contents of isoborneol, borneol, muscone, and cinnamaldehyde were determined by GC–MS/MS. 100 mg of three replicate SBP power was accurately weighted and 1 mL of acetidin was added. The sample was ultrasonically extracted for 15 min twice, and then centrifuged at 14,000 rpm for 10 min and filtered through a 0.22-μm membrane filter. All samples were dried with anhydrous Na_2SO_4 for more than 12 h, then filtered and diluted. Finally, 1 μL of filtrate was injected into the GC–MS/MS system. The results showed that the contents of isoborneol, borneol, muscone, and cinnamaldehyde were 46.53, 75.63, 0.38, and 1.43 mg/g in SBP, respectively.

10.3.1.4 Preparation of Standard and Quality Control (QC) Samples

The standard stock solution of isoborneol (2 mg/mL), borneol (2 mg/mL), muscone (200 μg/mL), cinnamaldehyde (200 μg/mL), and naphthalene (200 μg/mL) was prepared in methanol and stored at 4°C. Then, the four stock solutions were mixed and diluted with methanol to prepare a final mixed standard solution containing isoborneol (125 μg/mL), borneol (250 μg/mL), muscone (1500 ng/mL), and cinnamaldehyde (3750 ng/mL),

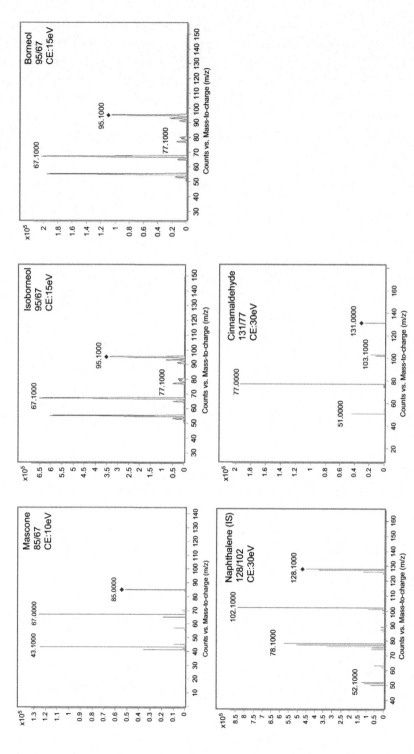

Fig. 10.13 Product ion mass spectra of the analytes and IS.

respectively. The mixture was subsequently diluted serially by blank rat plasma to prepare the nominal concentration range of 20–6250 ng/mL for isobornel, 40–12500 ng/mL for bornel, 0.24–75 ng/mL for muscone, and 0.60–187.5 ng/mL for cinnamaldehyde. Quality control (QC) samples of isoborneol, borneol, muscone, and cinnamaldehyde were respectively prepared at low (50, 100, 0.6, 1.5 ng/mL), medium (500, 1000, 6, 15 ng/mL) and high levels (6250, 12500, 75, 187.5 ng/mL) by spiking standard solutions to blank rat plasma with the required plasma concentrations.

10.3.1.5 Method Validation

The method was validated according to the USFDA guidelines.[27]

Specificity

The specificity of the method was evaluated by analyzing six different batches of blank rat plasma, plasma samples spiked with analytes at the concentration of the LLOQ and IS (500 ng/mL), and plasma samples after oral administration of the SBP.

Linearity, LLOQ, and LOD

The linearity of the method was evaluated by analysis of five calibration curves containing eight nonzero concentrations. The linearity of the calibration curve was confirmed by plotting peak-area ratios of each analyte to IS versus plasma concentrations using a $1/x^2$ weighted linear least squares regression model. The LLOQ was the lowest concentration of the calibration curve (S/N > 10). The LOD was defined as the amount that could be detected (S/N > 3).

Precision and Accuracy

The intraday precision and accuracy were evaluated by determining QC samples at three concentration levels containing five replicates on the same day while the interday precision and accuracy were estimated by assaying three validation batches on three consecutive days. The precision was calculated as RSD, and the accuracy was defined as the RE.

Recovery

The average recovery was determined as the amounts of extracted standards in blank plasma compared to standards in ultrapure water in three replicates at three QC levels.

Stability

The stability of the analytes in rat plasma was evaluated by analyzing five replicates of QC samples at low, medium, and high concentrations through three freeze-thaw cycles, at room temperature for 12 h, and at −20°C in the freezer for 30 days. The concentrations were compared with those of freshly prepared QC samples and the stability was expressed as a percentage of deviation.

PK Study in Rat Plasma

Seven male Sprague-Dawley rats (200 ± 20 g) were given unlimited access to standard laboratory food and water. They were fasted for 12 h but with access to water before the experiment. Each rat was given the SBP suspended in 0.5% carboxymethyl cellulose sodium salt (CMC-Na) aqueous solution at 11 g/kg (equivalent to 511.83 mg/kg of iso-borneol, 831.93 mg/kg of borneol, 4.18 mg/kg of muscone, and 15.73 mg/kg of cinnamaldehyde). Blood samples (about 250 μL) were collected in heparinized 1.5 mL polythene tubes at 0, 0.08, 0.17, 0.33, 0.5, 0.75, 1, 2, 3, 4, 6, 8, 12, and 24 h after oral administration. Then the samples were centrifuged at 14,000 rpm for 10 min at 4°C. The plasma samples were stored at −20°C until analysis.

Assay Application

PK parameters were calculated by WinNonlin 5.2 from Pharsight Corporation based on noncompartmental analysis of plasma concentration versus time data.

10.3.2 Results and Discussion

10.3.2.1 Method Development

Mass Spectrometry

The standard solutions of the analytes and IS were infused into the mass spectrometer separately to obtain detected ions and to optimize mass parameters. In the full scan mass spectra, 95.1 for borneol and isoborneol, 85.0 for muscone, 131.0 for cinnamaldehyde, and 128.1 for IS were chosen as the precursor ions, which were stable and exhibited higher abundance for MS/MS fragmentation analysis. The optimized mass transition ion pairs (m/z) for quantitation were 95.1/67.1 for borneol and isoborneol, 85.0/67.0 for muscone, 131.0/77.0 for cinnamaldehyde, and 128.1/102.1 for IS. The MRM transitions and collision energy were described in Fig. 10.13.

Optimization of SPDE Extraction Conditions

The number of extraction cycles was studied by varying the number in the range of 20–60 and optimum extraction cycles were found to be 40 with respect to peak response (Fig. 10.14A). Extraction temperature ranged between 60 and 100°C was investigated in this study and 90°C was chosen (Fig. 10.14B). SPDE extraction was performed at different incubation time ranging from 5–20 min and the optimum extraction time was found to be 5 min (Fig. 10.14C). Desorption time from 20–45 s was investigated and 20 s was found to be the optimum time to acquire the best peak shape and response. Optimum desorption volume was 1000 μL. The effect of pH was also studied at three pH levels: virgin pH of plasma, at neutral pH (by adding 0.1 M HCL), and at acidic pH = 5 (by adding 0.1 M HCl). The highest yield of cinnamaldehyde was obtained at pH = 5, and pH showed no obvious effect on the extraction efficiency of isoborneol, borneol, and muscone.

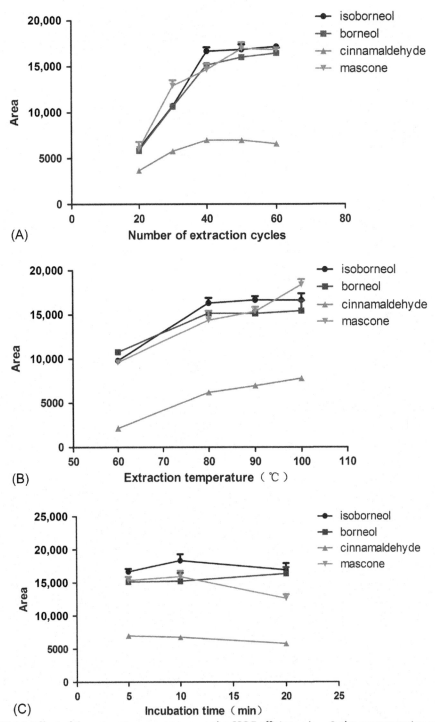

Fig. 10.14 Effect of the extraction parameters on the SPDE efficiency ($n = 3$, the concentration of each compound was 30 ng/mL, the peak areas of isoborneol and borneol were 1/10 of the actual areas): (A) number of extraction cycles, (B) extraction temperature, and (C) preincubation time.

10.3.2.2 Method Validation
Specificity, Calibration Curves, Linearity, LLOQ, and LOD

The representative MRM chromatograms of blank plasma, a blank plasma sample spiked with analytes and IS, and plasma samples after oral administration of the SBP were shown in Fig. 10.15, which presented that there were no interfering peaks in their peak region. The calibration curves of four compounds exhibited good linearity, and the LLOQs were sufficient for the assay of analytes in the PK studies, which were shown in Table 10.14.

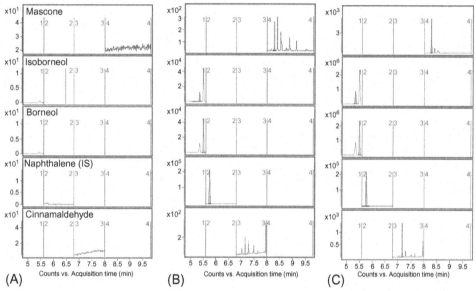

Fig. 10.15 Representative MRM chromatograms of the analytes and internal standards: (A) blank plasma sample, (B) blank plasma sample spiked with the analytes at the LLOQs and the level of the IS, and (C) plasma sample 1 h after the oral administration of SBP.

Table 10.14 Regression data, LLOQs, and LODs of the analytes

Analyte	Linear regression equation	r	Linear range (ng/mL)	LLOQ (ng/mL)	LLOD (ng/mL)
Isoborneol	$y = 0.00216x - 0.00584$	0.9986	20–6250	20	0.04
Borneol	$y = 0.00227x + 0.02881$	0.9993	40–12500	40	0.02
Muscone	$y = 0.00028x + 0.00004$	0.9998	0.24–75	0.24	0.10
Cinnamaldehyde	$y = 0.00012x + 0.00044$	0.9977	0.60–187.5	0.60	0.24

Precision and Accuracy

The accuracy (RE) of intraday and interday ranged from $-9.77.0\%$ to 9.87% and from -9.55% to 4.44%, and the precisions (RSD) were less than 9.79%. The results were summarized in Table 10.15 and indicated that the method was reliable.

Recovery

The mean recoveries of isoborneol, borneol, muscone, and cinnamaldehyde at three concentration levels were shown in Table 10.16. The recoveries of all QC samples were more than 79.57%, which was found to be within the acceptable range.

Stability

The stability of all the analytes under various conditions was presented in Table 10.16. The date indicated that these analytes were all stable in plasma at room temperature for 12 h, after three freeze/thaw cycles, and at $-20°C$ for 30 days, and determination with a concentration variation less than 15.0% of the initial values.

10.3.2.3 Application to Pharmacokinetic Study

The method was applied to the analysis of plasma samples obtained after oral administration of the SBP in rats. The mean plasma concentration-time profiles of the investigated components were shown in Fig. 10.16. The PK parameters were presented in Table 10.17. The C_{max} of isoborneol and borneol in rat plasma were 3360.01 ± 1432.56 and 5490.13 ± 2136.47 ng/mL, while T_{max} were 1.00 ± 0.52 h and 0.83 ± 0.58 h, respectively. It was demonstrated that isoborneol and borneol were absorbed easily and rapidly in rat plasma after oral administration of the SBP. However, C_{max} were 23.54 ± 4.33 ng/mL for muscone and 18.76 ± 2.11 ng/mL for cinnamaldehyde, which showed low plasma concentrations because of the low content of muscone and cinnamaldehyde in the SBP. Meanwhile, cinnamaldehyde was unstable in blood and oxidized to cinnamic acid in a short time after oral administration; only a little remained for 24 h in the blood,[37,38] which also leads to the low C_{max} and little concentration range.

10.3.3 Conclusion

The research shows that HS-SPDE-GC-MS/MS can be very successfully used for the determination of four volatile components in rat plasma. The main advantage of this method is the simple plasma sample preparation based on the HS-SPDE technique, and the LLOQs of muscone and cinnamaldehyde reach 0.24 and 0.6 ng/mL, respectively. The method in this study may be used for the assay of related volatile compounds or other similar TCMs in vivo. It is the first time to assess the PKs of these volatile components after oral administration of the SBP in rats. The results might be helpful for the clinical study of SBP in the future.

Table 10.15 Precision and accuracy for the analytes in rat plasma ($n = 3$ days, 5 replicates per day)

Analyte	Nominal concentration (ng/mL)	Intraday Concentration found (ng/mL) Mean	SD	Precision (%, RSD)	Accuracy (%, RE)	Interday Concentration found (ng/mL) Mean	SD	Precision (%, RSD)	Accuracy (%, RE)
Isoborneol	50	46.55	1.54	3.31	−6.89	46.23	1.67	3.61	−7.53
	500	529.09	43.90	8.30	5.82	522.20	36.00	6.89	4.44
	6250	6024.01	170.24	2.83	−3.61	5974.01	142.04	2.38	−4.41
Borneol	100	105.96	7.98	7.53	5.96	104.30	5.54	5.31	4.30
	1000	995.83	64.57	6.48	−0.42	964.48	52.57	5.45	−3.55
	12500	11278.17	422.25	3.74	−9.77	11306.13	820.87	7.26	−9.55
Muscone	0.6	0.62	0.04	6.45	2.67	0.62	0.03	4.84	2.28
	6	5.76	0.32	5.56	−4.00	5.87	0.24	4.09	−2.09
	75	74.42	5.20	6.99	−0.77	73.32	4.08	5.56	−2.24
Cinnamaldehyde	1.5	1.65	0.08	4.85	9.87	1.55	0.10	6.45	3.29
	15	13.79	1.35	9.79	−8.07	13.68	1.14	8.33	−8.78
	187.5	178.55	12.33	6.91	−4.77	175.28	9.99	5.70	−6.52

Table 10.16 Extraction recovery ($n = 3$) and stability of the analytes in rat plasma ($n = 5$)

	Nominal concentration (ng/mL)	Extraction recovery			At room for 12 h			Freeze-thaw cycles			at −20°C for 30 days		
		Concentration found (%)			Concentration found (%)			Concentration found (%)			Concentration found (%)		
		Mean	SD	RSD (%)	Mean	SD	RSD (%)	Mean	SD	RSD (%)	Mean	SD	RSD (%)
Isoborneol	50	97.81	8.33	8.52	98.28	2.93	2.98	92.00	5.53	6.01	95.89	6.59	6.87
	500	99.41	3.40	3.42	96.63	2.29	2.37	89.54	2.99	3.34	95.97	5.65	5.89
	6250	94.22	9.00	9.55	97.12	6.45	6.64	90.56	3.76	4.15	92.38	5.73	6.20
Borneol	100	100.97	4.98	4.93	100.74	2.03	2.01	94.27	4.21	4.47	97.56	2.76	2.83
	1000	98.46	6.30	6.40	98.09	8.60	8.77	92.64	6.25	6.75	91.53	6.99	7.64
	12500	99.09	10.11	10.20	97.92	6.96	7.11	93.77	6.84	7.29	94.10	8.14	8.65
Muscone	0.6	94.27	2.34	2.48	97.17	5.20	5.35	89.21	5.49	6.15	93.86	7.36	7.84
	6	90.49	2.74	3.03	99.34	2.01	2.02	93.47	5.72	6.12	95.99	2.73	2.84
	75	84.05	3.31	3.94	98.84	4.75	4.81	87.67	3.10	3.54	94.68	7.28	7.69
Cinnamaldehyde	1.5	83.87	6.59	7.86	85.72	5.60	6.53	85.68	6.03	7.04	92.46	9.21	9.97
	15	86.28	4.14	4.80	88.52	10.59	11.96	91.09	12.66	13.90	93.82	1.90	2.03
	187.5	79.57	2.47	3.10	88.74	4.40	4.96	87.06	9.70	11.14	93.31	6.12	6.56

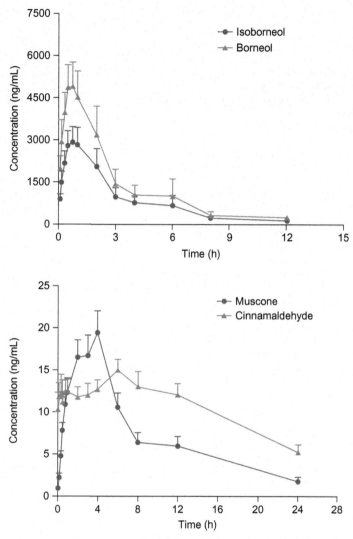

Fig. 10.16 Plasma concentration-time profiles of the analytes following oral administration of the SBP to rats.

Table 10.17 Pharmacokinetic parameters of the four analytes following single oral administration of the SBP to rats ($n = 7$)

	Isoborneol		Borneol		Muscone		Cinnamaldehyde	
Paramaters	Mean	SD	Mean	SD	Mean	SD	Mean	SD
T_{max} (h)	1.00	0.52	0.83	0.58	3.17	0.98	0.50	0.23
C_{max} (ng/mL)	3360.01	1432.56	5490.13	2136.47	23.54	4.33	18.76	2.11
AUC_{0-t} (ng/mL h)	11147.59	5864.04	17464.27	9093.13	176.33	61.35	262.22	63.92
$AUC_{0-\infty}$ (ng/mL h)	111559.23	5863.88	18293.54	9287.94	190.46	68.74	378.39	119.94
$T_{1/2}$ (h)	2.21	0.53	2.26	0.52	6.82	1.90	13.30	5.81
MRT_{0-t} (h)	3.02	0.76	2.87	0.84	6.95	0.86	9.80	0.66

REFERENCE

1. Zhang JW, Wang GJ, Sun J. Progress in pharmacodynamics and pharmacokinetics of ginsenoside Rg1. *J China Pharm Univ* 2007;**38**:283–8.
2. Huang HY. Research progress on pharmacology of ginsenoside Rg1. *J Pract Tradit Chin Med* 2012;**8**:608–9.
3. Chen CX, Zhang HY. Research progress of ginsenoside Re. *Foreign Med Sci* 2004;**31**:110–2 [Section of Pediatics].
4. Chu Y, Zhang HC, Li SM, Wang JM, Wang XY, Li W, et al. Determination of ginsenoside Rc in rat plasma by LC-MS/MS and its application to a pharmacokinetic study. *J Chromatogr B* 2013;**919–920**:75–8.
5. Xia CH, Wang GJ, Sun JG, Hao HP, Xiong YQ, Gu SH, et al. Simultaneous determination of ginsenoside Rg1, Re, Rd, Rb1 and ophiopogonin D in rat plasma by liquid chromatography/electrospray ionization mass spectrometric method and its application to pharmacokinetic study of 'SHENMAI' injection. *J Chromatogr B* 2008;**862**:72–8.
6. Zhao J, Su C, Yang C, Liu M, Tang L, Su W, et al. Determination of ginsenosides Rb1, Rb2, and Rb3 in rat plasma by a rapid and sensitive liquid chromatography tandem mass spectrometry method: application in a pharmacokinetic study. *J Pharm Biomed* 2012;**64–65**:94–7.
7. Joo KM, Lee JH, Jeon HY, Park CW, Hong DK, Jeong HJ, et al. Pharmacokinetic study of ginsenoside Re with pure ginsenoside Re and ginseng berry extracts in mouse using ultra performance liquid chromatography/mass spectrometric method. *J Pharm Biomed Anal* 2010;**51**:278–83.
8. Liu HF, Yang JL, FF D, Gao XM, Ma XT, Huang YH, et al. Absorption and disposition of ginsenosides after oral administration of *Panax notoginseng* extract to rats. *Drug Metab Dispos* 2009;**37**:2290–8.
9. Zhao J, Su C, Yang CP, Liu MH, Tang L, Su WW, et al. Determination of ginsenosides Rb1, Rb2, and Rb3 in rat plasma by a rapid and sensitive liquid chromatography tandem mass spectrometry method: application in a pharmacokinetic study. *J Pharm Biomed Anal* 2012;**64**:94–7.
10. Odani T, Tanizawa H, Takino Y. Studies on absorption, distribution, excretion and metabolism of ginseng saponins. II. The absorption, distribution and excretion of ginsenoside Rg1 in the rat. *Chem Pharm Bull* 1983;**31**:292–8.
11. Jiang B. The study on induction of traditional Chinese medicines on liver metabolic enzymes CYP3A4 and P-glycoprotein. Shanghai: Second Military Medical University, 2010. Available from: http://cdmd.cnki.com.cn/Article/CDMD-90024-2010150948.htm.
12. Graham MJ, Lake BG. Induction of drug metabolism: species differences and toxicological relevance. *Toxicology* 2008;**254**(3):184–91.
13. Jiang B, Cai F, Gao S, Meng L, Liang F, Dai X, et al. Induction of cytochrome P450 3A by Shexiang Baoxin Pill and its main components. *Chem Biol Interact* 2012;**195**(2):105–13.
14. Ma XC, Ning J, Ge GB, Liang SC, Wang XL, Zhang BJ, et al. Comparative metabolism of cinobufagin in liver microsomes from mouse, rat, dog, minipig, monkey, and human. *Drug Metab Dispos* 2011;**39**(4):675–82.
15. Ge GB, Ning J, LH H, Dai ZR, Hou J, Cao YF, et al. A highly selective probe for human cytochrome P450 3A4: isoform selectivity, kinetic characterization and its applications. *Chem Commun* 2013;**49**(84):9779–81.
16. Chen H, Deng S, Chang PR, Wang C, Ma X, Liu K, et al. Simultaneous determination of resibufogenin and its major metabolite 3-epi-resibufogenin in rat plasma by HPLC coupled with tandem mass spectrometry. *Chromatographia* 2012;**75**(3–4):103–9.
17. Li F, Weng Y, Wang L, He H, Yang J, Tang X. The efficacy and safety of bufadienolides-loaded nanostructured lipid carriers. *Int J Pharm* 2010;**393**(1):204–12.
18. Li G, Han W, Jiang W, Zhang D, Ye W, Chen X, et al. Quantitative determination of arenobufagin in rat plasma by ultra fast liquid chromatography-tandem mass spectrometry and its application in a pharmacokinetic study. *J Chromatogr B* 2013;**939**:86–91.
19. Liang Y, Liu AH, Qin S, Sun JH, Yang M, Li P, et al. Simultaneous determination and pharmacokinetics of five bufadienolides in rat plasma after oral administration of Chansu extract by SPE-HPLC method. *J Pharm Biomed Anal* 2008;**46**(3):442–8.

20. Xu W, Luo H, Zhang Y, Shan L, Li H, Yang M, et al. Simultaneous determination of five main active bufadienolides of Chan Su in rat plasma by liquid chromatography tandem mass spectrometry. *J Chromatogr B* 2007;**859**(2):157–63.

21. Zhang H, Yin Z, Sheng J, Jiang Z, Wu B, Su Y. A comparison study of pharmacokinetics between bufalin-loaded bovine serum albumin nanoparticles and bufalin in rats. *Zhong Xi Yi Jie He Xue Bao* 2012;**10**(6):674–80.

22. Zhang Y, Tang X, Liu X, Li F, Lin X. Simultaneous determination of three bufadienolides in rat plasma after intravenous administration of bufadienolides extract by ultra performance liquid chromatography electrospray ionization tandem mass spectrometry. *Anal Chim Acta* 2008;**610**(2):224–31.

23. Wang SW, Lin H, Tsai SC, Hwu CM, Chiao YC, CC L, et al. Effects of methanol extract of Chansu on hypothalamic-pituitary-testis function in rats. *Metabolism* 1998;**47**(10):1211–6.

24. Oberle RL, Amidon GL. The influence of variable gastric emptying and intestinal transit rates on the plasma level curve of cimetidine; an explanation for the double peak phenomenon. *J Pharmacokinet Biopharm* 1987;**15**(5):529–44.

25. Liu X, Xie L, Wang J, Zhou Y, Wang Z, Liu G. Two-site absorption model fits to pharmacokinetic data of gemfibrozil in man. *Acta Pharm Sin* 1996;**31**(10):737–41.

26. Morishita SI, Shoji M, Oguni Y, Ito C, Higuchi M, Sakanashi M. Pharmacological actions of "Kyushin", a drug containing toad venom: cardiotonic and arrhythmogenic effects, and excitatory effect on respiration. *Am J Chin Med* 1992;**20**(03–04):245–56.

27. Vaklavas C, Chatzizisis YS, Tsimberidou AM. Common cardiovascular medications in cancer therapeutics. *Pharmacol Ther* 2011;**130**(2):177–90.

28. Li HY, Xu W, Zhang X, Zhang WD, Hu LW. Bufalin inhibits CYP3A4 activity in vitro and in vivo. *Acta Pharmacol Sin* 2009;**30**(5):646–52.

29. Guo LA, Wang SP, Xiang L, Jiang P, Zhang WD, Liu RH. Identification of volatility components of Shexiang Baoxin pill in rat plasma by GC-MS. *J Pharm Pract* 2012;**30**:207.

30. Kataoka H, Saito K. Recent advances in SPME techniques in biomedical analysis. *J Pharm Biomed* 2011;**54**:926–50.

31. Jochmann MA, Kmiecik MP, Schmidt TC. Solid-phase dynamic extraction for the enrichment of polar volatile organic compounds from water. *J Chromatogr A* 2006;**1115**:208–16.

32. Jochmann MA, Yuan X, Schmidt TC. Determination of volatile organic hydrocarbons in water samples by solid-phase dynamic extraction. *Anal Bioanal Chem* 2007;**387**:2163–74.

33. Musshoff F, Lachenmeier DW, Kroener L, Madea B. Automated headspace solid-phase dynamic extraction for the determination of amphetamines and synthetic designer drugs in hair samples. *J Chromatogr A* 2002;**958**:231–8.

34. Lenz D, Kröner L, Rothschild MA. Determination of gamma-hydroxybutyric acid in serum and urine by headspace solid-phase dynamic extraction combined with gas chromatography-positive chemical ionization mass spectrometry. *J Chromatogr A* 2009;**1216**:4090–6.

35. Goodwin TE, Eggert MS, House SJ, Weddell ME, Schulte BA, Rasmussen L. *J Chem Ecol* 2006;**32**:1849.

36. Rossbach B, Kegel P, Letzel S. Application of headspace solid phase dynamic extraction gas chromatography/mass spectrometry (HS-SPDE-GC/MS) for biomonitoring of *n*-heptane and its metabolites in blood. *Toxicol Lett* 2012;**210**:232–9.

37. Yuan JH, Bucher JR, Goehl TJ, Dieter MP, Jameson CW. Quantitation of cinnamaldehyde and cinnamic acid in blood by HPLC. *J Anal Toxicol* 1992;**16**:359–62.

38. Yuan JH, Dieter MP, Bucher JR, Jameson CW. Toxicokinetics of cinnamaldehyde in F344 rats. *Food Chem Toxicol* 1992;**30**:997–1004.

CHAPTER 11

The Metabolomics Study of the Shexiang Baoxin Pill

Peng Jiang*, Runui Liu[†], Weidong Zhang[†]
*Shanghai Hutchison Pharmaceutical Limited Company, Shanghai, PR China
[†]Second Military Medical University, Shanghai, PR China

Abstract

A metabolomic method using reversed-phase liquid chromatography/quadrupole time-of-flight mass spectrometry (LC-Q-TOF-MS) was developed to obtain a systematic view of the development and progression of myocardial infarction (MI) and the treatment or protective effect of the Shexiang Baoxin Pill. By combining with partial least squares discriminant analysis (PLS-DA), 30 biomarkers in rat urine and serum were identified. A lot of pathways were regulated. The metabolomic results not only supplied a systematic view of the development and progression of MI but also provided the theoretical basis for the prevention or treatment of MI.

Keywords: Metabolomics study, The Shexiang Baoxin Pill, LC-Q-TOF-MS, Partial least squares discriminant analysis.

Cardiovascular diseases (CVDs), the world's largest killers, will claim 23.6 million lives by 2030, according to the World Health Organization. Most CVDs such as coronary heart diseases, angina, arrhythmias, and heart failure all trace to the formation of a myocardial infarction (MI). MI is a disease in which blood flow is obstructed through the coronary arteries that supply the heart with oxygen–rich blood. This obstruction leads to the imbalance between the supply and demand of myocardial oxygen.[1] Though previous studies have identified some important biomarkers such as troponin I and T for the prediction and treatment of MI,[2] the mortality induced by MI is still high. Therefore the biological processes of MI still need further investigation to find new biomarkers and illuminate disease mechanisms.

Medical treatment for MI in China includes not only modern medicines but also traditional Chinese medicine (TCM). The Shexiang Baoxin Pill (SBP), which is officially recorded in the Chinese pharmacopoeia 2010 edition and has been widely used in clinical practice for the treatment of MI for many years,[3–6] is a representative TCM. It consists of seven medicinal materials, including Moschus, Radix Ginseng, Calculus Bovis, Cortex cinnamomi, Styrax, Venenum Bufonis, and Borneolum Syntheticum. As there are complex components included in the SBP, it is hard to understand the remedial mechanisms completely.

As an important part of systems biology, metabolomics can be expected to provide new insights into the global effects of the disease related to metabolic pathways. In recent

Systems Biology and Its Application in TCM Formulas Research
https://doi.org/10.1016/B978-0-12-812744-5.00011-4

years, using a metabolomics approach to analyze disease-related biomarkers has attracted a great deal of interest, especially in the identification of MI-related biomarkers.[7–12] For example, Yao et al.[10] identified 24 metabolites in rat blood during the myocardial ische-mia. Those identified biomarkers gave a new insight into energy metabolism changes. Zhang et al.[11] demonstrated that most Lyso-PCs were downregulated in the serum of isoproterenol-induced MI rats. The results indicated that the pathway of phospholipase A2 could be activated in MI formation. The study of Lv[12] showed that the purine metab-olism was also an important process in an MI injury.

Though a lot of biomarkers have been successfully identified in the MI disease, the important biomarkers in urine have still not been studied using a metabolomics approach. To provide a new insight into the pathological processes of MI, an LC-Q-TOF-MS method based on a metabolomic strategy was developed. In addition, the reverse effects of the SBP and its mechanisms were also investigated by using a metabolomic approach for the first time.

11.1. THE TREATMENT EFFECTS OF SBP IN THE ACUTE MI IN A RAT USING A METABOLOMIC METHOD

11.1.1 Experimental

11.1.1.1 Materials

HPLC grade acetonitrile and formic acid were purchased from JT Baker (NJ, USA). Ultrapure water from a Milli-Q50 SP Reagent Water System (Millipore Corporation, MA, USA) was used for the preparation of samples and the mobile phase. The assay kits for lactate dehydrogenase (LDH) and creatine kinase (CK) were purchased from the Nanjing Jiancheng Bioengineering Institute (Nanjing, China). Commercial standards were purchased from Sigma/Aldrich (MO, USA). The SBP was kindly offered by the Shanghai Hutchison Pharmaceuticals Company (Shanghai China).

11.1.1.2 Animals

Twenty-five male Sprague-Dawley rats ($200 \pm 15\,g$) were purchased from the Slac Lab-oratory Animal Co., Ltd. (Shanghai, China). The rats were housed in stainless steel met-abolic cages with free access to food and tap water under standard conditions of humidity ($50 \pm 10\%$), temperature ($25 \pm 2°C$), and a 12 h light-dark cycle. The animals were accli-matized to the facilities for 5 days. All animals were handled with humane care through-out the experiment.

11.1.1.3 MI Model and Drug Administration

The MI model was established by the left anterior descending coronary artery (LADCA) ligation. The chest was opened by a middle thoracotomy under sterile conditions. After a pericardiotomy, the heart was rapidly exteriorized and a 4-0 black silk ligature was then placed under the LADCA to form an occlusion. Two rats died during the 24 h postoperative period. Twenty-three rats survived, including 13 MI rats and 10 control rats (without ligation). Seven of the 13 MI rats were treated with the SBP ($14 \, mg \, kg^{-1}$/ d) by oral gavage. The SBP was ground into a fine powder and dissolved in 0.5% carboxymethyl cellulose sodium salt (CMC-Na) aqueous solution ($0.56 \, mg \, mL^{-1}$). Isocyatic CMC-Na aqueous solution was orally administered to control ($n = 10$) and MI ($n = 6$) rats. All rats were consecutively oral administrated for 15 days.

11.1.1.4 Sample Collecting

The morning urine samples used for the metabolomic study were collected from the control group, the MI group, and the SBP treatment group on the 15th day (from 8 p.m. on the 14th day to 8 a.m. on the 15th day), respectively. Samples were stored at −80°C until analysis.

Blood was collected from the ophthalmic venous plexus for the analysis of serum concentrations of LDH and CK on the 15th day. In addition, all the rats' hearts were collected and weighed to investigate the infarct size of the MI. All histopathologic samples were used for the assessment of the validity of the MI model and the effect of the SBP treatment.

The experiment was carried out in accordance with guidelines of the Committee on the Care and Use of Laboratory Animals of the Institute of Laboratory Animal Resources of Shanghai, China. The study protocol was approved by the Animal Care and Use Committee of the Second Military Medical University.

11.1.1.5 Preparation of Metabolomic Samples

50 mL aliquots of urine were diluted with 100 mL of methanol. After vortex mixing for 30 s, these samples were centrifuged at 12,000 rpm for 10 min to remove particulate matters. The supernatant was then transferred to autosampler vials. The samples of the control group, MI group, and SBP treatment group were analyzed in the same working day.

A quality control (QC) sample was prepared by pooling the same volumes (20 mL) of each urine sample and then prepared in the same way as the samples. The pooled QC sample was analyzed randomly through the analytical run to monitor the stability of the sequence analysis. In addition, a random urine sample was divided into six parts and all the parts were treated in the same process to validate repeatability of the sample preparation method.

Blank sample (ultrapure water), which was treated exactly the same way as the samples, was used for needle washing following every five sample injections to minimize the carryover between injections.

11.1.1.6 Preparation of Histopathologic Samples

After standing for 30 min, blood samples were centrifuged at 3500 rpm for 10 min. Supernatant serum was then used for the analysis of LDH and CK. Serum concentrations of

LDH and CK were measured by a UV 1100 ultraviolet spectrophotometer (Beijing Rayleigh Analytical Instrument Corporation, Beijing, China). The intimate processes of detecting LDH and CK levels are shown in the ESI.

To investigate the infarct size of the MI, the left ventricles were dissected from the right ventricles and cut into five transverse slices from apex to base with each approximately 2–3 mm thick. These slices were then incubated in triphenyltetrazolium chloride solution (2% in phosphate buffer; pH 7.4) in a water bath at 37°C for 15 min to identify infarcted tissue. Finally, the stained tissue was removed and the unstained tissue was weighed. The results were expressed as the percentage of the infarcted heart weight to total heart weight and left ventricle weight.

11.1.1.7 LC-Q-TOF-MS Conditions

The LC-Q-TOF-MS analysis was performed on an Agilent-1200 LC system coupled with an electrospray ionization (ESI) source (Agilent Technologies, Palo Alto, CA, USA) and an Agilent-6520 Q-TOF mass spectrometer. The separation of all samples was performed on an Eclipse plus C_{18} column (1.8 μm, 2.1 mm × 100 mm, Agilent) with the column temperature set at 45°C. The flow rate was 0.3 mL min^{-1} and the mobile phase consisted of ultrapure water with 0.1% formic acid (A) and acetonitrile (B). The following gradient program was used: 0–2 min, 2% B; 2–3 min, 2%–20% B; 3–11 min, 20%–70% B; 11–12 min, 70%–95% B; and 12–17 min, washed with 100% B and followed by a reequilibration step of 4 min. The sample injection volume was 3 mL.

The mass detection was operated in both positive and negative ion modes with parameters set as follows: drying gas (N_2) flow rate, 8 L min^{-1}; gas temperature, 330°C; pressure of nebulizer gas, 35 psig; Vcap, 4000 V; fragmentor, 160 V; skimmer, 65 V; and scan range, m/z 50–1000. The MS/MS analysis was acquired in targeted MS/MS mode with collision energy from 5 to 20 V.

11.1.1.8 Analytical Method Assessment

The repeatability and stability of this experiment were tested for assessment of the newly developed LC-Q-TOF-MS method. According to different chemical polarities and m/z values, five ions including m/z 132.0783 (creatine, positive mode), 255.0376 (cysteine-homocysteine disulfide, positive mode), 146.0632 (glutamate, negative mode), 257.0943 (3-methyluridine, negative mode), and 343.2099 (11-dehydrocorticosterone, negative mode) were extracted for the assessment according to the variation of their peak areas and retention times (RT).

The six parallel samples, which were obtained from a random urine sample and extracted by the same method, were injected one by one to evaluate the sample preparation repeatability. In the sample analysis sequence, every time the injections of four unknown samples were finished, the prepared QC sample was then injected. As there were 23 unknown samples (10 from the control group, 6 from the MI group, and 7 from the SBP group), six batches of data from one QC sample could be obtained to evaluate the stability of the LC-Q-TOF-MS system for the large-scale sample analysis.

11.1.1.9 Statistical Analysis

For peak finding, alignment, and filtering, the raw LC-Q-TOF-MS data of all samples (excluding the data from blank samples) were first processed by the Agilent Mass Hunter Qualitative Analysis Software (Agilent Technologies, Palo Alto, CA, USA). A peak table was then created including the information of the RT, m/z, and ion intensity of all identified components. The filter parameters were used as follows: restrict RT, 0.3–12 min; restrict m/z, 80–1000 amu; peak relative height, $\geq 1.5\%$; mass tolerance, 0.05 Da; and RT windows, 0.1 min. Before multivariate analysis, the data of each sample were normalized to the total area to correct for the MS response shift from the first injection to the last injection. Then, PLS-DA in the software SIMCA-P (Ver 11, Umetrics, Umea, Sweden) was used for multivariate analysis. The significance was expressed by using one-way analyses of variance (ANOVAs) with a Bonferroni correction in the SPSS 13.0 for Windows (SPSS Inc., Chicago, IL, USA). P values less than 0.05 were considered significant.

11.1.2 Results and Discussion

11.1.2.1 Histopathology

The results of infarct size in control, MI, and SBP treatment groups are shown in Table 11.1. It can be seen that the infarct size accounted for $22.1 \pm 3.21\%$ weight of the cardiac muscle in the MI group and $27.9 \pm 3.61\%$ weight of the left ventricle. The infarct size was significantly decreased in the SBP group with $15.9 \pm 2.12\%$ weight of the cardiac muscle and $18.7 \pm 3.31\%$ weight of the left ventricle. The results indicated that the MI model produced by the coronary artery ligation was successful and the SBP could effectively protect the cardiac muscle in ischemic conditions.

The activities of serum enzymes such as LDH and CK have been cited as important parameters in the assessment of myocardial injury.[13] In this study, serum concentrations of LDH and CK were also analyzed to evaluate the validity of the MI model and the effect of the SBP treatment. As shown in Fig. 11.1, the concentrations of LDH and CK in MI model rats were significantly increased compared with the control rats ($P \leq 0.01$) while the effect could be reversed by the intervention of SBP administration ($P \leq 0.01$).

Table 11.1 The comparison of infarcted size in control, MI and SBP treatment groups

Group	Infarcted heart weight/total heart weight	Infarcted heart weight/left ventricle weight
Control	0	0
MI	22.1 ± 3.21	27.9 ± 3.61
SBP treatment	$16.5 \pm 4.12^*$	$20.7 \pm 3.31^*$

*Significant difference compared with MI group ($P < 0.05$).

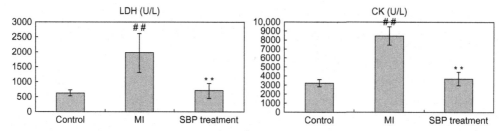

Fig. 11.1 Concentrations of major serum enzymes in control, MI, and SBP treatment groups. ##Significant difference compared with control group ($P<0.01$); **significant difference compared with MI groups ($P<0.01$).

Histopathology results demonstrated that the MI model was reliable and the SBP treatment had a positive effect on the MI model.

11.1.2.2 Assessment of the Repeatability and Stability of the LC-Q-TOF-MS Method

The data of system repeatability and stability are listed in Table 11.2. In the assessment of system repeatability, the RT and peak area of five selected ions in six batches of urinary samples varied with the RSD values within the range of 0.38%–0.74% (RT) and 8.44%–9.21% (peak area) in positive mode (0.12%–0.82% for RT and 6.55%–10.92% for peak area in negative mode). The assessment data acquired from the QC sample also showed good system stability. The RSD of RT and peak areas of five selected ions were 0.52%–0.78% and 6.23%–8.84% respectively in the positive mode (0.32%–0.97% for RT and 4.67%–13.33% for peak area in the negative mode).

All data indicated that the established sample analysis method is highly repeatable and stable, and could be used for analyzing large-scale samples in metabolomic experiments.

11.1.2.3 Biomarker Identification

The large amounts of signals obtained from the mass spectra included metabolites, adducts, ion fragments, noise, and so on. By using traditional statistical methods, it was hard to find the discriminating ions contributing to the classification of MI and sham

Table 11.2 The repeatability and stability data of the proposed method

| | | Repeatability ($n=6$) | | | | Stability ($n=6$) | | | |
| | | Retention time (min) | | Peak area | | Retention time (min) | | Peak area | |
Mode	Selected ion m/z	Mean	RSD (%)	Mean	RSD (%)	Mean	RSD (%)	Mean	RSD (%)
ESI(+)	253.1	1.41	0.78	1545	10.23	1.44	1.23	2105	11.25
	105.9	1.62	0.79	4728	10.71	1.62	0.18	8034	11.02
ESI(−)	243.1	1.37	0.64	2143	9.38	1.38	0.94	9864	10.03
	226.22	16.86	0.54	3721	9.24	16.88	0.54	4535	9.87

groups from thousands of signals. Thus PLS-DA, which is a well-established supervised method and has been widely used in metabolomic studies,[14,15] was adopted in this study. As Fig. 11.2A shows, there is a distinguishable classification between the clustering of MI and control groups.

To estimate the predictive ability of the model and thus ensure that the models are not over-fitted, a cross-validation was applied to the model. During cross-validation, a typical seven-round cross-validation was performed in Simca P 11.0. One seventh of the samples were excluded, a model was fitted to the remaining data, and subsequently the excluded data was predicted from the (reduced) model. This was repeated with each 1/7th of the samples until all samples had been predicted. Then the Predicted Residual Sum of Squares (PRESS) value was calculated. In Simca P 11.0, the value of PRESS is converted into Q^2Y. Good predictions will have low PRESS and so high Q^2Y. The established PLS-DA model using cross-validation could describe 66.4% of the variation in X ($R^2X=0.664$) and 92.3% of the variation in the response Y (class) ($R^2Y=0.923$), with a predictive ability of 78.7% ($Q^2Y=0.787$). The cross-validation results showed that a well-fitting PLS-DA model had been established. Latent variables (LVs) of the PLS-DA

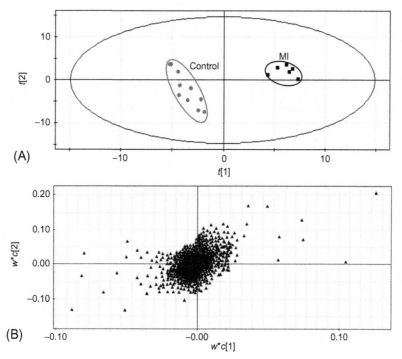

Fig. 11.2 PLS-DA model of the MI. (A) Scores plot of control *(circle)* and model *(square)* groups obtained from rat urine samples collected on day 15; (B) loadings plot obtained using Pareto scaling with mean centering. Each *triangle* represents an ion.

model were also determined during cross-validation in Simca P 11.0. The first LV was determined by maximizing the covariance between X and Y and thus to be a good predictor of Y, and then a new LV orthogonal to the first was then calculated from the updated X matrix and Y. When a new LV was used for the calculation, a PRESS value could be obtained. If the obtained PRESS value was significantly larger than the Residual Sum of Squares (RESS) value that was calculated before the new LV entered into the model, the new selected LV would be considered to be of no significance (did not contain the predictive information of Y), and then the calculation was stopped. In this model, two LVs were calculated during cross-validation in SIMCA P 11.0.

The corresponding loading plot (Fig. 11.2B) shows the contribution of different variables for the differences in the MI and control groups. Each triangle represents a variable. The more the variable deviates from the origin, the higher the value of variable importance projection (VIP) will be obtained. When VIP ≥ 1.0, the variable can be considered as a contributor for the classification of MI and control groups. According to the result of PLS-DA, a total of 44 (the value of VIP ≥ 1.0) out of 2430 variables (sum of variables detected in both positive mode and negative mode) contributed to the classification of the control and MI groups. Among these perturbed variables, 16 (6 in positive, 10 in negative) were predicted by comparing the accurate MS and MS/MS fragments with the metabolites by searching in databases (http://metlin.scripps.edu, http://www. hmdb.ca/) and then confirmed by the commercial standards (Table 11.3). Two of the identified biomarkers' MS/MS spectra (tryptophan and creatine) are shown in Fig. 11.3.

11.1.2.4 The Network of Identified Biomarkers and Their Functions

Among those 16 identified biomarkers, 8 were depressed in MI rats' urine and the other 8 were upregulated (Table 11.3). The related pathway of each biomarker was also recorded in Table 11.3 by searching the KEGG PATHWAY Database (http://www.genome.jp/ kegg/). Though the 16 biomarkers were distributed in 14 pathways, the interaction of these pathways still could be established. As shown in Fig. 11.4, except for 3-methyluridine and cystine-homocystine disulfide, the other 14 biomarkers could all participate in a metabolic network that was constructed by their related pathways. The established network includes the pathways of purine metabolism, glutamate metabolism, citric acid cycle, etc., which all play an important role in the formation of MI.[16–21] It can be seen from Fig. 11.4 that the citric acid cycle is the most important biological process in this network and energy metabolism is definitely disturbed after the formation of MI. The citric acid cycle related network of energy metabolism may play an important role in disease development.

Then the biological mechanisms of the identified biomarkers in the formation of MI were investigated in this study. It is well known that the obstruction of large coronary vessels can lead to myocardial ischemia as the oxygen requirement of the heart exceeds the oxygen supplied to the heart by coronary circulation. Ischemia can disturb the normal

Table 11.3 Sixteen identified biomarkers of MI detected by UPLC-Q-TOF-MS in both positive and negative ion modes[a]

Mode	Number	Retention time (min)	Exact mass	Formula	Compound	Trend[a]	Related pathway
Positive	1	0.8	214.0192	$C_5H_{11}O_7P$	2-Deoxy-D-ribose 5-phosphate	↓	Pentose phosphate pathway
	2	0.91	131.0762	$C_4H_9N_3O_2$	Creatine	↓	Arginine and proline metabolism
	3	1.18	244.0777	$C_9H_{12}N_2O_6$	Uridine	↑	Pyrimidine metabolism
	4	3.52	204.0965	$C_{11}H_{12}N_2O_2$	Tryptophan	↓	Tyrosine metabolism
	5	4.22	184.0300	$C_8H_8O_5$	3,4-Dihydroxymandelic acid	↓	Tryptophan metabolism
	6	6.07	254.0354	$C_7H_{14}N_2O_4S_2$	Cysteine–homocysteine disulfide	↑	Methionine degradation pathway
Negative	7	1.03	147.0597	$C_5H_9NO_4$	Glutamate	↓	Glutamate metabolism
	8	1.17	219.1180	$C_9H_{17}NO_5$	Pantothenic acid	↓	Pantothenate and CoA biosynthesis
	9	1.18	190.0179	$C_6H_6O_7$	Oxalosuccinic acid	↑	Citrate cycle (TCA cycle)
	10	1.21	193.0799	$C_{10}H_{11}NO_3$	Phenylacetylglycine	↑	Phenylalanine metabolism
	11	1.93	179.0648	$C_9H_9NO_3$	Hippuric acid	↑	Phenylalanine metabol
	12	3.48	344.2074	$C_{21}H_{28}O_4$	11-Dehydrocorticosterone	↑	Steroid hormone biosynthesis
	13	3.56	232.1278	$C_{13}H_{16}N_2O_2$	Melatonin	↓	Tryptophan metabolism
	14	6.73	334.0637	$C_{11}H_{15}N_2O_8P$	Nicotinamide mononucleotide	↑	Nicotinate and nicotinamide metabolism
	15	11.4	284.0824	$C_{10}H_{12}N_4O_6$	Xanthosine	↓	Purine metabolism
	16	14.2	258.0911	$C_{10}H_{14}N_2O_6$	3-Methyluridine	↑	DNA damage

[a] ↑ and ↓ represent the compound is up- and down-regulated in MI group compared with the control group, respectively.

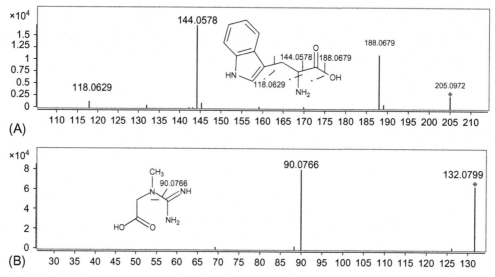

Fig. 11.3 MS/MS spectra of tryptophan (A) and creatine (B) in a urine sample.

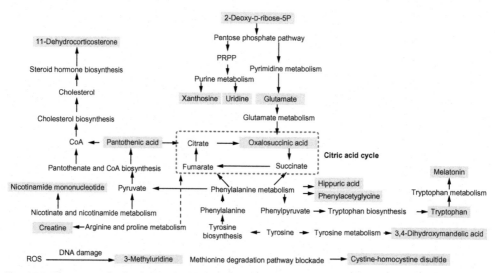

Fig. 11.4 The network of 16 identified biomarkers according to the KEGG PATHWAY Database. The *dashed area* denotes the identified metabolites.

function of cardiocytes, thus inducing the dysfunction of the myocardial energy metabolism. In this study, eight of the identified metabolites including creatine, uridine, glutamate, pantothenic acid, oxalosuccinic acid, nicotinamide mononucleotide, phenylacetylglycine, and xanthosine are all relevant to adenosine triphosphate (ATP) generation.[22–27]

For example, the level of glutamate was significantly decreased in this study. This result has been demonstrated by several lines of evidence.[22,28,29] As the degradation of glutamate delivers 20% of the ATP generated by the substrate level phosphorylation reaction, it can be estimated that the decreased glutamate level owes to the ATP requirement of the ischemic heart. It is well known that oxalosuccinic acid is an essential participant in the citric acid cycle for the production of ATP generated by glutamate. In hypoxic conditions, the level of oxalosuccinic acid can increase obviously and then promote the generation of ATP for the energy requirement of the ischemic heart. It has been demonstrated that uridine is a marker of myocardial viability after coronary occlusion and reperfusion and is capable of increasing myocardial ATP production by stimulating anerobic glycolsis.[30] As the ischemia induces injury to cardiocytes, the cellular RNA synthesis is disturbed, thus inducing the accumulation of uridine. Furthermore, creatine concentrations in serum and urine have also been described as markers for MI.[27] It was reported by Gordon et al.[31] that the level of creatine was depressed significantly in the conditions of MI. The result was also confirmed in our study. The seriously increased level of CK (Fig. 11.1) in serum could aggravate the conversion of creatine and consume ATP to create phosphocreatine. So the decreased level of creatine reflected the dysfunction of ATP production in MI.

In summary, perturbed energy metabolism was the significantly changed biological process in MI conditions. The citric acid cycle related network of energy metabolism might play an important role in the disease development. Sixteen identified biomarkers in MI rats also revealed a new insight into the MI network in vivo.

11.1.2.5 Metabolomic Study of SBP Treatment

The effective results of the SBP for the treatment of MI have been shown in Section 11.1.2.1, "Histopathology." To further evaluate the therapeutic effects of the SBP, a newly established PLS-DA model (Fig. 11.5) was applied and the variance in biomarkers was also investigated. The model of two PLS-components was significant according to cross-validation, that is, the model could describe 61.5% of the variation in X ($R^2X=0.615$) and 95.4% of the variation in the response Y (class) ($R^2Y=0.954$), with a predictive ability of 90.1% ($Q^2Y=0.901$).

According to the newly established PLS-DA model, the SBP treatment group was closer to the control group in 15 days, which might suggest SBP can reverse the pathological process of MI. Moreover, the SBP also could reverse the level of most biomarkers (except 3,4-dihydroxymandelic acid and 2-deoxy-D-ribose 5-phosphate) in the urine of MI rats. Five biomarkers, including creatine, uridine, glutamate, oxalosuccinic acid, and nicotinamide mononucleotide, which are all related to the energy metabolism as mentioned above, were completely reversed by SBP to normal levels (shown in Fig. 11.6).

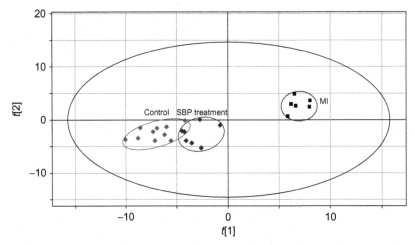

Fig. 11.5 Resulting scores plot from PLS-DA of LC-Q-TOF-MS data obtained from control rat *(circle)*; MI rat *(square)*; and SBP treatment rat *(diamond)* urine samples collected on day 15.

The results of histopathology and metabolomics demonstrated that the SBP had extensive effects in the treatment of MI through partially regulating the disturbed pathways of the energy metabolism.

11.1.3 Conclusion

In this study, a metabolomic approach based on LC–Q–TOF–MS detection has been successfully established for biomarker exploration in MI and mechanism studies of the SBP. As a result, 16 metabolites, which are distributed in 14 metabolic pathways, were identified as potential biomarkers of MI. Among these biomarkers, eight of them are related to the pathway of energy metabolism. The citric acid cycle related network of the energy metabolism was the significantly changed biological process after MI formation. SBP could reverse the pathological process of MI through regulating the disturbed pathway of the energy metabolism. The metabolomic results not only supply a systematic view of the development and progression of MI but also provide a theoretical basis for the prevention or treatment of MI.

11.2. THE PROTECTIVE EFFECTS OF THE SBP IN THE EARLY PERIOD OF ACUTE MI IN RATS USING A METABOLOMIC METHOD

11.2.1 Experimental

11.2.1.1 Materials

High performance liquid chromatography HPLC-grade acetonitrile and formic acid were purchased from JT Baker (NJ, USA). Ultrapure water from a Milli-Q50 SP reagent water system (Millipore Corporation, MA, USA) was used for the preparation of samples and the mobile phase. The assay kits for LDH and CK were purchased from Nanjing

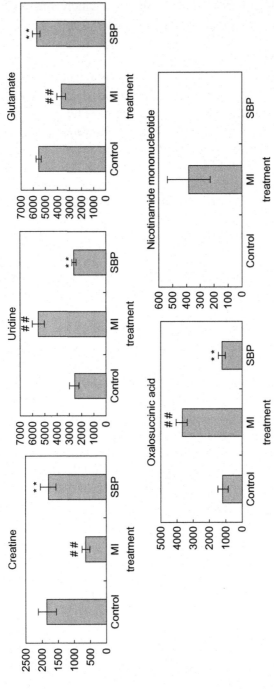

Fig. 11.6 Mean levels of five biomarkers completely reversed by the SBP in control, MI, and SBP treatment groups. #Significant difference compared with control group ($P < 0.01$); **significant difference compared with MI groups ($P < 0.01$).

Jiancheng Bio-engineering Institute (Nanjing, China). Commercial standards were purchased from Sigma/Aldrich (MO, USA). SBP was kindly offered by the Shanghai Hutchison Pharmaceuticals Company (Shanghai, China).

11.2.1.2 Animal and MI Model

Twenty male Sprague-Dawley rats (200 ± 15 g) were purchased from the Slac Laboratory Animal Co., Ltd. The animals were housed in stainless steel metabolic cages with free access to food and tap water under standard conditions of humidity ($50 \pm 10\%$), temperature ($25 \pm 2°C$), and 12 h light-dark cycle. The animals were acclimatized to the facilities for 5 days. All animals were handled with humane care throughout the experiment.

The AMI model was established by LADCA ligation, as described previously.[32] The chest was opened by a middle thoracotomy under sterile conditions. After pericardiotomy, the heart was rapidly exteriorized and a 4-0 black silk ligature was then placed under the LADCA to form an occlusion. Three rats died before collecting serum. Seventeen rats survived, including 11 AMI rats and 6 control rats (without ligation). All the rats were fixed on pad in a position on the back and two-lead electrocardiograms (ECGs) were recorded by the MPA 2000 biosignal analytical system (Shanghai Alcott Biotech Co., Ltd., Shanghai, China) after 5 h of the heart operation.

11.2.1.3 Drug Administration and Sample Collection

According to the clinical dosage of SBP ($2.25 \, \mathrm{mg\,kg^{-1}/d}$), 6 of 11 AMI rats were treated with the SBP at a dosage of $14 \, \mathrm{mg\,kg^{-1}/d}$ by oral gavage on 4 consecutive days before LADCA ligation.[33,34] SBP was ground into a fine powder and dissolved in 0.5% carboxymethyl cellulose sodium salt (CMC-Na) aqueous solution ($2.8 \, \mathrm{mg\,mL^{-1}}$). Isocyatic CMC-Na aqueous solution was administered orally to control ($n=6$) and AMI ($n=5$) rats. Serum was immediately collected from the ophthalmic venous plexus after recording ECGs. The collected serum was divided into two parts. One part was used for the analysis of serum concentrations of LDH and CK, and the other part was used for the metabolomic analysis. Serum concentrations of LDH and CK were measured by a UV 1100 ultraviolet spectrophotometer (Beijing Rayleigh Analytical Instrument Corp., Beijing, China).

The experiment was carried out in accordance with the guidelines of the Committee on the Care and Use of Laboratory Animals of the Institute of Laboratory Animal Resources of Shanghai, China. The study protocol was approved by the Animal Care and Use Committee of the Second Military Medical University.

11.2.1.4 Sample Preparation

For LC-MS analysis, 50 µL of rat serum was extracted with 150 µL acetonitrile. After vortex mixing for 30 s, these samples were centrifuged at 12,000 rpm for 10 min to remove proteins. The supernatant was then transferred to autosampler vials.

To ensure the stability of the sequence analysis, a QC sample was prepared by pooling the same volume (10 μL) from each serum sample and then preparing the pooled QC sample in the same way as the samples. The pooled QC sample was analyzed randomly through the analytical batch. In addition, six aliquots of serum sample from the same rat were treated in the same process to validate the repeatability of the sample preparation method.

11.2.1.5 Conditions of Liquid Chromatography-Quadrupole-Time of Flight-Mass Spectrometry (LC-Q-TOF-MS)

Metabolomic analysis was performed on an Agilent-1200 LC system that was coupled with an ESI source (Agilent Technologies, Palo Alto, CA, USA) equipped with an Agilent-6520 accurate-mass Q-TOF mass spectrometer. The separation of all samples was performed on an Eclipse Plus C_{18} column (1.8 μm, 2.1 mm × 100 mm, Agilent) with a column temperature maintained at 40°C. The flow rate was 0.3 mL min^{-1} and the mobile phase consisted of ultrapure water with 0.1% formic acid (A) and acetonitrile (B). The gradient program is shown in Table 11.4. The sample injection volume was 3 μL.

The mass spectrometer was operated in both positive and negative ion modes with parameters set as follows: drying gas (N_2) flow rate, 8 L min^{-1}; gas temperature, 330° C; pressure of nebulizer gas, 35 psig; Vcap, 4000 V; fragmentor, 160 V; skimmer, 65 V; and scan range, m/z 50–1000. The MS/MS analysis was acquired in the targeted MS/MS mode with collision energy ranging from 5 to 20 V.

11.2.1.6 Method Validation

The newly developed LC-Q-TOF-MS method needed to be validated. The stability and repeatability of this experiment were determined. According to the different chemical polarities and mass values, the five extracted ions of mass 184.0897 (epinephrine, positive mode), 125.0592 (5-methylcytosine, positive mode), 167.0292 (uric acid, negative mode), 329.2202 (deoxycorticosterone, negative mode), and 359.1938 (aldosterone, negative mode) were selected for validation.

Table 11.4 The gradient program of LC

Time (min)	A% (0.1% formic acid in H_2O)	B% (acetonitrile)
0	97	3
3	80	20
6	40	60
12	40	60
13	20	80
14	2	98
21	2	98

Extracts from six aliquots of a random serum sample were continuously injected to evaluate the repeatability. The data acquired from six QC samples (three unknown samples injected with one QC sample) were used to validate the LC-MS system stability for the large-scale sample analysis. The peak area and RT of five extracted ions were then analyzed to determine the variation.

11.2.1.7 Data Processing

The raw LC-MS data for all samples (exclude the data from blank samples) were firstly processed by the Agilent Mass Hunter Qualitative Analysis Software (Agilent Technologies, Palo Alto, CA, USA). The filter parameters were set as follows: restrict RT, 0.2–14 min; restrict mass, 80–1000 amu; peak relative height, $\geq 1.5\%$; mass tolerance, 0.05 Da; and RT windows, 0.1 min. After being filtered, a peak table was created that included the information of the RT, mass, and ion intensity for all identified components. The data from each sample were then normalized to total area and all data were imported into the software SIMCA-P (Ver. 11, Umetrics, Umea, Sweden) where multivariate analyses such as partial least squares-discriminate analysis (PLS-DA) were used for calculation. The significance was expressed by using one-way analyses of variance (ANOVAs) with a Bonferroni correction in the SPSS 13.0 for Windows (SPSS Inc., Chicago, IL, USA). P values less than 0.05 were considered significant.

11.2.2 Result and Discussion

11.2.2.1 ECG and Enzyme Test

In this study, typical ECG alterations such as oblique and upward ST segment elevation and broad T wave were detected in all AMI rats after 5 h of heart surgery. The changes in ECGs definitely demonstrated that the model was successful. Furthermore, the serum concentration of LDH and CK, which have been cited as important parameters in the assessment of myocardial injury[13], were also analyzed to evaluate the validity of the AMI model and the effect of the SBP pretreatment. As shown in Table 11.5, compared with control rats, the concentrations of LDH ($P < 0.01$) and CK ($P < 0.01$) in AMI model rats were significantly increased, an effect that can be reversed by the intervention of SBP administration. The enzymatic results demonstrated that the AMI model was reliable and the intervention of the SBP was positively effective.

11.2.2.2 Optimization of LC-MS

Metabolomics aims to pinpoint the interesting metabolites in a complex metabolite profile, so the process of sample pretreatment should be minimized to avoid the loss of potential biomarkers. To optimize the pretreatment method, deproteinating by adding acetonitrile was compared to deproteinating by adding methanol. Results showed that deproteinating by adding acetonitrile gave more ion information than adding

Table 11.5 Concentrations of major serum enzymes in the control, AMI and SBP treatment groups

Group	LDH(U/L)	CK(U/L)
Control	1778 ± 441	4242 ± 1070
AMI	$2673 \pm 669**$	$8828 \pm 2281**$
SBP treatment	$2058 \pm 588^{\#}$	$5406 \pm 1196^{\#\#}$

**Significant difference compared with control group ($P < 0.01$).
#Significant difference compared with AMI groups ($P < 0.05$).
##Significant difference compared with AMI groups ($P < 0.01$).

methanol. So serum samples were deproteinated by adding acetonitrile before LC-Q-TOF-MS analysis.

The flow rate was set at $0.3\,\mathrm{mL\,min^{-1}}$ because the chromatograms showed better resolution of adjacent peaks. The column temperature was set to 40°C to reduce the higher column pressure. Studies also showed that 0.1% formic acid added into the mobile phase (water) can obtain better separation of chromatographic peaks.

To obtain the full knowledge of the metabolite profile in rat serum, both positive and negative chromatograms were recorded in this study. The drying gas flow rate and gas temperature were set at $8\,\mathrm{L\,min^{-1}}$ and 330°C, respectively, to obtain the best ionization efficiency. The collision energy was optimized from 5 to 20 eV according to the chemical structure of potential biomarkers for MS/MS spectral analysis in both positive and negative mode.

11.2.2.3 LC-Q-TOF-MS Method Validation

The data for system repeatability and stability of the proposed method are listed in Table 11.6. In the validation of system repeatability, a stable RT for five selected ions in six batches of serum samples was observed with the variations less than 0.83% relative standard deviation (RSD) in positive mode and 0.77% RSD in negative mode. In

Table 11.6 The repeatability and stability data for the proposed method

Mode	Selected ion m/z	Repeatability ($n = 6$) Retention time (min) Mean	RSD (%)	Peak area Mean	RSD (%)	Stability ($n = 6$) Retention time (min) Mean	RSD (%)	Peak area Mean	RSD (%)
ESI(+)	184.1	1.83	0.83	5562	9.11	1.82	0.99	3187	10.79
	126.0	5.94	0.67	2533	10.04	5.94	0.48	3351	9.91
ESI(−)	167.0	5.82	0.77	7649	7.03	5.81	0.91	4569	5.61
	329.3	16.33	0.72	5124	8.29	16.34	0.67	3653	7.17
	359.3	16.99	0.69	1835	10.88	16.97	0.53	1307	12.74

addition, the RSD values for peak areas for the main ions were varied from 9.11% to 10.04% in positive mode and from 7.03% to 10.88% in negative mode.

The validation data acquired from the QC sample also showed good system stability. The RSD (%) of peak areas and RT of the main ions were 0.48%–0.99% for RT and 9.91%–10.79% for peak areas in the positive mode (0.53%–0.91% for RT and 5.61%–12.74% for peak areas in the negative mode).

All results indicated that the established LC-MS method could be used for analyzing the large-scale samples in the metabolomic studies.

11.2.2.4 Identification of Biomarkers in the Early Period of AMI in Rats

Because a large number of signals were obtained from the serum samples, a multivariate analysis method was needed to discriminate the ions that contribute to the classification of the control and AMI groups. Therefore, PLS-DA, a supervised projection method, was applied to the LC-MS data in this study. The established PLS-DA model using cross-validation could describe 72.8% of the variation in X ($R^2X = 0.728$) and 89.9% of the variation in the response Y (class) ($R^2Y = 0.899$) with a predictive ability of 85.1% ($Q^2Y = 0.851$). LVs of the PLS-DA model were also determined during cross-validation in Smica P 11.0. In this model, two LVs were calculated during cross-validation in SIMCA P 11.0. The cross-validation results showed that a well-fitting PLS-DA model had been established.

As shown in Fig. 11.7A, the score plot showed that AMI and the control groups could be classified clearly. The corresponding loading plot showed the contribution of the variables to the differences between AMI samples and the control groups (Fig. 11.7B). The more the variable deviates from the origin, the higher the value of the variable importance plot (VIP) that will be obtained. Therefore, the potential biomarkers in the early period of AMI are found in those variables that obviously deviate from the origin. In this study, a total of 42 variables (the value of VIP > 1.0) contributed to the metabolic variation. Among these variables, 14 (5 in positive mode, 9 in negative mode) were predicted by comparing the MS and MS/MS fragments with the metabolites found by searching in databases (http://metlin.scripps.edu, http://www.hmdb.ca/) and subsequently confirmed by the use of commercial standards (Table 11.7).

An identified biomarker produced the quasimolecular mass at mass 243.0920 (the RT was 5.76 min in the positive mode). $C_{10}H_{14}N_2O_5$ was subsequently calculated as the most probable molecular formula. The tandem MS fragment at mass 127.0899 yielded the molecular structure information (Fig. 11.8). The above information was also searched in the Internet databases mentioned above. Considering the molecular elemental composition, fragment information, and RT behavior together, the ion of mass 243.0920 was tentatively identified as thymidine. The identification was confirmed by comparison with

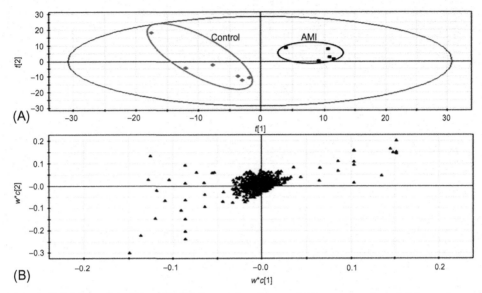

Fig. 11.7 PLS-DA model of the AMI. (A) Score plot of control *(diamond)* and model *(square)* groups obtained from rat serum samples. (B) Loading plot obtained using Pareto scaling with mean centering. Each *triangle* represents an ion.

the commercial standard. Using this iterative method, another 13 biomarkers were identified (Table 11.7).

11.2.2.5 Biomarkers and Their Pathways

Among those 14 identified biomarkers, three were depressed in AMI rat serum, and another 11 were elevated. The related pathway of every biomarker was also recorded in Table 11.7 by searching the KEGG PATHWAY Database (http://www.genome.jp/kegg/). Several lines of evidence have demonstrated that 11 of 14 identified biomarkers in this study play an important role in the formation of AMI. These 11 biomarkers mainly participate in three pathological processes, including inflammation, hypertrophy, and oxidative injury, which are all activated by AMI (Table 11.7).

The increasing level of homocysteine in the serum has been shown to be associated with an increased risk for occlusive vascular disease.[35,36] Welch and Losculzo[37] reported that homocysteine probably leads to oxidative damage of endothelial cells because of the reactive oxygen radicals that are produced during auto-oxidation of homocysteine in plasma. Poddar[38] demonstrated that homocysteine also promotes the recruitment of leucocytes, thereby enhancing the injury to the endothelial cells. MI is associated with tissue-specific activation of the myocardial aldosterone synthesis.[39] The increasing level of aldosterone may lead to the formation of hypertrophy, ventricular remodeling, and even heart failure.

Table 11.7 Related pathway and pathological processes for 14 identified biomarkers

Mode	Number	Retention time (min)	Exact mass	Formula	Compound	Trend	Related pathway	Disease meaning
Positive	1	1.34	160.0370	$C_6H_8O_5$	2-Oxoadipic acid	↓	Lysine degradation	–
	2	1.69	203.0247	$C_7H_9NO_4S$	Cystathionine ketimine	↑	Cysteine and methionine metabolism	Oxidative injury
	3	1.85	183.0891	$C_9H_{13}NO_3$	Epinephrine	↑	Tyrosine metabolism	Hypertrophy
	4	5.76	242.0913	$C_{10}H_{14}N_2O_5$	Thymidine	↓	Pyrimidine metabolism	–
	5	5.96	125.0584	$C_5H_7N_3O$	5-Methylcytosine	↓	Pyrimidine metabolism	–
Negative	6	1.58	268.0557	$C_8H_{16}N_2O_4S_2$	Homocystine	↑	Cysteine and methionine metabolism	Hypertrophy
	7	5.81	168.0288	$C_5H_4N_4O_3$	Uric acid	↑	Purine metabolism	Oxidative injury
	8	13.32	336.2303	$C_{20}H_{32}O_4$	12S-HPETE	↑	AA metabolism	Inflammation
	9	15.58	344.1984	$C_{21}H_{28}O_4$	11-Dehydrocorticosterone	↑	Steroid hormone biosynthesis	Hypertrophy
	10	15.83	320.2355	$C_{20}H_{32}O_3$	12S-HETE	↑	AA metabolism	Inflammation
	11	16.34	330.2197	$C_{21}H_{30}O_3$	Deoxycorticosterone	↑	Steroid hormone biosynthesis	Hypertrophy
	12	16.97	346.2147	$C_{21}H_{30}O_4$	Corticosterone	↑	Steroid hormone biosynthesis	Hypertrophy
	13	16.97	360.1932	$C_{21}H_{28}O_5$	Aldosterone	↑	Steroid hormone biosynthesis	Hypertrophy
	14	17.69	362.2091	$C_{21}H_{30}O_5$	Cortisol	↑	Steroid hormone biosynthesis	Hypertrophy

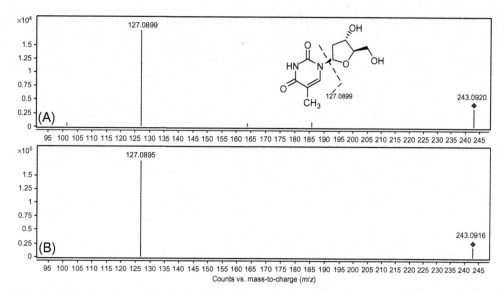

Fig. 11.8 MS/MS spectrum of thymidine (the precursor ion was mass 243.09; the major fragment was mass 127.08): (A) serum sample and (B) standard.

At present, aldosterone antagonists have been used widely for patients with post-MI heart failure in clinic. In addition, as the results of other studies showed, the higher serum levels of 11-dehydrocorticosterone, deoxycorticosterone, corticosterone, and cortisol, which all participate in the formation of hypertrophy, were also observed in this experiment. As aldosterone, 11-dehydrocorticosterone, deoxycorticosterone, corticosterone, and cortisol are in the pathway of steroid hormone biosynthesis, steroid hormone biosynthesis appears to be acutely perturbed in the early period of AMI. The hypertrophy-related biomarkers in the pathway of steroid hormone biosynthesis are shown in Fig. 11.9.

Several studies have demonstrated that ischemia results in the accumulation of unesterified arachidonic acid (AA) via the action of membrane-bound phospholipases.[40,41] The compounds 12(S)-hydroperoxyeicosatetraenoic acid (12(S)-HPETE) and 12(S)-hydroxyeicosatetraenoic acid (12(S)-HETE) are both metabolites of AA. The high levels of 12(S)-HPETE and 12(S)-HETE reflected the activation of the AA metabolism and contributed to the inflammatory reaction in AMI.

In summary, the 14 identified biomarkers in the early period of AMI rats not only revealed a new insight into the AMI network in vivo but also supplied the theoretical basis for the prevention or treatment of AMI. The multiple pathways included in this study also demonstrated the complicated mechanism of AMI.

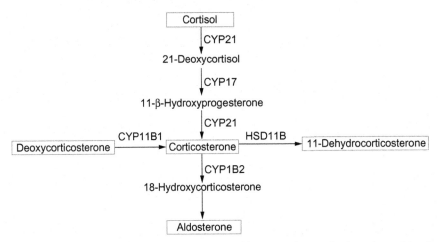

Fig. 11.9 Hypertrophy-related biomarkers in the steroid hormone biosynthesis pathway (the skeleton diagram represents identified biomarkers).

11.2.2.6 Metabolomic Study of SBP Pretreatment

The protective effects of the SBP for the treatment of AMI can be obtained not only from Section 3.1 but also can be demonstrated using metabolomic methods. The newly established PLS-DA model of two PLS-components was significant according to cross-validation ($R^2X = 0.646$, $R^2Y = 0.924$, and $Q^2Y = 0.879$).

The score plot of the PLS-DA model (Fig. 11.10) showed that control, AMI, and SBP pretreatment groups are classified clearly, and the SBP pretreatment group is closer to the control group than the AMI group, which might suggest that the SBP can reverse the pathological process of AMI.

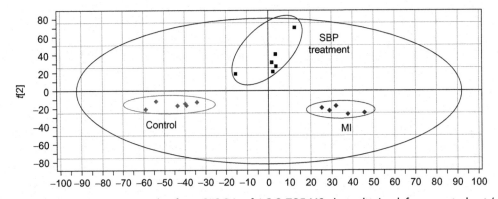

Fig. 11.10 Resulting scores plot from PLS-DA of LC-Q-TOF-MS data obtained from control rats' *(diamonds)*, AMI rats' *(dots)*, and the SBP pretreatment rats' *(squares)* serum samples.

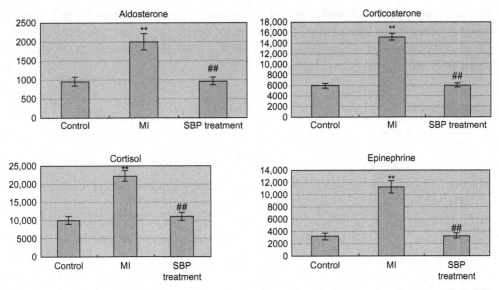

Fig. 11.11 Mean levels of four biomarkers completely reversed by SBP in control, AMI, and the SBP pretreatment groups. One-way ANOVA with a Bonferroni correction was used. **Significant difference compared with control group ($P < 0.01$); ##Significant difference compared with AMI groups ($P < 0.01$).

By comparing the identified biomarker level in AMI, control, and SBP pretreatment groups, four of the identified biomarkers, including corticosterone, aldosterone, cortisol, and epinephrine, are completely reversed by the SBP (shown in Fig. 11.11). All the reversed biomarkers are the metabolites of steroid hormone biosynthesis and contribute to the formation of hypertrophy. These results showed that the SBP pretreatment could depress the pathway of steroid hormone biosynthesis and decrease the level of hypertrophy-related metabolites, thereby inhibiting the pathological changes of hypertrophy and protecting the impaired heart.

The results of histopathology and metabolomics clearly demonstrate that the SBP has protective effects on AMI. The effects of SBP pretreatment partially depend on inhibiting the biosynthesis of steroid hormones.

11.2.3 Conclusion

In this study, 14 metabolites were identified as potential biomarkers in the early period of AMI in rat serum, and the steroid hormone biosynthesis (11-dehydrocorticosterone, deoxycorticosterone, corticosterone, aldosterone, and cortisol) was the acutely perturbed pathway in the early period of AMI. The identified biomarkers not only revealed a new insight into the AMI network in vivo but also supplied the theoretical basis for the prevention or treatment of AMI. The SBP could reverse the pathological changes of AMI through inhibiting the hypertrophy-related metabolites. Our study also demonstrates that the LC-MS-based metabolomic strategy is a powerful approach for biomarker exploration and mechanism elucidation of TCMs.

REFERENCES

1. Shimokawa H, Yasuda S. Myocardial ischemia: current concepts and future perspectives. *J Cardiol* 2008;**52**:67–78.
2. Apple FS, Wu AH. Myocardial infarction redefined: role of cardiac troponin testing. *Clin Chem* 2001;**47**:377–9.
3. *Editorial Committee of Pharmacopoeia of Ministry of Health P. R. China.* 2010. Beijing: China Chemical Industry Press; 2010. p. 1241–2 [Part 1].
4. Ye RY. Effect of heart-protecting Musk Pill on cardiac function of ischemic heart disease. *Zhejiang J Integr Tradit Chin West Med* 2006;**16**:734–5.
5. Wu DJ, Hong HS, Jiang Q. Effect of Shexiang Baoxin Pill in alleviating myocardial fibrosis in spontaneous hypertensive rats. *Chin J Integr Tradit West Med* 2005;**25**:350–3.
6. Song HT, Guo T, Zhao MH, Zhang RH, Hu HY, Chen XY. Pharmacodynamic studies on heart-protecting Musk Pills with myocardial blood flow perfusion in rats. *Pharm J Chin PLA* 2002;**18**:137–9.
7. Gika HG, Theodoridis G, Extance J, Edge AM, Wilson ID. High temperature-ultra performance liquid chromatography-mass spectrometry for the metabonomic analysis of Zucker rat urine. *J Chromatogr B Anal Technol Biomed Life Sci* 2008;**871**:279–87.
8. Wong MC, Lee WT, Wong JS, Frost G, Lodge J. An approach towards method development for untargeted urinary metabolite profiling in metabonomic research using UPLC/QTOF MS. *J Chromatogr B Anal Technol Biomed Life Sci* 2008;**871**:341–8.
9. Wang X, Lv H, Sun H, Liu L, Yang B, Sun W, et al. Metabolic urinary profiling of alcohol hepatotoxicity and intervention effects of Yin Chen Hao Tang in rats using ultra-performance liquid chromatography/electrospray ionization quadruple time-of-flight mass spectrometry. *J Pharm Biomed Anal* 2008;**48**:1161–8.
10. Yao H, Shi P, Zhang L, Fan X, Shao Q, Cheng Y. Untargeted metabolic profiling reveals potential biomarkers in myocardial infarction and its application. *Mol BioSyst* 2010;**6**:1061–70.
11. Zhang HY, Chen X, Hu P, Liang QL, Liang XP, Wang YM, et al. Metabolomic profiling of rat serum associated with isoproterenol-induced myocardial infarction using ultra-performance liquid chromatography/time-of-flight mass spectrometry and multivariate analysis. *Talanta* 2009;**79**:254–9.
12. Lv Y, Liu X, Yan S, Liang X, Yang Y, Dai W, et al. Metabolomic study of myocardial ischemia and intervention effects of Compound Danshen Tablets in rats using ultra-performance liquid chromatography/quadrupole time-of-flight mass spectrometry. *J Pharm Biomed Anal* 2010;**52**:129–35.
13. Zheng SY, Sun J, Zhao X, Xu JG. Protective effect of shen-fu on myocardial ischemia-reperfusion injury in rats. *Am J Chin Med* 2004;**32**:209–20.
14. Williams RE, Lenz EM, Evans JA, Wilson ID, Granger JH, Plumb RS, et al. A combined (1)H NMR and HPLC-MS-based metabonomic study of urine from obese (fa/fa) Zucker and normal Wistar-derived rats. *J Pharm Biomed Anal* 2005;**38**:465–71.
15. Bogdanov M, Matson WR, Wang L, Matson T, Saunders-Pullman R, Bressman SS, et al. Metabolomic profiling to develop blood biomarkers for Parkinson's disease. *Brain* 2008;**131**:389–96.
16. DeBoer LW, Ingwall JS, Kloner RA, Braunwald E. Prolonged derangements of canine myocardial purine metabolism after a brief coronary artery occlusion not associated with anatomic evidence of necrosis. *Proc Natl Acad Sci U S A* 1980;**77**:5471–5.
17. Flameng W, Vanhaecke J, Van Belle H, Borgers M, De Beer L, Minten J. Relation between coronary artery stenosis and myocardial purine metabolism, histology and regional function in humans. *J Am Coll Cardiol* 1987;**9**:1235–42.
18. Thomassen AR, Mortensen PT, Nielsen TT, Falstie-Jensen N, Thygesen K, Henningsen P. Altered plasma concentrations of glutamate, alanine and citrate in the early phase of acute myocardial infarction in man. *Eur Heart J* 1986;**7**:773–8.

19. Niemann CU, Saeed M, Akbari H, Jacobsen W, Benet LZ, Christians U, et al. Close association between the reduction in myocardial energy metabolism and infarct size: dose-response assessment of cyclosporine. *J Pharmacol Exp Ther* 2002;**302**:1123–8.

20. Sernov LN, Snegireva GV, Gatsura VV. The effect of Krebs cycle intermediates on the size of the necrotic zone and on the course of early postocclusion arrhythmia in experimental myocardial infarct in rats. *Farmakol Toksikol* 1989;**52**:47–9.

21. Rumpf KD, Grögler F, Beddermann C, Frank G, Zazvorka FZ. Anaerobic glycolysis and citrate cycle during temporary myocardial ischemia. *Res Exp Med (Berl)* 1972;**157**:172–4.

22. Wiesner RJ, Deussen A, Borst M, Schrader J, Grieshaber MK. Glutamate degradation in the ischemic dog heart: contribution to anaerobic energy production. *J Mol Cell Cardiol* 1989;**21**:49–59.

23. Halestrap AP. The mitochondrial pyruvate carrier. Kinetics and specificity for substrates and inhibitors. *Biochem J* 1975;**148**:85–96.

24. Berger F, Lau C, Dahlmann M, Ziegler M. Subcellular compartmentation and differential catalytic properties of the three human nicotinamide mononucleotide adenylyltransferase isoforms. *J Biol Chem* 2005;**280**:36334–41.

25. Vemuri R, Willem de Jong J, Hegge JA, Huizer T, Heller M, Pinson A. Studies on oxygen and extra-cellular fluid restrictions in cultured heart cells: high energy phosphate metabolism. *Cardiovasc Res* 1989;**23**:254–61.

26. Rosenfeldt FL, Richards SM, Lin Z, Pepe S, Conyers RA. Mechanism of cardioprotective effect of orotic acid. *Cardiovasc Drugs Ther* 1998;**12**:159–70.

27. Taes YE, Lameire NH, De Buyzere ML, Shoja A, De Backer G, Delanghe JR. Exercise-induced myocardial ischemia is accompanied by increased serum creatine concentrations. *Clin Chem* 2003;**49**:684–6.

28. Saifutdinov RI, IAI K, Tikhaze AK, Lankin VZ. Changes in antioxidative enzyme activity in patients with chronic heart failure. *Kardiologiia* 1990;**30**:65–8.

29. Pisarenko OI, Solomatina ES, Ivanov VE, Studneva IM, Kapelko VI, Smirnov VN. On the mechanism of enhanced ATP formation in hypoxic myocardium caused by glutamic acid. *Basic Res Cardiol* 1985;**80**:126–34.

30. Yaoita H, Fischman AJ, Strauss HW, Saito T, Sato E, Maruyama Y. Uridine: a marker of myocardial viability after coronary occlusion and reperfusion. *Int J Card Imaging* 1993;**9**:273–80.

31. Gordon A, Hultman E, Kaijser L, Kristjansson S, Rolf CJ, Nyquist O, et al. Creatine supplementation in chronic heart failure increases skeletal muscle creatine phosphate and muscle performance. *Cardiovasc Res* 1995;**30**:413–8.

32. Wang JW, Liu XL, Ren B, Rupp H, Takeda N, Dhalla NS. Modification of myosin gene expression by imidapril in failing heart due to myocardial infarction. *J Mol Cell Cardiol* 2002;**34**:847–57.

33. Wang DY, Li Y, Fan WH. Effect of decreasing infarct area and stimulating angiogenesis of Shexiang-baoxin Pills in rat with coronary occlusion. *Chin Tradit Patent Med* 2004;**26**:912–5.

34. SY H, Tian DK, Chen GL, Liu J, Ke Y, Bian K. Protective effect of heart protecting Musk Pill on heart in spontaneously hypertensive rats. *Lishizhen Med Mater Med Res* 2009;**20**:2458–61.

35. Olszewski AJ, Szostak WB. Homocysteine content of plasma proteins in ischemic heart disease. *Atherosclerosis* 1988;**69**:109–13.

36. Chambers JC, Kooner JS. Homocysteine: a novel risk factor for coronary heart disease in UK Indian Asians. *Heart* 2001;**86**:121–2.

37. Welch GN, Loscalzo J. Homocysteine and atherothrombosis. *N Engl J Med* 1998;**338**:1042–50.

38. Poddar R. Homocystine induced expression and secretion of monocyte chemoattractant protein 1 and IL-8 in human aortic endothelial cells, implication for vascular disease. *Circulation* 2001;**103**:2717–23.

39. Silvestre JS, Heymes C, Oubénaïssa A, Robert V, Aupetit-Faisant B, Carayon A, et al. Activation of cardiac aldosterone production in rat myocardial infarction: effect of angiotensin II receptor blockade and role in cardiac fibrosis. *Circulation* 1999;**99**:2694–701.

40. Gross GJ, Falck JR, Gross ER, Isbell M, Moore J, Nithipatikom K. Cytochrome P450 and arachidonic acid metabolites: role in myocardial ischemia/reperfusion injury revisited. *Cardiovasc Res* 2005;**68**:18–25.

41. Hjelte LE, Nilsson A. Arachidonic acid and ischemic heart disease. *J Nutr* 2005;**135**:2271–3.

CHAPTER 12

Network Pharmacology Study of the Shexiang Baoxin Pill

Jing Zhao*, Peng Jiang[†], Runui Liu[‡], Weidong Zhang[‡]
*Shanghai University of Traditional Chinese Medicine, Shanghai, PR China
[†]Shanghai Hutchison Pharmaceutical Limited Company, Shanghai, PR China
[‡]Second Military Medical University, Shanghai, PR China

The *Shexiang Baoxin Pill* (SBP) is a formula of traditional Chinese medicine (TCM) that is composed of seven ingredients: Moschus, total gingenoside ginseng root, Styrax, Cinnamomi Cortex, Bufonis Venenum, Bovis Calculus Artifactus, and Borneolum Syntheticum. A TCM formula usually includes multiple chemical components. When these components are absorbed by plasma, they achieve their effects of inhibiting the disease by targeting and regulating corresponding proteins. In other words, the TCM formulae realize synergistic efficacy by acting on multicomponents and multitargets. In China, the SBP has clinical application in the treatment of complex cardiovascular diseases (CVD) such as myocardial ischemia, angina pectoris, and myocardial infarction, etc. Cardiovascular diseases are a collection of complex chronic disorders that appear in the cardiovascular system. The pathogenesis of CVD involves the dysfunction of hundreds of genes, encoded proteins, and signal pathways. In fact, those dysfunctional proteins tend to interact with each other and thus form a complex disease-affected subnetwork. Therefore, it is helpful for us to utilize network pharmacology as a methodology to systematically analyze how the multiple components in the SBP regulate CVD-related signal pathways as well as CVD-related disease networks. At last, it is possible for us to uncover the therapeutic mechanism of the SBP.

In this chapter, we combine bioinformatics analysis with pharmacology experiments and employ network pharmacology to study the therapeutic mechanism of the SBP on CVD. At first, through retrieving and reading numerous literatures, we collect and summarize related signal pathways, drug targets, and intervention methods of Western medicine for coronary heart disease. Next, using bioinformatics and the network modeling method, we identify CVD-related signal pathways that are synergistically regulated by components in the SBP. Moreover, we validate the computational results by a gene expression experiment. Finally, using the Western medicine polypill, which has clear therapeutic mechanism as a contrast according to experimental results obtained from a yeast cell experimental platform, we identify genes significantly affected by the small molecules in the SBP. We then construct a drug-affected subnetwork as well as a target-affected subnetwork. We further study these subnetworks and the pathways regulated by drug small molecules so as to elucidate the therapeutic mechanism of the SBP on the molecular level.

12.1. A SURVEY ON CORONARY HEART DISEASE-RELATED SIGNAL PATHWAYS

Abstract

Coronary heart disease (CHD), the most common form of cardiovascular disease, is a chronic, multifactorial disease. With significant advances in our understanding of the pathophysiological process of CHD in recent years, more and more drug targets have been identified and adopted in drug discovery for CHD. In this review, a comprehensive perspective of pathological and pharmacological development of CHD was introduced through searching in multiple bibliographic sources. CHD-related signal pathways (including 409 proteins), drug targets (including 101 proteins), and pharmacological interventions were summarized and visualized. The knowledge of these signal pathways and drug targets may facilitate new drug discovery and medicine intervention for CHD in the future.

Keywords: Coronary heart disease, Pathophysiological process, Signal pathways

12.1.1 Introduction

Cardiovascular disease (CVD) is the most common cause of death worldwide. It was estimated that around 23.6 million people will die from CVDs by 2030 and approximately half of these occurrences are directly related to coronary heart disease (CHD).[1,2] CHD is the consequence of atherosclerosis with accumulation of atheromatous plaques within walls of coronary arteries that supply the myocardium with oxygen and nutrients. The progress of CHD is characterized by its chronicity. It is particularly insidious in initial stages. Several risk factors such as cigarette smoking, hypercholesterolemia, hypertension, hyperglycemia, and work stress have been demonstrated to be closely related to the processing of CHD. Acute myocardial infarction, arrhythmia, angina pectoris, and heart failure are major clinical manifestations of CHD.

In the formation of atherosclerosis and CHD, endothelial cells (ECs), vascular smooth muscle cells (VSMCs), macrophages, T leukomonocytes, monocytes, mast cells, dendritic cells, platelets, and cadiocytes interact with each other to damage normal functions of the coronary artery and heart muscle.[3–10] Multiple intracellular and extracellular signal pathways containing hundreds of proteins participate in these interactions. A total of 413 CHD-associated proteins were listed in Supplementary Table S1. Some of these proteins, such as 3-hydroxy-3-methylglutaryl-coenzyme A reductase (HMG-CoA reductase), angiotensin-convertion enzyme (ACE), and the angiotensin (Ang II) receptor, have been identified as drug targets. Drugs designed according to these targets have played important roles in the treatment of CHD.

In this section, we summarize CHD-related signal pathways through searching in multiple bibliographic sources. By doing so, a comprehensive knowledge of ligands and targets relevant to CHD can be shown, further facilitating drug discovery.

12.1.2 Cells, Pathways, and Proteins Related to CHD

CHD is a chronic disease in which blood flow is obstructed through coronary arteries that supply the heart with oxygen–rich blood. As shown in Fig. 12.1, this obstruction is caused by atherosclerosis, the development of which is a lifelong process. According to the "response to injury" hypothesis of atherosclerosis, endothelial dysfunction is the first step in atherosclerosis.[11] Subsequently, monocytes gather at the site of the injury and in turn provoke an inflammatory immune response that causes further damage to the arterial wall. Over time, low–density lipoprotein (LDL) penetrates into the arterial wall and is modified by oxidasis, then combines with the monocyte-derived macrophages to form a foam cell. Simultaneously, T lymphocytes, dendritic cells, mast cells, and platelets can enter the intima of the arterial wall through an injured endothelial layer and induce the releasing of cytokines. With the participation of these cytokines such as matrix metallo-proteinases (MMPs) and platelet-derived growth factors (PDGF), VSMCs can proliferate and migrate through intermediate lesions via the degradation of extracellular matrix components, thus promoting the formation of atherosclerosis plaque. Once plaque ruptures, some pieces of the plaque can travel through arteries until they cause a blockage. Then, myocardial infarction happens and leads to the dysfunction of cadiocytes. Finally, injured vascular and heart muscles lead to the occurrence of CHD.

In this section, we mainly introduce the functions of related cells in the formation of CHD, including ECs, VSMCs, T lymphocytes, dendritic cells, monocytes, macrophage, mast cells, platelets, and cadiocytes.

12.1.2.1 ECs

ECs are inert barriers of rowing blood and underlying tissue. They play important roles in regulating hemostasis, tracking cellular and nutrient. Under normal conditions, ECs are a well-aligned, tight junction with very low rates of death and are permeable to some macromolecules such as LDL. ECs can produce numerous vasoactive factors such as nitric oxide (NO), prostaglandin, endothelin (ET-1), and Ang II. Vascular dysfunction due to endothelial cell injury alters these normal homeostatic properties. For example, the synthesis of NO is reduced while the expression of vasoconstrictive molecules such as ET-1 is upregulated.[12,13]

Hyperlipidemia, hypertension, hyperglycemia, and smoking are the main causes for EC injury. Because of the increased permeability of ECs induced by injury, atherogenic matter LDL transmigrates through the endothelial layer and transforms into ox-LDL.[14] As shown in Fig. 12.2, once ox-LDL enters the intima, an oxidized low-density lipoprotein receptor 1 (LOX) can be activated, thus inducing NF-κb activation and leading to the upregulation of adhesion molecules such as Eselectin, P-selectin, the platelet-endothelial cell adhesion molecule (PECAM), the intercellular adhesion molecule (ICAM), and chemotatic factors such as C–C motif chemokine 2 (MCP-1) and

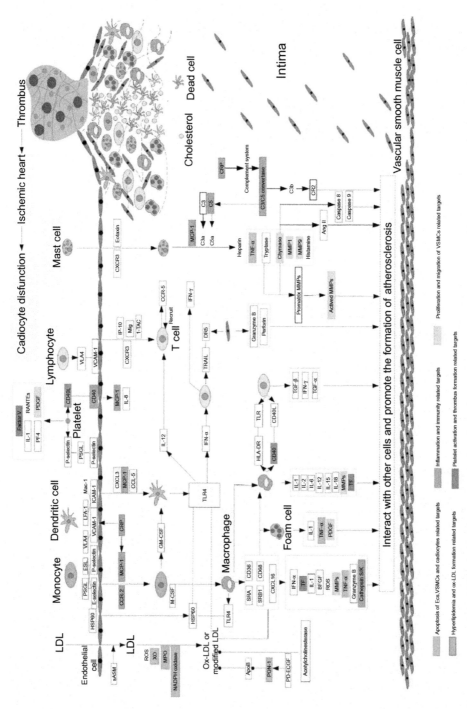

Fig. 12.1 Interaction of different cells in the formation of ischemic heart. All the shadow rectangles were signed by rectangles. All proteins were signed by rectangles. All the shadow rectangles were potential drug targets.

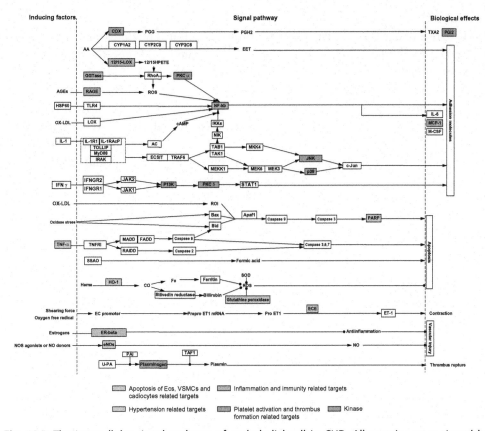

Fig. 12.2 The intracellular signal pathway of endothelial cell in CHD. All proteins were signed by rectangles. All the shadow rectangles were potential drug targets.

macrophage colony-stimulating factor 1 (M-CSF). In fact, except for ox-LDL, HSP 60, and cytokines such as arachidonic acid (AA), protein geranylgeranyltransferase type-1 (GGTase), advanced glycation endoproducts (AGEs), immunoreactive fibronectin-γ (IFN-γ), and interleukin-1 (IL-1) can also promote ECs to secrete adhesion molecules and chemotatic factors. With the help of these adhesion molecules and chemotatic factors, the atherosclerotic cells such as monocytes, lymphocytes, dendritic cells, mast cells, and platelets begin to accumulate and enter intima, thus increasing the likelihood of plaque formation.[14-16]

Apoptosis of ECs is an important event in ECs injury. As Fig. 12.2 shows, ox-LDL not only promotes the accumulation of atherogenic cells but also participates in the apoptosis of ECs by activating the caspase pathway. Oxidative stress and tumor necrosis factor-α (TNF-α) are also important factors leading to the apoptosis of ECs through regulating the caspase pathway.

12.1.2.2 VSMCs

VSMCs are essential for vascular contraction and relaxation. They alter the luminal diameter and enable blood vessels to maintain an appropriate blood pressure. The increased vascular contractility, migration, proliferation, and apoptosis of VSMCs are all important factors for the formation of atherosclerotic plaque.

(1) *Contractility*: The activation of the renin-angiotensin system (RAS) is an important event for contractility of VSMCs. Once RAS is activated, the level of renin in the blood is evaluated, thus promoting the production of Ang II. By combining with Ang II receptors (AgtR1 and AgtR2), the vascular contraction increases significantly (shown in Fig. 12.3).[17] ET-1, the strongest vasoconstrictor peptide secreted by impaired ECs, also can stimulate contraction of VSMCs.[18] In addition, as shown in Fig. 12.3, 5-hydroxytryptamine (5-HT) and AA metabolites such as hydroxy-eicosatetraenoic acids (HETEs) also make a contribution to the contraction of VSMCs.

(2) *Migration and proliferation*: As shown in Fig. 12.3, PDGF secreted by foam cells and activated platelets is the most important factor for migration and proliferation of VSMCs.[19] MMPs that can digest the extracellular matrix (ECM) in the intima also supply convenient conditions for migration of VSMCs. In addition, the urokinase-type plasminogen activator (U-PA) and the leukotriene B4 receptor 1 (BLT1) also can aggravate the migration of VSMCs through activating focal adhesion kinase 1 (FAK) and upregulating the production of MMPs (shown in Fig. 12.3).[20,21]

In the aspect of proliferation of VSMCs, except PDGF, Ang II and ET-1 are also important factors for the proliferation for VSMCs (shown in Fig. 12.3). In recent years, some studies demonstrated that urotensin II can also inducing the proliferation of VSMCs.[22,23]

(1) *Apoptosis*: Proliferation and apoptosis of SMCs are coincidence events which not only contribute to vessel remodeling but also lead to VSMCs destabilization of VSMCs fibrous cap in arteriosclerotic lesions.[24,25] Various stimuli, including oxidized lipoproteins, altered hemodynamic stress, and free radicals, can precipitate macrophage and T lymphocytes to secrete apoptosis factors. TNF-a and IFN-γ are typical factors that contribute to the apoptosis of VSMCs and ECs[24] (shown in Fig. 12.2). T lymphocytes can also induce apoptosis of VSMCs via the release of perforin and granzyme B (shown in Fig. 12.1). In addition, Fas-mediated apoptosis of VSMCs could be another important pathway as reported[26] (shown in Fig. 12.3).

12.1.2.3 Monocytes and Macrophages

Monocytes can enter intima and differentiate into macrophages in the formation of atherogenesis. As shown in Fig. 12.1, with the continuing expression of adhesion molecules on injured ECs, monocytes are initially attracted to lesion-prone sites. The initial adhesion involves selectins, which mediate a rolling interaction, and is followed by firmer attachment by means of integrins. Adherent monocytes migrate into intima with the help of chemo-attractant molecules MCP-1.[4,27] After migrating into the subendothelial space,

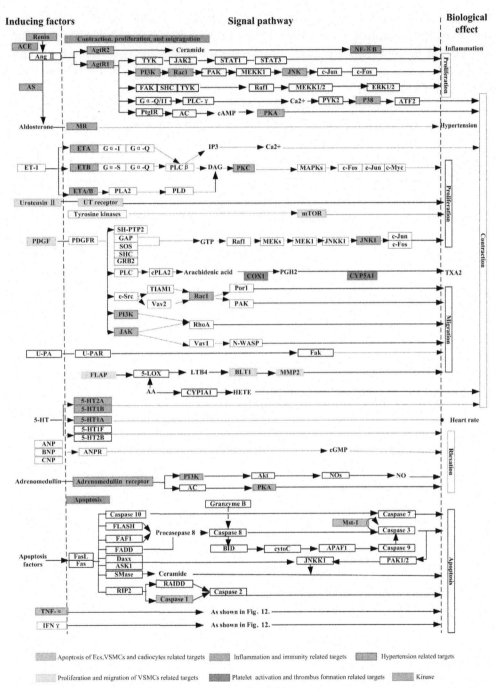

Fig. 12.3 The intracellular signal pathway of vascular smooth muscel cell in CHD. All proteins were signed by rectangles. All the shadow rectangles were potential drug targets.

monocytes differentiate into activated macrophages via the existence of M-CSF.[28] Once differentiation is finished, scavenger receptors such as scavenger receptor class A (SRA) and platelet glycoprotein 4 (CD36) on the surface of macrophages will phagocytose ox-LDL or other modified LDL, thus inducing the formation of foam cells and fatty streak in atherosclerosis.

Macrophages are considered to be major inflammatory mediators during atherosclerosis progression. As shown in Figs. 12.1 and 12.4, through combination of the CD40 ligand with its receptor, macrophages can express amounts of chemokines and cytokines such as MCP-1, RANTES, IL-1, IFN-γ, MMPs, TNF-α, and tissue factor.[29] Once macrophages develop into foam cells, they also secret an amount of cytokines. These factors continually augment in the flammatory reaction in vessels and promote the development of atherosclerosis[5,15] (Fig. 12.1). In addition to playing an important role in inflammation, macrophages also mediate the immunity reaction in atherosclerosis. Macrophages that contain phagotrophic ox-LDL particles act as antigen-presenting cells to T-cells[6] (Fig. 12.1).

Besides, a number of recent studies have demonstrated that macrophages also play an important role in reverse cholesterol transport.[30,31] Ox-LDL can be decomposed into cholesterol and oxysterol in macrophages. Cholesterol is further modified into cholesterol ester with the help of acyl–CoA cholesterol acyl transferase (ACAT) and this leads to the formation of foam cells. Oxysterol can activate the liver X receptor (LXR) in macophages, thus promoting cholesterol efflux through apolipoprotein A-1 (ApoAI). By upregulating the ATP-binding cassette transporter 1 (ABCA1) and ApoAI, the retinoic acid X activated peroxisome proliferator activated receptor (PPAR) also participates in the reverse transport of cholesterol in macrophages. In addition, the nuclear receptor ROR, the farnesoid X receptor (FXR) and the ADPribosylation factor-related protein 1 (ARP1) in macrophages can also regulate the transportation of cholesterol through activating or inhibiting ApoAI.

12.1.2.4 T Lymphocytes

T lymphocytes are the most important immune cells in atherosclerosis plaque. The transendothelial process of lymphocytes is similar to that of monocytes except using different chemo-attractants. Known chemo-attractants for T lymphocytes include inducible protein-10 (IP-10), monokine induced by IFN-γ (Mig), and IFN-inducible T-cell α-chemo-attractant (I-TAC).[15,32] These chemokines bind to C-X-C chemokine receptor type 3 (CXCR3), which is expressed by T lymphocytes in atherosclerotic lesion, and facilitate the migration of T lymphocytes (Fig. 12.1).

Once in the arterial intima, T lymphocytes have chances to interact with antigen-presenting cells (APCs) such as macrophages. More and more studies demonstrated that the CD40 ligand (CD40L) and its receptor CD40, which can be expressed in macrophages and T cells, play an important role in antigen presentation and autoimmunity as costimulatory factors.[33,34] Except macrophages, VSMCs are another kind of APCs that

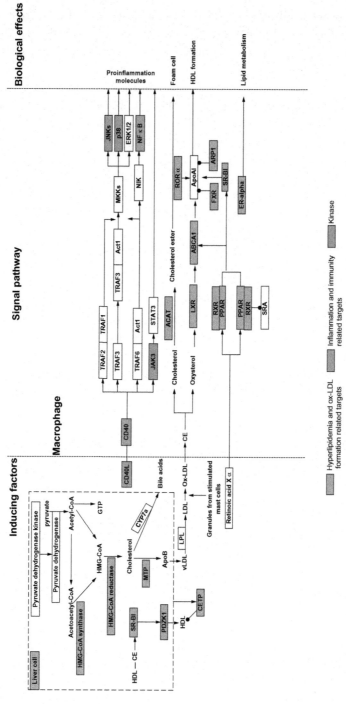

Fig. 12.4 The intracellular signal pathway of macrophage in CHD. All the shadow rectangles were signed by rectangles. All proteins were signed by rectangles. All the shadow rectangles were potential drug targets.

can be recognized by T cells. By binding to an HLA class II histocompatibility antigen (DR5), which is expressed by VSMCs, T cells are activated and then secrete granzyme B and perforin, both of which can induce apoptosis of VSMCs[8,26] (Fig. 12.1). In some studies, oxidized LDL and heat-shock protein 60 (HSP60) also have been identified as antigens for T lymphocytes.[35,36]

As can be seen in Fig. 12.1, activated T cells also predominate the production of proinflammatory cytokines such as IFN-γ, TNF α and β, and chemokines such as the C–C chemokine receptor type 5 (CCR5). These cytokines can augment the inflammatory and immune response.[37]

12.1.2.5 Mast Cells

Mast cells, an inflammatory cell type, contain highly enriched proteases, tryptase, and chymase in intracellular granules. They have been found to participate in the inflammatory reaction of atherosclerotic lesions.

As shown in Fig. 12.1, the transendothelial migration of mast cells is mediated by a chemo-attractant named eotaxin, which interacts with the chemokine receptor CXCR3 expressed on the surface of mast cells.[32] After entering intima and then being activated by complement system components such as complement C3a, complement C5a, and chemokines such as MCP-1,[38,39] mast cells become degranulated and release a number of inflammatory mediators including histamine, tryptase, chymase, and a variety of cytokines, which can promote vascular inflammation, endothelial dysfunction, and foam cell formation.[40] The subendothelial LDL can be modified by binding to the granule remnants from activated mast cells. These binding particles can be phagocytosed by macrophages more likely than LDL alone, thus promoting the formation of foam cells[41] (Fig. 12.4). A study has demonstrated that granules from stimulated mast cells can also degrade the capability of removing cholesterol from macrophages.[42] Therefore, mast cells not only promote LDL aggregation but also interfere with cholesterol removal, both of which contribute to foam cell formation.

Mast cells can also weaken the fibrous cap in different ways as follows (Fig. 12.1): (1) Activated mast cells may release MMPs, such as MMP-1 and MMP-9, both of which directly cause matrix degradation.[43,44] (2) Secreted tryptase and chymase precipitate the pro-MMPs forming active MMPs.[40,45] (3) Stimulated mast cells can express TNF-α, which is able to enhance the apoptosis of VSMCs, macrophages, and ECs, and subsequently weaken and rupture the atherosclerotic plaques.[46] (4) Chymase released from mast cells is reported to activate caspase-8 and caspase-9, two key effector molecules in apoptotic cascade.[47]

12.1.2.6 Dendritic Cells

DCs are also antigen-presenting cells with the unique ability to initiate a primary immune response by activating native T lymphocytes. Though, DCs are typically localized in the subendothelial space as indigenous residents of healthy arteries; circulating DCs in blood can evade into an injury site with the help of chemokines and adhesion molecules in the progress of atherosclerosis.[48] As shown in Fig. 12.1, adhesion molecules such as P-selectin, E-selectin, and VCAM-1 and chemokines such as C-X-C motif chemokine 3 (CXCL3) and C–C motif chemokine 5 (CCL5) are all potential candidates for recruiting DCs to transendothelium.[49,50] The granulocyte/macrophage colony-stimulating factor (GM-CSF), which may facilitate the transformation of transendothelial monocytes into DCs, is another factor to increasing the number of DCs in the atherosclerotic area.[51]

Subendothelium DCs express toll-like receptors (TLRs) to recognize dangerous signals and phagocytize antigens such as oxidized LDL and heat-shock proteins. Once finishing the process of phagocytosis, DCs become activated and produce vast amounts of cytokines such as IFN-α and interleukin-12 (IL-12). IFN-α can upregulate the expression of the proapoptotic protein TRAIL on T lymphocytes, thereby multiplying their ability to kill plaque resident cells.[8,52] IL-12 can upregulate the expression of the chemokine receptor CCR5 on T lymphocytes, which in turn leads to the accumulation of T lymphocytes in the atherosclerotic plaque.[53]

12.1.2.7 Platelets

Platelets play an important role in the hemostatic process and thrombus formation as well as in the inflammation reaction in atherosclerotic plaque.

After the injury of ECs, the endothelial cells' barrier is lost. Extracellular matrix leaks from the intima and triggers the formation of a hemostatic thrombus. In this event, platelets participate in three successive and closely integrated biological processes, that is, adhesion, activation, and aggregation[54] (Fig. 12.5).

(1) At impaired vascular lesions, extracellular matrix components such as von Willebrand factor (vWF) and collagen are exposed to the blood. Platelets can detect these changes in blood circulation and adhere to collagen via the membrane adhesion receptor GPVI (platelet glycoprotein VI), which leads to further combination of vWF with integrin receptors GpIb-IX-V (platelet glycoprotein IX-V) and collagen with α2β1 (integrin alpha-2) in platelets, thus resulting in fast adhesion.[55–58]

(2) Once adhesive receptors combine with their ligands on extracellular matrix components, the activation of platelets will start. This process can be further strengthened by thrombin, adenosine diphosphate (ADP), epinephrine, and thromboxane A2 (TXA2), all of which are synthesized by stimulated platelets.[54,59–61]

(3) Aggregation is mediated by adhesive substrates bounding to membranes of activated platelets. Among adhesive substrates, activated GPIIb/IIIa (integrin beta-3/integrin alpha-IIb) is one of the most important factors contributing to the stable adhesion and recruiting of more platelets.[54,62] Platelets are also mediators of inflammation involved in the development of atherosclerosis. As shown in Fig. 12.1, (1) activated platelets can release P-selectin, which promotes monocyte recruitment via platelet-monocyte

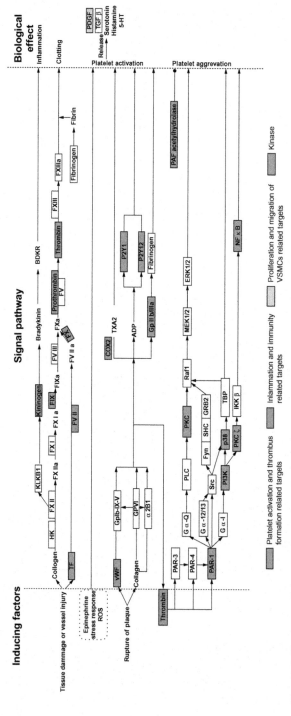

Fig. 12.5 The intracellular signal pathway of platelet in CHD. All proteins were signed by rectangles. All the shadow rectangles were potential drug targets.

interactions and delivers platelets' proinflammatory factors to monocytes; (2) activated platelet surfaces also express CD40L, which further binds to CD40 on the surface of ECs to upregulate the expression of adhesion molecules and chemokines in ECs[63]; and (3) activated platelets can release an amount of proinflammatory cytokines, chemokines, growth factors, and blood coagulation factors, thus promoting leukocytes recruitment and proliferation of VSMCs 17 (Fig. 12.2).

12.1.2.8 Cadiocytes

Once obstruction happens in coronary vessels, myocardial ischemia takes place and disturbs the normal function of cadiocytes, including dysfunction of the myocardial energy metabolism, abnormal intracellular Ca2+ handling, cadiocytes hypertrophy, and apoptosis.

(1) Dysfunction of the energy metabolism

During ischemia, the cardiac energy metabolism is dramatically altered, resulting in fatty acid oxidation as the dominant source of oxidative metabolism at the expense of glucose oxidation.[64] As shown in Fig. 12.6, the proteins in the AMPK (5′-AMP-activated protein kinase) pathway such as carnitine palmitoyl tranferase 1 (CPT-1), acetyl CoA carboxylase (ACC), and malonyl CoA decarboxylase (MCD) are important modifier factors in the energy metabolism of fatty acid.[65]

Except with the imbalance of the energy metabolism between fatty acid and glucose in the ischemic heart, the other proteins related to energy such as the F1F0 ATPase also become abnormal.[66] F1F0 ATPase is a critical enzyme to release ATP from the catalytic F1 domain. But under ischemic conditions, this enzyme became an ATP hydrolase leading to an undesirable hydrolysis of ATP in the ischemic heart.[67,68]

To overcome myocardial ischemia, an endogenic reimbursement mechanism is activated. Hypoxia-inducible factor 1-alpha (HIF-α) may function as a master regulator of oxygen homeostasis.[69,70] By enhancing the transport of glucose, HIF-α increases the oxidation of pyruvate participating in the production of ATP in mitochondrion.

(2) Abnormal intracellular Ca2+ handling

Once heart ischemia happens, the concentration of noradrenaline/adrenaline, Ang II, ET-1, dopamine, acetylcholine, and histamine in circulation significantly increases. By binding to their receptors on cadiocytes, these factors induce abnormal intracellular Ca2+ handling. In cadiocytes, both calcium release channel ryanodine receptor (RyR) and sarcoplasmic reticulum Ca2+-ATPase (SERCA2) can mediate Ca2+ releasing into the sarcoplasmic reticulum, thus inducing the decrease of the intracellular Ca2+ concentration. An L-type Ca2+ channel (LTCC) is a Ca2+ inRow channel that may induce the increase of intracellular Ca2+ concentration[71,72] (Fig. 12.6). The dysfunction of these proteins will directly result in abnormal Ca2+ handling.

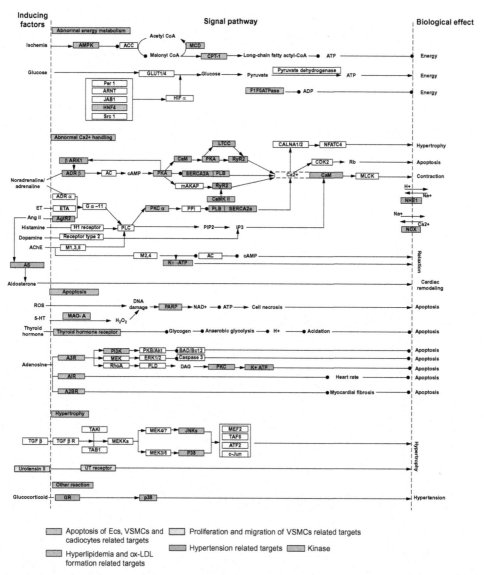

Fig. 12.6 The intracellular signal pathway of cadiocyte in CHD. All proteins were signed by rectangles. All the shadow rectangles were potential drug targets.

(3) Hypertrophy of cadiocytes

Hypertrophy is another significant pathological change as the result of ischemia. Elevated Ca2+ concentration is an important factor for cadiocytes hypertrophy. High levels of Ang II and ET-1 after ischemia can seriously affect Ca2+ concentration in cadiocytes (Fig. 12.6). There are some other upregulated cytokines that contribute to cadiocytes hypertrophy. For example, both transforming growth factor beta-1 (TGF-β) and urotensin II can combine with their receptors on the surface of cadiocytes and then induce hypertrophy (Fig. 12.6).

(4) Cell apoptosis in the ischemic heart

While the dysfuction of the energy metabolism and abnormal intracellular Ca2+ handling can induce the apoptosis of cadiocytes, some other factors can also contribute to this process. As Fig. 12.6 shows, with the help of monoamine oxidase, 5-HT can produce H_2O_2. H_2O_2 and another noxious substances reactive oxygen species (ROS) both can lead to DNA strand breakage.[73,74] Subsequently, poly(ADPribose) polymerase (PARP) induces an inefficient cellular metabolic cycle and promotes cadiocyte death.[75,76]

On the other side, some endogenous factors such as the thyroid hormone and adenosine are beneficial to cadiocytes in the hypoxia condition. For example, adenosine is released by ischemic cadiocytes and subsequently reduces cellular injury and restores energetic homeostasis by binding to its receptors.[77,78] The single pathway of adenosine and thyroid hormone are shown in Fig. 12.6.

12.1.3 Conclusion

CHD is a chronic and multifactorial disease. As hundreds of complex signal pathways are contained in the CHD formation, it is important to construct a biological network and protein database about CHD. In this review, we not only compiled CHD-related signal pathways and a protein database, but also provided a comprehensive knowledge of drug targets and their application in the clinic for the treatment of CHD. As the protein database includes potential drug targets for the treatment of CHD, it may help drug discovery in the future. With the development of drug discovery, it can be anticipated that more and more efficient medicinal solutions would be applied in clinic for the treatment of CHD.

12.2. THERAPEUTIC MECHANISM OF THE SHEXIANG BAOXIN PILL ON CARDIOVASCULAR DISEASES FROM THE PERSPECTIVE OF PROTEIN INTERACTION NETWORKS AND SIGNALING PATHWAYS

Abstract

The *Shexiang Baoxin Pill* (SBP) is commonly used to treat cardiovascular disease (CVD) in China. However, the complexity of composition and targets has deterred our understanding of its mechanism of action. Using network pharmacology-based approaches, we established the mechanism of action for SBP to treat CVD by analyzing protein-protein interactions and pathways. The computational results were confirmed at the gene expression level in microarray-based studies. Two of the SBP's targets were further confirmed at the protein level by Western blot. In addition, we validated the theory that the SBP's plasma-absorbed compounds play a major therapeutic role in treating CVD.

Keywords: Network pharmacology, Protein-protein interaction networks, Signaling pathways, Gene expression, Western blot

12.2.1 Introduction

Cardiovascular disease (CVD) is a group of disorders that affects heart and blood vessels. It mainly includes coronary heart disease,[79] atherosclerosis,[80] myocardial ischemia,[81] myocardial fibrosis,[82] cerebrovascular disease,[83] peripheral arterial disease,[84] congenital heart disease, and deep vein thrombosis.[85,86] In comparison to common acute diseases (e.g., influenza), complex chronic diseases such as CVD cannot be completely cured. Drugs mainly regulate disease progression and relieve the symptoms. The treatment goal for these complex chronic diseases is to regulate the pathological state, thus controlling disease manifestation and retarding progression.[87]

In China, the *Shexiang Baoxin Pill* (SBP) has a long history of clinical application to treat coronary heart disease,[79] atherosclerosis,[80] myocardial ischemia,[81] and myocardial fibrosis,[82] with significant curative effects. Earlier studies investigated the SBP's activities in cells and animal models.[88–91] Recent studies revealed that the SBP exerts a range of pharmacological activities, including increasing the level of NO,[92] enhancing the expression of endothelial NO synthase,[89] alleviating damage to blood vessels,[93] decreasing MMP-2 expression,[94] and promoting myocardial ischemia caused by myocardial necrosis.[95] Although the SBP has been extensively evaluated for clinical efficacy, its mechanism of function remains unresolved.

The SBP is composed of seven medicinal materials, including Moschus, total ginosenoside ginseng root, Styrax, Cinnamomi Cortex, Bufonis Venenum, Bovis Calculus Artifactus, and Borneolum Syntheticum. Each ingredient contains a large number of chemical compounds. Like all TCM formulae, SBP is a multicomponent and multitarget agent from the molecular perspective. As a result, its mode of action is most likely to be illustrated by network pharmacology-based approaches.

Based on the TCM formula's characteristics of complex components, unclear targets, and holistic regulation, we have proposed a workflow for a network-based TCM pharmacology study.[87] It starts with the identification of compounds present in the TCM formula and corresponding targets, and ends with discovering the signaling pathways and subnetworks regulated by the TCM formula and evaluating its effects on the disease network. Several studies have been conducted following this flow diagram, revealing the modes of action for different TCM formulae.[95]

It is clear that the identification of compounds contained in the TCM formula constitutes the basis of the network-based TCM pharmacology study. Two different strategies have been used regarding compound selection. Some studies included all the identified compounds in every single component of the TCM formula. For example, Zhang et al. studied all 451 compounds from the five Chinese herbs of the TCM formula Wu-tou decoction.[96] On the other hand, considering that most TCM formulae are taken orally, it is assumed that only the compounds that appear in blood are biologically active.

Therefore, other studies only included compounds detected in the plasma after the administration of the TCM formula.[97,98] We used this strategy to analyze the antirheumatic effects of the TCM formula Huang-Lian-Jie-Du-Tang (HLJDT), in which only 14 active compounds from HLJDT were examined.[99] However, very few studies have compared the effects of plasma-absorbed compounds of a TCM formula with that of a full compound set.

This study is to investigate the mechanism of action for the SBP to treat CVD using network pharmacology-based methods, and to elucidate if the plasma-absorbed compounds are responsible for the SBP's anti-CVD therapeutic effects. Following extensive data mining, we assembled a list of CVD-related disease genes, two sets of SBP compounds, and their corresponding targets. The algorithm of random walk with restart (RWR) was applied to calculate the regulation scores of disease genes and to target proteins to the human protein-protein interaction (PPI) network and pathways, respectively. The computational results were verified by microarray-based experiments and two SBP targets were validated by Western blot.

12.2.2 Materials and Methods

12.2.2.1 Data Preparation

CVD associated genes. DisGeNet is a plugin of Cytoscope,[100] which has collected various classes of disease-associated genes. On the settings window of "Diseasegene Network" in Cytoscope, we set "select source" as "All," "select association type" as "Any," and "select disease class" as "Cardiovascular Disease." In this way, we obtained 301 CVD associated genes (see Table S2 in Supplementary).

All compounds included in the SBP and their corresponding targets. The SBP contains seven medicinal materials that include Moschus, total ginsenoside ginseng root, Styrax, Cinnamomi Cortex, Bufonis Venenum, Bovis Calculus Artifactus, and Borneolum Syntheticum. We used several TCM databases, including TCMDS,[101] HIT,[102] TCM Database@Taiwan,[103] TCMID,[104] and 3D-MSDT,[105] to collect information about all compounds in the SBP. Using the name of each SBP individual medicinal material as input, we searched these databases and acquired the names and chemical structures of compounds from the corresponding medicinal ingredient as output. The outputs from these databases were combined to assemble a list of all identified SBP compounds. There are 166 chemically distinct compounds in total (see Table S3 in Supplementary). These are considered as full compounds included in the SBP. For each compound, we searched its putative targets in the following two databases:

(1) *Herbal Ingredients' Targets Database (HIT)*[102]: HIT is a comprehensive and fully curated database that contains information on the protein targets of compounds found in Chinese herbs. Based on over 3250 papers in the literature, HIT includes 1301 protein targets affected by 586 herbal compounds found in more than 1300

Chinese herbs (http://lifecenter.sgst.cn/hit/). By searching the database with the name of the chemical compound, we will be able to obtain information on its target proteins if this compound is included in the HIT.

(2) *Search Tool for Interactions of Chemicals (STITCH)*[106]: STITCH is a collective database from 1133 organisms (http://stitch.embl.de/), composed of interactions existing between 300,000 small molecules and 2.6 million proteins. The biggest asset of STITCH is the huge amount of data and the structural similarity comparison tool it provides. In the event that we cannot find the targets of a compound in HIT and STITCH, we can input its structure into STITCH and identify similar chemical molecules with a similarity score greater than 0.9. Targets of these chemically similar compounds are considered putative targets of the queried compound.

At the end, 522 distinct protein targets of the SBP were obtained after integrating HIT and STITCH search results, in which 86 were identified from HIT, 416 were from STITCH, and 20 are included in both databases (see Table S4 in Supplementary).

SBP's plasma absorbed compounds and their targets. Our earlier serum medicinal chemistry and pharmacokinetic studies identified 34 compounds in the plasma after oral administration of the SBP,[92,107] 26 of which were the original chemical compounds found in SBP, and 8 of which were metabolites. Among the 26 compounds from SBP, 1 is from Moschus, 7 are from the total gingenoside ginsenoside ginseng root, 8 are from Bufonis Venenum, 5 are from Bovis Calculus Artifactus, 3 are from Styrax, and 2 are from Borneolum Syntheticum. Mining HIT and STITCH databases, we identified 113 distinct targets for these 26 original chemical compounds. Targets of the eight metabolites cannot be found, thus they are not pursued in this study. The detailed information is provided in Table S5 of Supplementary.

For convenience, we named all compounds included in the SBP and SBP's plasma-absorbed compounds as SBPac and SBPpc, respectively. When studying TCM pharmacology at the molecular level, all compounds identified in a TCM formula are considered to be equivalent to the formula itself. Thus in this study, we think SBPac is equivalent to the SBP itself.

Protein-protein interaction data. Protein-protein interactions in the human genome were extracted from version 9.05 of STRING,[108] a weighted interaction database with physical and functional interactions that are integrated from multiple data sources (such as experimental data, computation-based prediction, and literature mining). STRING gives each interaction a confidence score (which was normalized to the interval of [0, 1]) by a scoring system to weigh the reliability of the interaction.

In order to construct a background PPI network with high confidence edges, we first filtered the STRING with threshold 0.9. Only interactions with weight above the threshold were selected for the newly constructed background network. We also checked whether CVD disease genes and the SBP's target proteins are covered in the new network. In case of existing disease or target genes that are included in STRING but not in the new network, we lowered the threshold for these genes and their interactions until all these genes were included in the background network. As a result, a weighted PPI background network with 9289 nodes and 57,179 edges was obtained.

Data of pathway gene sets. A total of 4722 pathway gene sets was derived from the C2: CP collection of the MSigDB database,[109] which is a comprehensive integration of certain online pathway databases such as BioCarta, Reactome, and KEGG.

12.2.2.2 Microarray Experiment and Significantly Expressed Genes

Cell lines and treatment. The cell line we used in this study is MCF7, one of the five cell lines used in the connectivity map (CMAP) database as reference cells to connect biology, chemistry, and different clinical conditions including CVD.[110–112] MCF7 cells were obtained from the American Type Culture Collection (ATCC) and maintained in MEM/EBSS (Hyclone), supplemented with 10% fetal bovine serum, 1mM sodium pyruvate, 0.1mM MEM nonessential amino acids, 100unit/mL penicillin, and 100mg/mL streptomycin in a humidified environment under 5% CO_2:95% Air at 37°C. MCF7 cells were treated with SBP extract at 1 μg/mL for 12h. Stock solutions of the SBP were prepared in DMSO. Solvent (DMSO) treated cells were used as control, the same as most microarray experiments.[112,113]

RNA isolation. Total RNA samples were extracted from MCF7 cells using Trizol reagent (Life technologies, Carlsbad, CA, USA). The integrity and purity of total RNA samples were monitored by formaldehyde agarose gel electrophoresis, and quantified by spectrophotometry (NanoDrop, Wilmington, DE, USA).

Microarray analysis. RNA samples were purified from cells using the QIAGEN RNeasy Kit (GmBH, Germany). Biological replica was included for each cell line. cRNA products, generated from the fragmentation of double-stranded cDNA and biotin-labeled cRNA, were pooled to perform microarray experiments using the Affymetrix chip (Human U133 A 2.0), by Shanghai Biotechnology Corporation following the Affymetrix technical manual.

The SBP-related microarray experiments yielded 621 differentially expressed genes, with mean expression ratios between the SBPac group and the control group greater than 4 or lower than 0.25. The detailed results are shown in Table S6 of Supplementary.

12.2.2.3 RWR-Based Evaluation of Drug's Effect

The hypothesis for analyzing polygenic diseases and corresponding intervention in the molecule network is that genes and their products do not fulfill their biological functions independently but through prevalent interactions among different genes, and these interactions constitute a molecular network. Single gene alteration(s) incurred by diseases or drugs will affect its neighboring genes, forming a subnetwork impacted by diseases or drugs. Fig. 12.7 shows the flow diagram of determining a drug's effect based on random walk with restart (RWR).

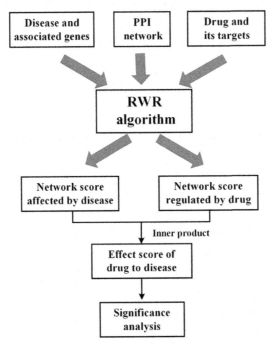

Fig. 12.7 Flow diagram to evaluate the effect of a drug based on RWR.

RWR Algorithm

Random walk with restart (RWR) is an improved algorithm derived from the random walk algorithm.[114] It simulates a random walker that starts from nodes in the seed set. At any time, the walker can either randomly move to a neighboring node from the current position or return to a seed node at a relatively low probability.

RWR effectively measures the proximity of a node to a seed set so that nodes adjacent to the seed set can be prioritized. In view of this utility, RWR has been applied to predict potential disease genes by employing part of known disease genes to detect novel disease genes.[115–117] To be more specific, causative disease genes are considered as a seed set while candidate genes in the PPI network are ranked based on their proximity to the seed set scored by RWR in descending order. The genes with the highest score are most likely to be disease-relevant.

In this study, disease genes and drug target genes were selected as seed nodes, respectively. The extent of each gene in the network affected by the disease or drug is determined by way of scoring each gene by RWR. In general, the higher score a gene receives, the more pronounced the effect by the disease or drug. Specifically, a node's score at the $t+1$ step is calculated as:

$$x^{t+1} = (1-r)Px^t + rx^0 \qquad (12.1)$$

P is the column–normalized adjacent matrix of the PPI network that represents the connectivity between nodes, x^0 is the initial probability vector indicating a preference to the seed set, and r is the restart probability that generally has a low value. For a nonbipartite and undirected graph, the equation is deemed to converge. Thus, node scores can be obtained after performing the iteration in Eq. (12.1). It is obvious that the closer the nodes connected to the seed set, the higher the scores, and vice versa. The r in Eq. (12.1) is a parameter that varies with practical prioritization needs. In order to choose the optimal r, Erten et al. altered r values to determine how RWR affects candidates' rank.[117] It was found that an r value of 0.3 outperforms others. Thus, r denoted by 0.3 is generally adopted in the ranking of sound disease genes. We set r as 0.3 in this research.

Scoring Disease's Effect on the Human PPI Network

Scoring a disease's effect on the human PPI network is a process that estimates the proximity between each gene and disease genes by the RWR algorithm. Disease-associated genes are viewed as the seed set. If there are m diseases genes in total, the corresponding initial component of a disease gene in Eq. (12.1) is $x_0(i) = 1/m$, otherwise, $x_0(i) = 0$. By iterating Eq. (12.1), the steady solution $x_{disease}$ that represents the disease's effect on the human PPI network is obtained.

Scoring Drug's Effect on the Human PPI Network

To obtain the scores measuring the effect(s) of a drug on the background network, drug target proteins are used as the seed set.

If gene i is the target gene of active ingredients in the TCM formula, its corresponding component in the initial vector is set as $x_0(i) = 0.01$, otherwise $x_0(i) = 0$.

The reason for the initial vector selection is that active ingredients in the TCM formula are natural products with generally weaker effects on target proteins in comparison to chemically defined drug molecules. Moreover, our previous study found that the FDA-approved drug has around two orders of inhibition effect on target proteins ACE and CN than the natural compound Astragaloside, when applied at the same dose.[118]

For each drug, their respective effect scores on the PPI network x_{drug} are acquired with Eq. (12.1).

In order to evaluate TCM formulae in a statistically significant fashion, we set up 1000 random counterpart sets of target proteins, each of which includes the same number of proteins randomly selected from the network. We reran the RWR process on each of these random seed sets.

Scoring Effects of a Drug to Disease

In the network, the easier a node can be influenced by the seed set, the higher the score it will gain and vice versa. Therefore, genes with high scores and ranked above a defined threshold form a disease-affected subnetwork that is vulnerable to diseases. A similar definition is used to establish a drug-affected subnetwork. The extent of overlap between the two subnetworks is used to predict whether the drug can effectively exert its influence on the disease. This overlap can be quantitatively measured by an inner product of $x_{disease}$ and x_{drug} so as to evaluate the performance of the drug in the treatment of the disease.[119] The equation is

$$s = \left\langle x_{disease}, x_{drug} \right\rangle \tag{12.2}$$

Scoring Effects of a Drug or Disease on Pathways

Signaling pathways are relatively independent biomolecule subsystems or interaction subnetworks that carry out important biological tasks and complex information processing between molecules. Scoring signaling pathways allows us to identify biological processes influenced by diseases or regulated by drugs.

As shown in Fig. 12.8, we score the effects of a drug or disease on pathways by mapping network scores of genes calculated onto the pathway gene sets. The details are provided below.

(1) Using RWR to score the effect(s) of a disease or drug on all genes in the PPI network;

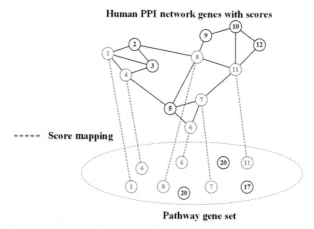

Fig. 12.8 Map network genes' scores to the pathway gene set.

(2) Mapping gene scores generated in step (1) to the corresponding genes in pathways. For genes on the pathways that are not included in the background network, their scores are assigned as zero (Fig. 12.8).

(3) Adding up the scores in each pathway and denoting the average scores as a disease's or drug's effect scores on the pathway.

Evaluation Measures

To determine if the TCM formula exerts significant effect(s) on the network, we generate a wide spectrum of random seed sets (e.g., 1000 sets). Each seed set is randomly generated, containing the same number of target proteins as that of the original seed set. For each random counterpart, we compute its effect scores on each gene of the background network by Eq. (12.1).

Here Z-score is introduced to quantify the score difference existing between the original seed set and its counterparts. It is expressed as follows:

$$Z = \frac{s - \bar{s}_r}{\Delta s_r} \tag{12.3}$$

where s is the antidisease effect score of the TCM formula, while $\bar{s}_r$ and Δs_r represent mean and standard deviation of the scores stemming from random counterparts, respectively.

Then, for each disease and drug, we take pathways with the highest 5% scores, respectively. These are considered as pathways significantly influenced by the disease or regulated by the drug. The common pathways influenced by the disease and drug are used to measure drug efficacy from the biological perspective.

12.2.2.4 Target Validation by Western Blot

Drug Preparation

SBP samples were ground into fine powder. Four grams of accurately weighed sample powder were transferred to a 250 mL round bottom flask, extracted with 52 mL mixed solvent (methanol:dichlormethane:water = 4:2:0.5, v/v) by ultrasonic extraction (30 min), filtered, and the filtrate collected. The detailed extraction method was described in Ref.[120] The filtrated extract sample was dried by rotation evaporation under 55°C. A stock solution of 50 mg/mL was prepared by dissolving a 5 mg extract sample in 100 µL DMSO.

A total number of 26 SBP compounds detected in plasma were used to prepare SBPpc. Specifically, the stock solution of SBP's plasma-absorbed compounds was prepared by dissolving the mixture of all 26 compounds in DMSO at a concentration of 100 mg/mL. See Table 12.1 for contents of the compounds in the solution.

Table 12.1 Content of the 26 bioactive compounds in the SBPpc solution

No.	Compound	Content (mg)
S-1	Muscone	1.05
S-2	Bufalin	4.95
S-3	Resibufogenin	3.33
S-4	Cinobufogenin/cinobufagin	0.64
S-5	Gamabufagin	0.63
S-6	Arenobufagin	0.62
S-7	Telocinobufagin	0.09
S-8	Bufotalin	0.23
S-9	Cinbufotalin	0.15
S-10	Cholic acid	5.1
S-11	Deoxycholic acid	0.88
S-12	Chenodeoxycholic acid	0.57
S-13	Hyodeoxycholic acid	0.44
S-14	Ursodeoxycholic acid	1.48
S-15	Cinnamic aldehyde	1.43
S-16	Cinnamic acid	0.36
S-17	Ginsenoside Rb_1	7.65
S-18	Ginsenoside Rb_2	4.64
S-19	Ginsenoside Rb_3	2.43
S-20	Ginsenoside Rc	7.26
S-21	Ginsenoside Rd	4.73
S-22	Ginsenoside Re	7.27
S-23	Ginsenoside Rg_1	8.75
S-24	Borneol	82.37
S-25	(+)-Borneol	31.63
S-26	Benzyl benzonate	8.37

Western Blot Analysis in Human Umbilical Vein Endothelial Cells

Human Umbilical Vein Endothelial Cells (HUVEC) were purchased from AllCells (Emeryville, CA, USA). The antibodies used for Western blot analysis are: rabbit anti-human intercellular adhesion molecule-1, rabbit antihuman cyclooxygenase 2, and mouse antihuman GAPDH (Beyotime, Shanghai, China). Human tumor necrosis factor alpha (TNFα) was from PeproTech (Rocky Hill, NJ, USA).

HUVECs were seeded into 60 mm cell culture plates with complete endothelial growth medium (AllCells). After reaching 80% confluence, cells were exposed to the SBP extract and SBPpc in the presence or absence of TNFα (25 ng/mL) for 16 h. The conditioned media were removed, HUVECs washed and lysed, and protein concentrations determined using the BCA protein assay kit (Beyotime, Shanghai, China). The lysate samples were stored in −80°C.

Samples containing equal amounts of proteins were separated by SDS–PAGE electrophoresis (10% SDS-polyacrylamide gel), and transferred onto polyvinyl membranes. The membranes were blocked with 5% dry milk in TRIS-buffered saline containing 0.1%

Tween 20 (room temperature, 1 h), incubated with the specified primary antibodies (dilutions: COX-2 1:500, ICAM-1 1:1000, and GAPDH 1:1000) overnight at 4°C. The membranes were visualized using Odessey (LI-COR, Lincoln, NE, USA).

12.2.3 Results and Discussion

12.2.3.1 Overlap of CVD Disease Genes With the SBP's Target Genes

From the pharmaceutical perspective, proteins encoded by disease genes may serve as potential drug targets for treatment. Earlier network analysis of the DrugBank database revealed that certain FDA-approved drugs, including those that treat cardiovascular diseases, preferentially target disease genes.[121] To determine if the SBP acts in a similar manner, we counted the number of CVD disease genes that are also SBP target genes. Among the 522 target genes of SBPac, 46 are CVD disease genes, which is 15.3% of the total disease genes. However, SBPpc targeted only 11 CVD disease genes, ~3.7% of the total disease genes. Table 12.2 summarizes the 11 common genes and their functions.

All 11 genes are associated with the functions of heart or blood vessels that are important in the etiology of CVD. Given the fact that there are 301 CVD-associated genes, targeting 46 or 11 out of 301 genes is not sufficient to explain the SBP's efficacy in treating CVD.

12.2.3.2 Network Analysis of SBP on CVD

To quantitatively display the effect of the SBP on CVD treatment from a network perspective, we applied the RWR algorithm to measure the impact of seed nodes on other nodes in the background network.

By setting CVD disease genes and target genes of SBPac and SBPpc as seed nodes, respectively, we first used Eq. (12.1) to calculate the effect score vectors of CVD, SBPac,

Table 12.2 CVD disease genes targeted by the SBP's plasma-absorbed compounds (SBPpc)

No.	Gene symbol	Gene function
1	COL1A1	Platelet–derived growth factor binding protein[122]
2	CYP2C9	Heme binding protein[123]
3	ESR2	A group of heme-thiolate monooxygenases[124]
4	ICAM1	Ligands for the leukocyte adhesion protein LFA-1 (integrin alpha-L/beta-2)[125]
5	LDLR	Receptor of low-density lipoprotein (plasma cholesterol apolipoprotein)[126]
6	MMP9	May play an essential role in local proteolysis of the extracellular matrix and in leukocyte migration[127]
7	NOS3	Modulate angiogenesis, blood pressure, and calcium channel[128]
8	COX-2	Regulate vasoconstriction and blood pressure[129]
9	TGFB1	Regulation of vascular endothelial cell migration[130]
10	TLR4	Immune response and inflammatory process regulation[131]
11	VCAM1	Involved in calcium-mediated signaling pathways of intracellular calcium source[132]

Table 12.3 The effect scores of SBPac and SBPpc on CVD

Name	Target number	Effect score	Z-score
The SBP's all compounds (SBPac)	522	0.4452	12.1930
The SBP's plasma-absorbed compounds (SBPpc)	113	0.1138	7.7493

and SBPpc on the background network. Eq. (12.2) was subsequently applied to calculate the inner products between affected vectors of CVD and SBPac and CVD and SBPpc. The network effect scores of SBPac and SBPpc on CVD were 0.4452 and 0.1138, respectively.

To determine whether the network effect scores of the drug to disease are significant, we compared their scores with the scores obtained from random seed sets. Based on the 522 targets of SBPac and 113 targets of SBPpc, we generated 1000 random target gene sets from the background network, respectively. Each of these sets contained the same number of targets as SBPac and SBPpc, respectively. The scores from random seed sets could be obtained using Eqs. (12.1), (12.2). The average and standard deviation values of effect scores for the 1000 random counterparts of each group were calculated. The Z-scores of the effect scores of SBPac and SBPpc to CVD were obtained using Eq. (12.3). As shown in Table 12.3, the Z-score values are 12.193 and 7.749 of SBPac and SBPpc, suggesting that the subnetworks regulated by them overlap significantly with the CVD-impacted subnetwork. This is because a Z-score value greater than 3 often indicates a statistically significant deviation between the actual value and the random ones. Therefore, we can conclude that both SBPac and SBPpc have significant effects to CVD.

12.2.3.3 Pathways Significantly Regulated by SBP

We mapped the network scores of genes from the calculation above to the 4722 pathways from the C2:CP collection of the MSigDB database. For those genes on the pathways that cannot be mapped, their scores were assigned zero. The average value of all genes on each pathway was obtained. Using this approach, we acquired effect scores of CVD disease genes and SBPac and SBPpc target genes on each pathway, respectively.

We defined pathways significantly regulated by the disease or drug as those with scores ranked in the top 5% of the 4722 pathways. This classification led to 236 pathways affected by CVD, SBPac, and SBPpc, respectively. Among the 236 pathways significantly impacted by CVD, 113 and 97 are also regulated by SBPac and SBPpc (Fig. 12.9), constituting 47.8% and 41% of the CVD pathways, respectively. The observation that nearly half of CVD-affected pathways are regulated by the SBP supports the therapeutic effect of the SBP on CVD.

There are 81 pathways that are significantly affected by CVD and regulated by SBPac and SBPpc both, constituting 71.7% of the SBPac-regulated CVD affected pathways. Since SBPac is considered as equivalent to the SBP itself, these results suggest that the SBP's plasma-absorbed compounds play major roles in the SBP's treatment of CVD.

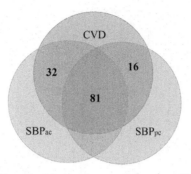

Fig. 12.9 The Venn diagram of the coinciding pathway number from CVD, SBPac, and SBPpc regulated pathways.

12.2.3.4 Microarray Experiment Validation

Microarray-based studies were performed to verify the network analysis results. A total of 621 genes with mean expression ratios of the SBP group to the control group greater than 4 or less than 0.25 were considered differentially expressed genes.

Among these 621 genes, only 31 and 9 genes are target genes of SBPac and SBPpc, respectively, identified by the bioinformatics method. Meanwhile, 29 of the 621 genes are CVD disease genes, among which two genes—ICAM1 and COX-2—are also target genes of SBPac and SBPpc. Both ICAM1 and COX-2 are important disease genes associated with CVD.

The 621 significantly expressed genes were set as the seed nodes and the corresponding component of the gene in the initial vector as the normalized differential expression ratio. Using an approach similar to that described earlier, we calculated the differentially expressed genes' network effect scores on CVD and on each of the 4722 pathways from the C2:CP collection of the MSigDB database. This led to the identification of 236 pathways significantly regulated by these 621 genes with scores in the top 5%. Among them, 119 pathways are affected by CVD, which is 50.4% of all 236 pathways. These gene expression data further support the therapeutic effect of the SBP on CVD.

We compared the 113 and 97 CVD-affected pathways, which are also regulated by SBPac and SBPpc, with the 119 CVD-affected pathways regulated by significantly expressed genes under the SBP treatment, respectively. It was found that 80 of the 113 SBPac-affected pathways and 70 of the 97 SBPpc-affected pathways also appeared in these 119 pathways, corresponding to 67.2% and 58.8%, respectively. Specifically, 63 CVD-affected pathways are also regulated by SBPac, SBPpc, and altered gene expression significantly upon the SBP treatment. These results validate the reliability of the SBP's target genes and their regulating pathways identified by our bioinformatics methods.

Fig. 12.10 shows the number of genes in different intersection sets of the four gene sets, and the number of pathways affected by genes in these intersections. It could be seen that, although the SBP directly acts on only a few CVD disease genes, through network

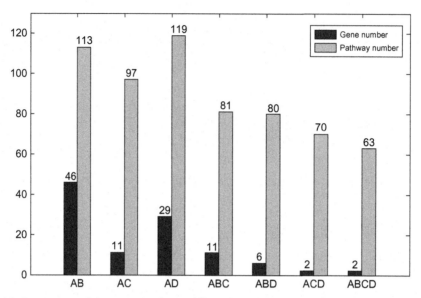

Fig. 12.10 Comparison of the gene number in different intersection sets of the four gene sets and the number of pathways affected by corresponding genes, where A, B, C, and D denote CVD disease genes, SBPac's target genes, SBPpc's target genes, and significantly expressed genes upon the SBP treatment, respectively. AB denotes the intersection set between A and B, and so on.

interactions, SBPac, SBPpc, and significantly expressed genes under SBP treatment regulate a greater number of common CVD-related signaling pathways. Although the 11 CVD genes targeted by SBPpc (AC in Fig. 12.10) are only 24% of the 46 CVD genes targeted by SBPac (AB in Fig. 12.10), the number of CVD-associated pathways regulated by SBPpc (AC in Fig. 12.10, 97) is 86% of the number of the CVD-associated pathways regulated by SBPac (AB in Fig. 12.10, 113). Meanwhile, only a few CVD disease genes targeted by SBPac and SBPpc were validated in the gene expression experiment, that is, 6 and 2 genes, respectively (ABD and ACD in Fig. 12.10). In contrast, more CVD-affecting pathways regulated by SBPac and SBPpc were verified in the gene expression study, that is, 80 and 70 pathways, respectively (ABD and ACD in Fig. 12.10). That is to say, about 70% of CVD-associated pathways affected by SBPac and SBPpc were validated in the microarray-based studies.

These results suggest that the SBP regulates the CVD-associated network through multicomponents and multitargets to achieve its clinical efficacy. The high consistency between the pathways identified by the bioinformatics methods and the microarray confirmation studies exemplifies the reliability of our data mining and analytical methods. It also reveals that the SBP's plasma-absorbed components exert nearly the same function as that of the SBP's full compound set for CVD treatment.

Among the 63 experimentally validated CVD pathways regulated by both SBPac and SBPpc (ABCD in Fig. 12.10 and Table S7 of Supplementary), most are directly associated

Table 12.4 List of selected CVD-affecting pathways regulated by both the SBP and the SBP's plasma-absorbed components

ID	Pathway name	The association with CVD
1	AT1R_PATHWAY	Vasodilator and myocardial hypertrophy[133]
2	SPPA_PATHWAY	Vasoconstriction and platelet activation
3	EPO_PATHWAY	Increasing erythrocyte[134]
4	HIF_PATHWAY	Vascular remodeling and thrombopoietin[135]
5	IL4_PATHWAY	Hematopoietic association[136]
6	IL6_PATHWAY	Hematopoietic association[137]
7	CARDIACEGF_PATHWAY	Cardiac hypertrophy and angiotensin[138]
8	TPO_PATHWAY	Thrombopoietin[139]
9	ANGIOPOIETINRECEPTOR_PATHWAY	Angiopoietin[140]
10	S1P_S1P1_PATHWAY	Endothelial cell induction[141]
11	VEGFR1_PATHWAY	Vascular endothelial growth factor receptor[142]
12	LYMPHANGIOGENESIS_PATHWAY	Angiogenesis[143]
13	HEMATOPOIESIS_STAT3_TARGETS	Hematopoietic[144]

with CVD, further supporting the effectiveness of the SBP to treat CVD. Table 12.4 lists some of these pathways that are associated with CVD.

12.2.3.5 Target Validation in Cell-Based Studies

Based on the above analysis, genes ICAM-1 and COX-2 are included in four different gene sets under study, that is, CVD disease genes, SBPac's target genes, SBPpc's target genes, and significantly expressed genes under the SBP treatment. Moreover, their encoded proteins are readily available. Thus we chose protein ICAM-1 and COX-2 for experimental validation.

To validate the SBP's effects on ICAM-1 and COX-2, we conducted Western blot experiments in HUVECs. As shown in Fig. 12.11, the SBP extract (1 µg/mL) and SBPpc (0.1 µg/mL) each induced the expression of the COX-2 protein while inhibiting the expression of the TNFα-induced ICAM-1 protein.

Both ICAM-1 and COX-2 are expressed in endothelial cells and play important roles in the initiation and progression of cardiovascular disease. ICAM-1 facilitates the transmigration of leukocytes across the vascular wall during the inflammatory response. COX-2 converts arachidonic acid to various metabolites, including prostacyclin (PGI2), a major COX-2 metabolite found in endothelial cells and an effective vasodilator. These observations support the notion that SBP and its plasma-absorbed compounds (SBPpc) exert their anti-CVD effects by vasodilation and antiinflammatory action, through the upregulation of COX-2 and downregulation of ICAM-1.

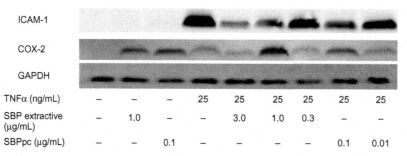

Fig. 12.11 Expression of ICAM-1 and COX-2 proteins in HUVECs treated with the SBP extract and SBPpc samples for 16h in the presence or absence of TNFα (25 ng/mL). Specific proteins were detected by Western blot as described in Section 12.2.2. Each blot is representative of three independent experiments.Fig. 12.11

12.2.4 Conclusions

This study investigated the therapeutic effect of the SBP on CVD in depth using a network pharmacological approach. First, we calculated the network effect score of the disease and drug on genes in the background network and further analyzed the score's significance to determine whether the SBP significantly impacts CVD. Second, we mapped the scores of all genes in the background network obtained through RWR to 4722 pathways and calculated the regulation scores of CVD, all compounds of the SBP and plasma-absorbed compounds of the SBP to these pathways. As a result, we identified biological processes significantly regulated by the SBP's different compound sets and found that most of them are associated with CVD. Finally, we validated our bioinformatics results in microarray- and Western blot-based studies.

We found that, unlike FDA-approved CVD drugs that mainly target specific disease genes, the SBP only targets a very small fraction of CVD disease genes. However, from the perspective of network regulation, the subnetwork regulated by the SBP and most signaling pathways significantly regulated by the SBP are overlapped with those influenced by CVD disease genes, respectively. These results suggest that SBP achieves its efficacy on CVD treatment by regulating the disease network though interactions between genes, instead of directly acting on CVD disease genes. When compared to the anti-CVD effects of all compounds included in the SBP, the SBP's plasma-absorbed compounds acquired a significant anti-CVD effect score. Approximately 70% of CVD-associated pathways affected by both the SBP's full compound set and the SBP's plasma-absorbed compound set were validated in microarray-based studies, indicating that the SBP's plasma-absorbed compounds play a major role in the SBP's treatment of CVD. Finally, two important CVD-associated disease genes that are targeted by the SBP were validated at the protein expression level by Western blot.

In summary, this study applied a network pharmacology approach to determine the SBP's anti-CVD effect. It shed lights on the modern approaches to investigating TCM pharmacology and to promoting the development of traditional medicine.

Table S1 Proteins associated with CHD

Short name	Unit prot ID	Recommended name
12-LOX	P18054	Arachidonate 12-lipoxygenase, 12S-type
15-LOX	P16050	Arachidonate 15-lipoxygenase
5-HT1A	P08908	5-Hydroxytryptamine receptor 1A
5-HT1B	P28222	5-Hydroxytryptamine receptor 1B
5-HT2A	P28223	5-Hydroxytryptamine receptor 2A
5-HT1F	P30939	5-Hydroxytryptamine receptor 1F
5-HT2B	P41595	5-Hydroxytryptamine receptor 2B
5-LOX	P09917	Arachidonate 5-lipoxygenase
ABCA1	O95477	ATP-binding cassette subfamily A member 1
ACAT	P24752	Acetyl-CoA acetyltransferase, mitochondrial
ARP1	Q13795	apoA-I regulatory protein 1
AC	Q08828	Adenylate cyclase type 1
ACC2	O00763	Acetyl-CoA carboxylase 2
ACC1	Q13085	Acetyl-CoA carboxylase 1
ACE	P12821	Angiotensin-converting enzyme
AChE	P22303	Acetylcholinesterase
Act1	O43734	Adapter protein CIKS
A3R	P33765	Adenosine receptor A3
A1R	P30542	Adenosine receptor A1
A2BR	P29275	Adenosine receptor A2b
Adrenomedullin receptor	O15218	G-protein coupled receptor 182
ADRα1A	P35348	Alpha-1A adrenergic receptor
ADRα1B	P35368	Alpha-1B adrenergic receptor
ADRα2A	P08913	Alpha-2A adrenergic receptor
ADRα2B	P18089	Alpha-2B adrenergic receptor
ADRβ2	P07550	Beta-2 adrenergic receptor
ADRβ1	P08588	Beta-1 adrenergic receptor
AgtR1	P30556	Type-1 angiotensin II receptor
AgtR2	P50052	Type-2 angiotensin II receptor
Akt1 = PKBα	P31749	RAC-alpha serine/threonine-protein kinase
Akt2 = PKBβ	P31751	RAC-beta serine/threonine-protein kinase
Akt3 = PKBγ	Q9y243	RAC-gamma serine/threonine-protein kinase
AS	P19099	Cytochrome P450 11B2, mitochondrial
AMPK beta-1 chain	Q9Y478	5′-AMP-activated protein kinase subunit beta-1
Ang II	P01019	Angiotensinogen
ANP	P01160	Atrial natriuretic factor
ANPR-A	P16066	Atrial natriuretic peptide receptor 1
ANPR-B	P20594	Atrial natriuretic peptide receptor 2
ANPR-C	P17342	Atrial natriuretic peptide receptor 3
APAF1	O14727	Apoptotic protease-activating factor 1
ApoAI	P02647	Apolipoprotein A-I
ApoB	P04114	Apolipoprotein B-100

Continued

Table S1 Proteins associated with CHD—cont'd

Short name	Unit prot ID	Recommended name
ARNT	P27540	Aryl hydrocarbon receptor nuclear translocator
ARP1	P24468	COUP transcription factor 2
Ask1 = MEKK5	Q99683	Mitogen-activated protein kinase kinase kinase 5
ATF2	P15336	Cyclic AMP-dependent transcription factor ATF-2
BAD	Q92934	Bcl2 antagonist of cell death
Bax	Q07812	Apoptosis regulator BAX
Bcl2	P10415	Apoptosis regulator Bcl-2
BFGF	P09038	Heparin-binding growth factor 2
BID	P55957	BH3-interacting domain death agonist
Bilivedin reductase A	P53004	Biliverdin reductase A
BLT1	Q15722	Leukotriene B4 receptor 1
BNP	P16860	Natriuretic peptides B
C3	P01024	Complement C3
C3/C5 convertase	P06681	Complement C2
C5	P01031	Complement C5
CALNA2	P16298	Serine/threonine-protein phosphatase 2B catalytic subunit beta isoform
CALNA1	Q08209	Serine/threonine-protein phosphatase 2B catalytic subunit alpha isoform
Calmodulin	P62158	Calmodulin
CaMKIIδ	Q13557	Calcium/calmodulin-dependent protein kinase type II delta chain
CaMKIIγ	Q13555	Calcium/calmodulin-dependent protein kinase type II gamma chain
CaMKIIβ	Q13554	Calcium/calmodulin-dependent protein kinase type II beta chain
CaMKIIα	Q9UQM7	Calcium/calmodulin-dependent protein kinase type II alpha chain
Caspase 2	P42575	Caspase-2
Caspase3	P42537	Caspase-3
Caspase 6	P55212	Caspase-6
Caspase 7	P55210	Caspase-7
Caspase 8	Q14790	Caspase-8
Caspase 9	P55211	Caspase-9
Caspase1	P29466	Caspase-1
Caspase10	Q92851	Caspase-10
Cathepsin K	P43235	Cathepsin K
Cathepsin S	P25774	Cathepsin S
CCR-2	P41597	C–C chemokine receptor type 2
CCR-5	P51681	C–C chemokine receptor type 5
CCL-5	P13501	C–C motif chemokine 5

Table S1 Proteins associated with CHD—cont'd

Short name	Unit prot ID	Recommended name
CD36	P16671	Platelet glycoprotein 4
CD40	P25942	Tumor necrosis factor receptor superfamily member 5
CD40L	P29965	CD40 ligand
CD68	P34810	Macrosialin
CDK2	Q9BW66	Cyclin-dependent kinase 2-interacting protein
CETP	P11597	Cholesteryl ester transfer protein
c-Fos	A8K4E2	V-fos FBJ murine osteosarcoma viral oncogene homolog, isoform CRA_b
Chymase	P23946	Chymase
c-Jun	P05412	Transcription factor AP-1
c-Myc	P01106	Myc proto-oncogene protein
CNP	P23582	C-type natriuretic peptide
COX1	O97554	Prostaglandin G/H synthase 1
COX2	P35354	Prostaglandin G/H synthase 2
cPLA2	P47712	Cytosolic phospholipase A2
CPT-1	Q92523	Carnitine O-palmitoyltransferase 1, muscle isoform
CR2	P20023	Complement receptor type 1
CRP	P02741	C-reactive protein
c-Src	P12931	Proto-oncogene tyrosine-protein kinase Src
CXCL16	Q9H2A7	C-X-C motif chemokine 16
CXCR3	P49682	C-X-C chemokine receptor type 3
CXCL3	P19876	C-X-C motif chemokine 3
CYP1A1	P04798	Cytochrome P450 1A1
CYP1A2	P05177	Cytochrome P450 1A2
CYP2C8	P10632	Cytochrome P450 2C8
CYP2C9	P11712	Cytochrome P450 2C9
CYP5A1	P24557	Thromboxane-A synthase
CYP7a	P22680	Cholesterol 7-alpha-monooxygenase
cytoC	P99999	Cytochrome c
Daxx	Q9uer7	Death domain-associated protein 6
Dopamine receptor type 2	P14416	D(2) dopamine receptor
DR5	P20039	HLA class II histocompatibility antigen, DRB1-11 beta chain
ECE	P42892	Endothelin-converting enzyme 1
ECSIT	Q9BQ95	Evolutionarily conserved signaling intermediate in Toll pathway, mitochondrial
Eotaxin	P56171	Eotaxin
ERK2(MAPK1/2)	P28482	Mitogen-activated protein kinase 1
ERK1(MAPK3)	P27361	Mitogen-activated protein kinase 3
E-selectin	P16581	E-selectin

Continued

Table S1 Proteins associated with CHD—cont'd

Short name	Unit prot ID	Recommended name
ESL	Q92896	Golgi apparatus protein 1
ER α	P03372	Estrogen receptor
ER β	Q92731	Estrogen receptor beta
ET-1	P05305	Endothelin-1
ETA	P25101	Endothelin-1 receptor
ETB	P24530	Endothelin B receptor
F1F0ATPase (d)	O75947	ATP synthase subunit d, mitochondrial
F1F0ATPase (g)	O75964	ATP synthase subunit g, mitochondrial
F1F0ATPase (f)	P56134	ATP synthase subunit f, mitochondrial
FII(thrombin)	P00734	Prothrombin
FV	P12259	Coagulation factor V
FVII	P08709	Coagulation factor VII
FVII	P00451	Coagulation factor VIII
FIX	P00740	Coagulation factor IX
FX	P00743	Coagulation factor X
FXIII	Q9BX29	Coagulation factor XIII, A1 polypeptide
FXIIIa	P00488	Coagulation factor XIII A chain
FXI	P03951	Coagulation factor XI
FXII	P00748	Coagulation factor XII
FADD	Q13158	Protein FADD
FAF1	Q549F0	Fas (TNFRSF6) associated factor 1
FAK	Q05397	Focal adhesion kinase 1
Fas	P25445	Tumor necrosis factor receptor superfamily member 6
FasL	P48023	Tumor necrosis factor ligand superfamily member 6
Ferritin heavy chain	P02794	Ferritin heavy chain
Ferritin light chain	P02792	Ferritin light chain
Fibrinogen α	P02671	Fibrinogen alpha chain [Cleaved into: Fibrinopeptide A]
Fibrinogen β	P02675	Fibrinogen beta chain [Cleaved into: Fibrinopeptide B]
Fibrinogen γ	P02679	Fibrinogen gamma chain
FXR	B6ZGS9	Farnesoid X receptor
FLAP	P20292	Arachidonate 5-lipoxygenase-activating protein
FLASH	Q9UKL3	CASP8-associated protein 2
Fyn	P06241	Tyrosine-protein kinase Fyn
GAP	P20936	Ras GTPase-activating protein 1
GGTase	P49354	Protein farnesyltransferase/ geranylgeranyltransferase type-1 subunit alpha
GR	P04150	Glucocorticoid receptor

Table S1 Proteins associated with CHD—cont'd

Short name	Unit prot ID	Recommended name
GLUT1	P11166	Solute carrier family 2, facilitated glucose transporter member 1
GLUT4	P14672	Solute carrier family 2, facilitated glucose transporter member 4
Glutathine peroxidase	P07203	Glutathione peroxidase 1
GM-CSF	P04141	Granulocyte-macrophage colony-stimulating factor
GpIIb	P08514	Integrin alpha-Iib
GpIIIa	P05106	Integrin beta-3
GpIb-V	P40197	Platelet glycoprotein V
GpIb-IX	P14770	Platelet glycoprotein IX
GpVI	Q9HCN6	Platelet glycoprotein VI
Granzyme B	P10144	Granzyme B
GRB2	P62993	Growth factor receptor-bound protein 2
Gα-13	Q14344	Guanine nucleotide-binding protein subunit alpha-13
Gα-12	Q03113	Guanine nucleotide-binding protein subunit alpha-12
Gα-I alpha-3	P08754	Guanine nucleotide-binding protein G(k) subunit alpha
Gα-I alpha-2	P04899	Guanine nucleotide-binding protein G(i) subunit alpha-2
Gα-I alpha-1	P63096	Guanine nucleotide-binding protein G(i) subunit alpha-1
Gα-Q	P50148	Guanine nucleotide-binding protein G(q) subunit alpha
Gα-11	P29992	Guanine nucleotide-binding protein subunit alpha-11
Gα-S	Q5JWF2	Guanine nucleotide-binding protein G(s) subunit alpha isoforms Xlas
HO-1	P09601	Heme oxygenase 1
HIFα	Q16665	Hypoxia-inducible factor 1 alpha
Histamine H1 receptor	P35367	Histamine H1 receptor
HK1	P19367	Hexokinase-1
HK2	P52789	Hexokinase-2
HK3	P52790	Hexokinase-3
HLA-DRA	P01903	HLA class II histocompatibility antigen, DR alpha chain
HMG-CoA reductase	P14891	3-Hydroxy-3-methylglutaryl-coenzyme A reductase 1
HMG-CoA synthase	P54868	Hydroxymethylglutaryl-CoA synthase, mitochondrial

Continued

Table S1 Proteins associated with CHD—cont'd

Short name	Unit prot ID	Recommended name
HNF4α	P41235	Hepatocyte nuclear factor 4-alpha
HNF4γ	Q14541	Hepatocyte nuclear factor 4-gamma
HSP60	P10809	60 kDa heat shock protein, mitochondrial
ICAM-1	P05362	Intercellular adhesion molecule 1
IFNGR1	P15260	Interferon gamma receptor 1
IFNGR2	P38484	Interferon gamma receptor 2
IFN-α 1/13	P01562	Interferon alpha-1/13
IFN-α 2	P01563	Interferon alpha-2
IFN-α 4	P05014	Interferon alpha-4
IFN-α 5	P01569	Interferon alpha-5
IFN-α 6	P05013	Interferon alpha-6
IFN-α 7	P01567	Interferon alpha-7
IFN-α 8	P32881	Interferon alpha-8
IFN-α 10	P01566	Interferon alpha-10
IFN-α 14	P01570	Interferon alpha-14
IFN-α 16	P05015	Interferon alpha-16
IFN-α 17	P01571	Interferon alpha-17
IFN-α 21	P01568	Interferon alpha-21
IKKα	O15111	Inhibitor of nuclear factor kappa-B kinase subunit alpha
IKKβ	O14920	Inhibitor of nuclear factor kappa-B kinase subunit beta
IKKγ	Q9Y6K9	NF-kappa-B essential modulator
IKKepsilon	Q14164	Inhibitor of nuclear factor kappa-B kinase subunit epsilon
IL-1 alpha	P01583	Interleukin-1 alpha
IL-1 beta	P01584	Interleukin-1 beta
IL-12 alpha	P29459	Interleukin-12 subunit alpha
IL-12 beta	P29460	Interleukin-12 subunit beta
IL-15	P40933	Interleukin-15 (IL-15)
IL-18	Q14116	Interleukin-18
IL-2	P60568	Interleukin-2
IL-1R1	P14778	Interleukin-1 receptor type 1
IL-1RAcP	Q9NPH3	Interleukin-1 receptor accessory protein
IL-6	P05231	Interleukin-6
IL-8	P10145	Interleukin-8
IP-10	P02778	C-X-C motif chemokine 10
IRAK1	P51617	Interleukin-1 receptor-associated kinase 1
IRAK2	O43187	Interleukin-1 receptor-associated kinase-like 2
IRAK3	Q9Y616	Interleukin-1 receptor-associated kinase 3
IRAK4	Q9NWZ3	Interleukin-1 receptor-associated kinase 4
I-TAC	O14625	C-X-C motif chemokine 11

Table S1 Proteins associated with CHD—cont'd

Short name	Unit prot ID	Recommended name
JAB1	Q92905	COP9 signalosome complex subunit 5
JAK1	P23458	Tyrosine-protein kinase JAK1
JAK2	O60674	Tyrosine-protein kinase JAK2
JAK3	P52333	Tyrosine-protein kinase JAK3
JNK1	P45983	Mitogen-activated protein kinase 8
JNK2	P45984	Mitogen-activated protein kinase 9
JNK3 = MAPK10	P53799	Mitogen-activated protein kinase 10
JNKK1 = MKK4 = MEK4	P45985	Dual specificity mitogen-activated protein kinase kinase 4
K+-ATP	Q09428	ATP-binding cassette subfamily C member 8
Kininogen	P01042	Kininogen-1
KLKB1	P03952	Plasma kallikrein
LFA-1	P20701	Integrin alpha-L
LOX	P78380	Oxidized low-density lipoprotein receptor 1
LPL	P06858	Lipoprotein lipase
LTCC	Q13936	Voltage-dependent L-type calcium channel subunit alpha-1C
LXRα	Q13133	Oxysterols receptor LXR-alpha
LXRβ	P55055	Oxysterols receptor LXR-beta
M1	P11229	Muscarinic acetylcholine receptor M1
M2	P08172	Muscarinic acetylcholine receptor M2
M3	P20309	Muscarinic acetylcholine receptor M3
M4	P08173	Muscarinic acetylcholine receptor M4
M5	P08912	Muscarinic acetylcholine receptor M5
MAO-A	P21397	Amine oxidase [flavin-containing] A
MADD	Q8WXG6	MAP kinase-activating death domain protein
Makap	Q13023	A-kinase anchor protein 6
MAPK4	P31152	Mitogen-activated protein kinase 4
MAPK6	Q16659	Mitogen-activated protein kinase 6
MCD	O95822	Malonyl-CoA decarboxylase, mitochondrial
MCP-1	P13500	C–C motif chemokine 2
M-CSF	P09603	Macrophage colony-stimulating factor 1
MEF2	Q02078	Myocyte-specific enhancer factor 2A
MEK1	Q02750	Dual specificity mitogen-activated protein kinase kinase
MEK2	Q63932	Dual specificity mitogen-activated protein kinase kinase 2
MEK3	P46734	Dual specificity mitogen-activated protein kinase kinase 3
MEK5	Q13163	Dual specificity mitogen-activated protein kinase kinase 5

Continued

Table S1 Proteins associated with CHD—cont'd

Short name	Unit prot ID	Recommended name
MEK6	P52564	Dual specificity mitogen-activated protein kinase kinase 6
MEK7	O14733	Dual specificity mitogen-activated protein kinase kinase 7
MEKK1	Q13233	Mitogen-activated protein kinase kinase kinase 1
MEKK2	Q9Y2U5	Mitogen-activated protein kinase kinase kinase 2
MEKK3	Q99759	Mitogen-activated protein kinase kinase kinase 3
MEKK4	Q9Y6R4	Mitogen-activated protein kinase kinase kinase 4
Mig	Q07325	C-X-C motif chemokine 9
MR	P08235	Mineralocorticoid receptor
MLCK1	Q15746	Myosin light chain kinase, smooth muscle
MLCK2	Q9H1R3	Myosin light chain kinase 2, skeletal/cardiac muscle
MLCK3	Q32MK0	Putative myosin light chain kinase 3
MLCK4	Q86YV6	Myosin light chain kinase family member 4
MMP12	P39900	Macrophage metalloelastase
MMP2	P08253	72 kDa type IV collagenase
MMP7	P09237	Matrilysin
MMP8	P22894	Neutrophil collagenase
MMP9	P14780	Matrix metalloproteinase-9
MPO	P05164	Myeloperoxidase
Mst-1	Q13043	Serine/threonine-protein kinase 4
mTOR	P42345	Serine/threonine-protein kinase mTOR
MTP	P55157	Microsomal triglyceride transfer protein, large subunit
MyD88	Q99836	Myeloid differentiation primary response protein MyD88
NADPH oxidase	Q9NRD9	Dual oxidase 1
NCX	P32418	Sodium/calcium exchanger 1
NHE1	P19634	Sodium/hydrogen exchanger 1
NFATC4	Q14934	Nuclear factor of activated T-cells, cytoplasmic 4
NF-κB	Q04206	Transcription factor p65
NIK	Q99558	Mitogen-activated protein kinase kinase kinase 14
eNOs	P29474	Nitric oxide synthase, endothelial
N-WASP	A4D0Y1	Wiskott-Aldrich syndrome-like
P2Y1	P47900	P2Y purinoceptor 1
P2Y12	Q9H244	P2Y purinoceptor 12
PAF acetylhydrolase	Q13093	Platelet-activating factor acetylhydrolase
PAI-1	P05121	Plasminogen activator inhibitor 1
PAK1	Q13153	Serine/threonine-protein kinase PAK 1
PAK2	Q13177	Serine/threonine-protein kinase PAK 2
PAR1	P25116	Proteinase-activated receptor 1

Table S1 Proteins associated with CHD—cont'd

Short name	Unit prot ID	Recommended name
PAR3	O00254	Proteinase-activated receptor 3
PAR4	Q96RI0	Proteinase-activated receptor 4
PARP	P09874	Poly [ADP-ribose] polymerase 1
PD-ECGF	P19971	Thymidine phosphorylase
PDGFA	P04085	Platelet-derived growth factor subunit A
PDGFB	P01127	Platelet-derived growth factor subunit B
PDGFC	Q9NRA1	Platelet-derived growth factor C
PDGFD	Q9GZP0	Platelet-derived growth factor D
PDGFRA	P16234	Alpha-type platelet-derived growth factor receptor
PDGFRB	P09619	Beta-type platelet-derived growth factor receptor
PDZK1	O60450	Na(+)/H(+) exchange regulatory cofactor NHE-RF3
Per1	O15534	Period circadian protein homolog 1
Perforin	P14222	Perforin-1
PF4	P02776	Platelet factor 4
PI3K gamma	P48736	Phosphatidylinositol-4,5-bisphosphate 3-kinase catalytic subunit gamma isoform
PI3K beta	P42338	Phosphatidylinositol-4,5-bisphosphate 3-kinase catalytic subunit beta isoform
PI3K delta	O00329	Phosphatidylinositol-4,5-bisphosphate 3-kinase catalytic subunit delta isoform
PI3K alpha	P42336	Phosphatidylinositol-4,5-bisphosphate 3-kinase catalytic subunit alpha isoform
PKA	Q9FAB3	Serine/threonine-protein kinase A
PKC eta	P24723	Protein kinase C eta type
PKC gamma	P05129	Protein kinase C gamma type
PKC β	P05771	Protein kinase C beta type
PKCα	P17252	Protein kinase C alpha type
PKCδ	Q05513	Protein kinase C delta type
PLA2	P04054	Phospholipase A2
Plasminogen	P00747	Plasminogen
PLB	P26678	Cardiac phospholamban
PLC Gamma 1	P19174	1-Phosphatidylinositol-4,5-bisphosphate phosphodiesterase gamma-1
PLC Gamma 2	P16885	1-Phosphatidylinositol-4,5-bisphosphate phosphodiesterase gamma-2
PLC β1	Q9NQ66	1-Phosphatidylinositol-4,5-bisphosphate phosphodiesterase beta-1
PLC β2	Q00722	1-Phosphatidylinositol-4,5-bisphosphate phosphodiesterase beta-2

Continued

Table S1 Proteins associated with CHD—cont'd

Short name	Unit prot ID	Recommended name
PLC β3	Q01970	1-Phosphatidylinositol-4,5-bisphosphate phosphodiesterase beta-3
PLC β4	Q15147	1-Phosphatidylinositol-4,5-bisphosphate phosphodiesterase beta-4
PLD2	O14939	Phospholipase D2
PLD1	O13393	Phospholipase D1
PLD3	Q8IV08	Phospholipase D3
PLD 5	Q8N7P1	Inactive phospholipase D5
PLD6	Q8N2A8	Phospholipase D6
PLD4	Q96BZ4	Phospholipase D4
PON-1	P27169	Serum paraoxonase/arylesterase 1
Por1	P53365	Arfaptin-2
PP1 alpha	P62136	Serine/threonine-protein phosphatase PP1-alpha catalytic subunit
PP1 beta	P62140	Serine/threonine-protein phosphatase PP1-beta catalytic subunit
PP1 gamma	P36873	Serine/threonine-protein phosphatase PP1-gamma catalytic subunit
PPARα	Q07869	Peroxisome proliferator-activated receptor alpha
PPARγ	P37231	Peroxisome proliferator-activated receptor gamma
P-selectin	P16109	P-selectin
PSGL	Q14242	P-selectin glycoprotein ligand 1
PtgIR	P43119	Prostacyclin receptor
PYK2	Q14289	Protein tyrosine kinase 2 beta
Pyruvate dehydrogenase	Q968X7	Pyruvate dehydrogenase [NADP +]
Pyruvate dehydrogenase kinase	Q15118	[Pyruvate dehydrogenase [lipoamide]] kinase isozyme 1, mitochondrial
Rac1	A4D2P2	Ras-related C3 botulinum toxin substrate 1
Raf1	P04049	RAF proto-oncogene serine/threonine-protein kinase
RAGE	Q15109	Advanced glycosylation end product-specific receptor
RAIDD	B5BU44	Death domain-containing protein CRADD
Renin	P00797	Renin
RhoA	P61586	Transforming protein RhoA
RIP2	O43353	Receptor-interacting serine/threonine-protein kinase 2
RORα	P35398	Nuclear receptor ROR-alpha
RXR α	P19793	Retinoic acid receptor RXR-alpha
RXR β	P28702	Retinoic acid receptor RXR-beta
RXR γ	P48443	Retinoic acid receptor RXR-gamma

Table S1 Proteins associated with CHD—cont'd

Short name	Unit prot ID	Recommended name
RyR2	Q92736	Ryanodine receptor 2
SCD-1	O00767	Acyl-CoA desaturase
Serca2a	P16615	Sarcoplasmic/endoplasmic reticulum calcium ATPase 2
SHC1	P29353	SHC-transforming protein 1
SH-PTP2	Q06124	Tyrosine-protein phosphatase nonreceptor type 11
Smase 3	Q9NY59	Sphingomyelin phosphodiesterase 3
Smase 2	O60906	Sphingomyelin phosphodiesterase 2
SMase	P17405	Sphingomyelin phosphodiesterase
SOS1	A8K2G3	cDNA FLJ76778, highly similar to Homo sapiens son of sevenless homolog 1
SOS2	B7ZKT5	Son of sevenless homolog 2
SRA	Q9H7N4	Splicing factor, arginine/serine-rich 19
SRBI	Q8WTV0	Scavenger receptor class B member 1
Src	Q76P87	Proto-oncogene tyrosine-protein kinase Src
Src1	Q15788	Nuclear receptor coactivator 1
SSAO	Q16853	Membrane primary amine oxidase
STAT1	B2RCA0	Signal transducer and activator of transcription 1, 91 kDa, isoform CRA_a
STAT3	P40763	Signal transducer and activator of transcription 3
TAB1	Q15750	Mitogen-activated protein kinase kinase kinase 7-interacting protein 1
TAF6	P49848	Transcription initiation factor TFIID subunit 6
TAF1	P21675	Transcription initiation factor TFIID subunit 1
TAK1 = MAP3K7	O43318	Mitogen-activated protein kinase kinase kinase 7
TBP	P20226	TATA-box-binding protein
TF	P13726	Tissue factor
TGFβ1	P01137	Transforming growth factor beta-1
TGFβ2	P61812	Transforming growth factor beta-2
TGFβ3	P10600	Transforming growth factor beta-3
TGFβR1	P36897	TGF-beta receptor type-1
TGFβR2	P37173	TGF-beta receptor type-2
TGFβR3	Q03167	TGF-beta receptor type III
Thyroid hormone α	P10827	Thyroid hormone receptor alpha
Thyroid hormone β	P10828	Thyroid hormone receptor beta
TIAM1	Q13009	T-lymphoma invasion and metastasis-inducing protein 1
TLR4	O00206	Toll-like receptor 4
TNFR1	P19438	Tumor necrosis factor receptor superfamily member 1A
TNFα	P01375	Tumor necrosis factor

Continued

Table S1 Proteins associated with CHD—cont'd

Short name	Unit prot ID	Recommended name
TOLLIP	Q9H0E2	Toll-interacting protein
TRAF1	Q13077	TNF receptor-associated factor 1
TRAF2	Q12933	TNF receptor-associated factor 2
TRAF3	Q13114	TNF receptor-associated factor 3
TRAF6	Q9Y4K3	TNF receptor-associated factor 6
TRAIL	P50591	Tumor necrosis factor ligand superfamily member 10
Tryptase alpha1	P15157	Tryptase alpha-1
Tryptase beta1	Q15661	Tryptase beta-1
Tryptase beta2	P20231	Tryptase beta-2
Tryptase gamma	Q9NRR2	Tryptase gamma
Tryptase delata	Q9BZJ3	Tryptase delta
TYK	P29597	Nonreceptor tyrosine-protein kinase TYK2
Tyrosine kinases	Q06187	Tyrosine-protein kinase BTK
u-PA	P00749	Urokinase-type plasminogen activator
u-PAR	Q03405	Urokinase plasminogen activator surface receptor
Urotensin II	O95399	Urotensin-2
UT receptor	Q9UKP6	Urotensin-2 receptor
Vav1	P15498	Proto-oncogene vav
Vav2	P52735	Guanine nucleotide exchange factor VAV2
VCAM-1	P19320	Vascular cell adhesion protein 1
VLA4	P13612	Integrin alpha-4
Vwf	P04275	von Willebrand factor
XO	P47989	Xanthine dehydrogenase/oxidase
$\alpha 2\beta 1$	P17301	Integrin alpha-2
Bark1	P25098	Beta-adrenergic receptor kinase 1

Table S2 Genes associated with CVD

Entrez ID	GENE symbol
26298	EHF
338	APOB
197	AHSG
114805	GALNT13
3553	IL1B
390174	OR9G1
4837	NNMT
7980	TFPI2
441911	OR10J3
5465	PPARA
283189	OR9G4

Table S2 Genes associated with CVD—cont'd

Entrez ID	GENE symbol
2646	GCKR
5139	PDE3A
339479	FAM5C
9201	DCLK1
57698	KIAA1598
118	ADD1
51083	GAL
56259	CTNNBL1
6364	CCL20
151	ADRA2B
1907	EDN2
1524	CX3CR1
5743	PTGS2
4023	LPL
57761	TRIB3
2696	GIPR
5791	PTPRE
2161	F12
54873	PALMD
10911	UTS2
2688	GH1
84059	GPR98
3479	IGF1
1401	CRP
9619	ABCG1
6696	SPP1
9955	HS3ST3A1
10221	TRIB1
2876	GPX1
8858	PROZ
120406	FAM55B
3992	FADS1
3569	IL6
3784	KCNQ1
116519	APOA5
2894	GRID1
4313	MMP2
337	APOA4
7450	VWF
221692	PHACTR1
2695	GIP
11132	CAPN10

Continued

Table S2 Genes associated with CVD—cont'd

Entrez ID	GENE symbol
91137	SLC25A46
63826	SRR
7124	TNF
7054	TH
22926	ATF6
3484	IGFBP1
54769	DIRAS2
285195	SLC9A9
2243	FGA
2099	ESR1
348	APOE
9365	KL
153241	CEP120
10891	PPARGC1A
6462	SHBG
10257	ABCC4
2056	EPO
4288	MKI67
3557	IL1RN
81833	SPACA1
1435	CSF1
3673	ITGA2
4153	MBL2
26059	ERC2
6774	STAT3
22843	PPM1E
585	BBS4
1559	CYP2C9
167465	ZNF366
5169	ENPP3
183	AGT
4852	NPY
4056	LTC4S
128821	CST9L
5950	RBP4
5739	PTGIR
1002	CDH4
7412	VCAM1
2852	GPER
1813	DRD2
3600	IL15
9575	CLOCK

Table S2 Genes associated with CVD—cont'd

Entrez ID	GENE symbol
814	CAMK4
5328	PLAU
128822	CST9
129684	CNTNAP5
60412	EXOC4
4524	MTHFR
2159	F10
9415	FADS2
6144	RPL21
1113	CHGA
5480	PPIC
7048	TGFBR2
23310	NCAPD3
4016	LOXL1
4878	NPPA
3667	IRS1
79001	VKORC1
1234	CCR5
2212	FCGR2A
2897	GRIK1
255520	ELMOD2
6403	SELP
4881	NPR1
53942	CNTN5
2152	F3
5891	MOK
5144	PDE4D
57580	PREX1
2786	GNG4
23118	TAB2
2784	GNB3
1012	CDH13
152330	CNTN4
1278	COL1A2
3039	HBA1
91074	ANKRD30A
5142	PDE4B
376497	SLC27A1
1585	CYP11B2
3576	IL8
8091	HMGA2
7351	UCP2

Continued

Table S2 Genes associated with CVD—cont'd

Entrez ID	GENE symbol
284040	CDRT4
5627	PROS1
1952	CELSR2
222553	SLC35F1
104	ADARB1
6347	CCL2
5468	PPARG
51741	WWOX
57531	HACE1
55720	TSR1
2100	ESR2
23345	SYNE1
3630	INS
6720	SREBF1
54332	GDAP1
4208	MEF2C
6401	SELE
3123	HLA-DRB1
185	AGTR1
1557	CYP2C19
7040	TGFB1
3586	IL10
9745	ZNF536
55247	NEIL3
25924	MYRIP
213	ALB
26047	CNTNAP2
154	ADRB2
2138	EYA1
1404	HAPLN1
6331	SCN5A
127385	OR10J5
2168	FABP1
57863	CADM3
79068	FTO
1805	DPT
325	APCS
3084	NRG1
2244	FGB
23671	TMEFF2
3240	HP
9370	ADIPOQ

Table S2 Genes associated with CVD—cont'd

Entrez ID	GENE symbol
257194	NEGR1
7881	KCNAB1
177	AGER
56606	SLC2A9
54914	KIAA1797
7839	LSL
133	ADM
22795	NID2
8792	TNFRSF11A
3297	HSF1
3952	LEP
10060	ABCC9
948	CD36
23263	MCF2L
1471	CST3
4018	LPA
9771	RAPGEF5
55703	POLR3B
2200	FBN1
4846	NOS3
160777	CCDC60
3690	ITGB3
23293	SMG6
7143	TNR
7421	VDR
4982	TNFRSF11B
9388	LIPG
5327	PLAT
153	ADRB1
2952	GSTT1
5314	PKHD1
9962	SLC23A2
54212	SNTG1
84236	RHBDD1
345	APOC3
3753	KCNE1
7391	USF1
5350	PLN
2878	GPX3
6262	RYR2
6558	SLC12A2
10516	FBLN5

Continued

Table S2 Genes associated with CVD—cont'd

Entrez ID	GENE symbol
875	CBS
387119	CEP85L
58191	CXCL16
7099	TLR4
26476	OR10J1
5054	SERPINE1
219493	OR5AR1
2155	F7
7941	PLA2G7
2266	FGG
8600	TNFSF11
64241	ABCG8
9312	KCNB2
1906	EDN1
5444	PON1
3762	KCNJ5
84722	PSRC1
6532	SLC6A4
9353	SLIT2
3383	ICAM1
3077	HFE
3329	HSPD1
6288	SAA1
79991	OBFC1
2053	EPHX2
3075	CFH
6638	SNRPN
9631	NUP155
726	CAPN5
341	APOC1
5742	PTGS1
2169	FABP2
2205	FCER1A
54504	CPVL
3757	KCNH2
79698	ZMAT4
55668	C14orf118
27303	RBMS3
5445	PON2
137492	VPS37A
5992	RFX4
1573	CYP2J2

Table S2 Genes associated with CVD—cont'd

Entrez ID	GENE symbol
192343	NEWENTRY
7486	WRN
1071	CETP
3481	IGF2
164781	WDR69
7408	VASP
5781	PTPN11
7139	TNNT2
1047	CLGN
9948	WDR1
161357	MDGA2
7422	VEGFA
131096	KCNH8
3570	IL6R
64410	KLHL25
10217	CTDSPL
1356	CP
4314	MMP3
54433	GAR1
1636	ACE
335	APOA1
11107	PRDM5
10082	GPC6
1277	COL1A1
4318	MMP9
6843	VAMP1
3606	IL18
9722	NOS1AP
255738	PCSK9
1520	CTSS
9905	SGSM2
338675	OR5AP2
10003	NAALAD2
6894	TARBP1
3949	LDLR
6649	SOD3
56729	RETN
4879	NPPB

Table S3 The SBP's medicinal materials and chemical compounds

Medicinal material	Chemical compound
Moschus	Muscone
	Normuscone
	Muscopyridine
	Muscol
	Muscopyran
	Hydroxymuscopyridine A
	Hydroxymuscopyridine B
	3-Methylcyclotridecan-1-one
	Cyclotetradecanone
	Cholest-4-en-3-one
	Cholesterol
	Testosterone
	Estradiol
	5-Alpha-androstan-3,17-dione
Total gingenoside ginseng root	Panaxadiol
	Panaxatriol
	Oleanolic acid
	Ginsenoside Fc
	Ginsenoside Ra_1
	Ginsenoside Ra_2
	Ginsenoside Ra_3
	Ginsenoside Rb_1
	Ginsenoside Rb_2(20-[(6-O-alpha-L-arabinopyranosyl-beta-D-glucopyranosyl)oxy]-12beta-hydroxydammar-24-en-3beta-yl 2-O-beta-D-glucopyranosyl-beta-D-glucopyranoside)
	Ginsenoside Rb_3 (dammarane,β-D-glucopyranoside deriv)
	Ginsenoside Rd
	Ginsenoside Rc
	Ginsenoside Re
	Ginsenoside Rf (dammarane,β-D-glucopyranoside deriv)
	Ginsenoside Rg_1
	Ginsenoside Rg_2
	Ginsenoside Rg_3
	Ginsenoside Rh_1
	Ginsenoside Rh_2
	Ginsenoside Ro
	Ginsenoside Rs_1
	Ginsenoside Rs_2
	Notoginsenoside R_1
	Notoginsenoside R_2
	Notoginsenoside Fa
	Quinquenoside R_1

Table S3 The SBP's medicinal materials and chemical compounds—cont'd

Medicinal material	Chemical compound
Bufonis Venenum	Cinobufagin 3-acetate
	Resibufogenin
	Resibufagin
	Cinobufagin
	1-Hydroxy-cinobufagin
	Gamabufotalin (gamabufogenin)
	Arenobufagin
	Bufalin
	1β-Hydroxybufalin
	Bufotalin
	Bufarenogin
	Ψ-Bufarenogin (psi-bufarenogin)
	Desacetylbufotalin
	Telocinobufagin
	Cinobufotalin
	19-Oxo-desacetyl-cinobufotalin
	Resibufogenol
	Cinobufaginol
	19-Oxo-cinobufotalin
	Marinobufagenin
	Desacetyl-cinobufagin
	Desacetylcinobufaginol
	Bufotalidin (hellebrigenin)
	Bufotalinin
	Marinobufagin
	Nicotinamide
	Butanoic acid
	Bufoserotonins A
	Bufoserotonins B
	Bufoserotonins C
	2-Piperidinecarboxylic acid
	6-Oxo-methylester
	Adenine
	Uracil
	5-Hydroxyindoleacetic acid (5-HIAA)(5-hydroxyindole-3-acetic acid)
	Bufothionine
Bovis Calculus Artifactus	Ursodeoxycholic acid
	Cholic acid
	Deoxycholic acid
	Chenodeoxycholic acid
	Hyodeoxycholic acid
	Taurocholic acid
	Glycocholic acid
	Cholesterol
	Bilirubin

Continued

Table S3 The SBP's medicinal materials and chemical compounds—cont'd

Medicinal material	Chemical compound
Styrax	Benzyl benzoate (Ascabin)
	Oleanonic acid
	3-Epioleanolic acid
	Pimaric acid
	Isopimaric acid
	Dehydroabietic acid
	Abietatriene-3β-Ol
	Methyl 4-hydroxcinnamate(methyl p-Couma)
	Vanillin
	Vanillic acid
	5-Hydroxymethyl-2-furaldehyde
	Cinnamyl acetate
	Benzyl cinnamate
	Alpha-pinene
	Beta-pinene
	Myrcene
	Camphene
	Limonene
	L, 8-Cineole
	p-Cymene
	Terpinolene
	Linalool
	4-Terpineol
	α-Terpineol
	Cinnamaldehyde
	4-Ethyphenol
	2-Ethyphenol
	3-Ethyphenol
	Allylphenol
	N-Propyl cinnamate
	β-Phenylpropionic acid
	L-Benzoyl-3-phenylpropyne
	Benzoic acid
	Palmitic acid
	Linoleic acid
	Dihydrocoumarone
	Epoxycinnamyl cinnamate
	cis-Cinnamic acid
	cis-Cinnamylcinnamate
Cinnamomi Cortex	Cinnamaldehyde
	Cinnamyl acetate

Table S3 The SBP's medicinal materials and chemical compounds—cont'd

Medicinal material	Chemical compound
	Ethylcinnamate
	Benzyl benzoate
	Benzaldehyde
	Coumarin
	β-Cadinene
	Calamenene
	B-Elemane
	Protocatechuic acid
	Transcinnamic acid
	3′-O-Methyl-(−)-epicatechin
	5,3′-Di-O-methylate-(−)-epicatechin
	5,7,3′-Tri-O-methylate-(−)-epicatechin
	(4′-O-Methyl-(+)-catechin)
	(7,4′-Di-O-methylate-(+)-catechin)
	(5,7,4′-Tri-O-methylate-(+)-catechin)
	((−)-Epicatechin 3-O-β-D-glucopyranoside)
	((−)-Epicatechin 8-C-β-D-glucopyranoside)
	((−)-Epicatechin 6-C-β-D-glucopyranoside)
	(−)-Epicatechin
	Cinnamtannin A2
	Cinnamtannin A3
	Procyanidin
	(Procyanidin B-2 6-C-β-D-glucopyranoside)
	Cinnzeylanine
	Cinncassiols
	Cinncassiols A
	Cinncassiols B
	Cinncassiols C3
	Cinncassiols D1
	Cinncassiols D3
	Cinncassiols D4
	Lyoniresinol-3A-O-β-D-glucopyranoside
	3,4,5-Trimethoxyphenol-β-D-apiofuranosyl(1 → 6)-β-D-glucopyranoside
	Syringaresinol
	5,7-Dimethyl-3′,4′-di-O-methylene-(±)-epicatechin
	Cinnamic aldehydecyclicglycerol-1,3-acetal(9,2′-*trans*)
	Cinnamic aldehydecyclicglycerol-1,3-acetal(9,2′-*cis*)
	Cassioside
	Cinnamoside
Borneolum Syntheticum	D-Borneol
	Isoborneol

Table S4 SBP's target proteins

Compounds	Gene symbol	Entrez	Database
β-Phenylpropionic acid	GOT1	2805	STITCH
β-Phenylpropionic acid	GOT2	2806	STITCH
β-Phenylpropionic acid	HADHA	3030	STITCH
β-Phenylpropionic acid	LPO	4025	STITCH
β-Phenylpropionic acid	MPO	4353	STITCH
β-Phenylpropionic acid	EPX	8288	STITCH
β-Phenylpropionic acid	GOT1L1	137362	STITCH
B-Elemane	LTA4H	4048	STITCH
β-Cadinene	TRIO	7204	STITCH
β-Cadinene	KALRN	8997	STITCH
β-Cadinene	ARHGEF25	115557	STITCH
Vanillin, vanillic acid, *cis*-cinnamic acid, *cis*-cinnamylcinnamate, 3′-*O*-methyl-(−)-epicatechin, 5,3′-di-*O*-methylate-(−)-epicatechin, 5,7,3′-tri-*O*-methylate-(−)-epicatechin, (4′-*O*-methyl-(+)-catechin), (7,4′-di-*O*-methylate-(+)-catechin), (5,7,4′-tri-*O*-methylate-(+)-catechin), 5,7-dimethyl-3′,4′-di-*O*-methylene-(±)-epicatechin	CA2	760	STITCH
Vanillin, *cis*-cinnamic acid, *cis*-cinnamylcinnamate, 3′-*O*-methyl-(−)-epicatechin, 5,3′-di-*O*-methylate-(−)-epicatechin, 5,7,3′-tri-*O*-methylate-(−)-epicatechin, (4′-*O*-methyl-(+)-catechin), (7,4′-di-*O*-methylate-(+)-catechin), (5,7,4′-tri-*O*-methylate-(+)-catechin), 5,7-dimethyl-3′,4′-di-*O*-methylene-(±)-epicatechin	CA1	759	STITCH
Vanillin	OR1G1	8390	STITCH
Vanillin	TRPV3	162514	STITCH
Ursodeoxycholic acid, cholic acid, glycocholic acid	FABP6	2172	HIT,STITCH
Ursodeoxycholic acid	E2F1	1869	HIT
Ursodeoxycholic acid	NCOA1	8648	HIT
Uracil	CD69	969	STITCH
Uracil	CDA	978	STITCH
Uracil	DPYD	1806	STITCH
Uracil	DPYS	1807	STITCH
Uracil	TYMP	1890	STITCH
Uracil	GPR17	2840	STITCH
Uracil	TDG	6996	STITCH
Uracil	TYMS	7298	STITCH
Uracil	UNG	7374	STITCH

Table S4 SBP's target proteins—cont'd

Compounds	Gene symbol	Entrez	Database
Uracil	UPP1	7378	STITCH
Uracil	CCNO	10309	STITCH
Uracil	SMUG1	23583	STITCH
Uracil	UCKL1	54963	STITCH
Uracil	AICDA	57379	STITCH
Uracil	PUS3	83480	STITCH
Uracil	UPRT	139596	STITCH
Uracil	TRUB1	142940	STITCH
Uracil	UPP2	151531	STITCH
Testosterone, estradiol, ginsenoside Fc, ginsenoside Ra_1, ginsenoside Ra_2, ginsenoside Ra_3, ginsenoside Rb_2(20-[(6-O-alpha-L-arabinopyranosyl-beta-D-glucopyranosyl)oxy]-12beta-hydroxydammar-24-en-3beta-yl 2-O-beta-D-glucopyranosyl-beta-D-glucopyranoside), ginsenoside Rb_3(dammarane,β-D-glucopyranoside deriv), ginsenoside Rs_1, ginsenoside Rs_2, notoginsenoside Fa, quinquenoside R1, (−)-epicatechin, cinnamtannin A2, cinnamtannin A3, (procyanidin B-2 6-C-β-D-glucopyranoside), cinncassiols C3, cinnamoside	AKT1	207	STITCH,HIT
Testosterone, estradiol, (−)-epicatechin	CYP19A1	1588	STITCH,HIT
Testosterone, estradiol, (−)-epicatechin	ABCG2	9429	STITCH,HIT
Testosterone, estradiol	IGF1	3479	STITCH
Testosterone, estradiol	IGFBP3	3486	STITCH
Testosterone, estradiol	PRL	5617	STITCH
Testosterone, estradiol	SHBG	6462	STITCH
Testosterone, bufoserotonins A, bufoserotonins B	POMC	5443	STITCH
Testosterone, bilirubin, D-borneol	UGT1A1	54658	STITCH
Testosterone, bilirubin	UGT1A6	54578	STITCH
Testosterone	HSD3B1	3283	STITCH
Testosterone	HSD17B3	3293	STITCH
Testosterone	HSD17B6	8630	STITCH
Taurocholic acid, (−)-epicatechin	JUN	3725	HIT,HIT
Taurocholic acid	GSR	2936	HIT
Taurocholic acid	NR3C2	4306	HIT
Taurocholic acid	VEGFA	7422	HIT
Syringaresinol	NOS1	4842	STITCH
Sulfadiazine	BRD2	6046	STITCH

Continued

Table S4 SBP's target proteins—cont'd

Compounds	Gene symbol	Entrez	Database
Resibufogenin, resibufagin, gamabufotalin (gamabufogenin), 1β-hydroxybufalin, bufotalin, 19-oxo-desacetyl-cinobufotalin, resibufogenol, cinobufaginol, desacetyl-cinobufagin, desacetylcinobufaginol, bufotalinin	SERPINA6	866	STITCH
Resibufogenin, resibufagin, gamabufotalin (gamabufogenin), 1β-hydroxybufalin, bufotalin, 19-oxo-desacetyl-cinobufotalin, resibufogenol, cinobufaginol, desacetyl-cinobufagin, desacetylcinobufaginol, Bufotalinin	DRG1	4733	STITCH
Resibufogenin, resibufagin, gamabufotalin (gamabufogenin), 1β-hydroxybufalin, bufotalin, 19-oxo-desacetyl-cinobufotalin, resibufogenol, cinobufaginol, desacetyl-cinobufagin, desacetylcinobufaginol, bufotalinin	PGK1	5230	STITCH
Resibufogenin, resibufagin, gamabufotalin (gamabufogenin), 1β-hydroxybufalin, bufotalin, 19-oxo-desacetyl-cinobufotalin, resibufogenol, cinobufaginol, desacetyl-cinobufagin, desacetylcinobufaginol, bufotalinin	PHKA1	5255	STITCH
Resibufogenin, resibufagin, gamabufotalin (gamabufogenin), 1β-hydroxybufalin, bufotalin, 19-oxo-desacetyl-cinobufotalin, resibufogenol, cinobufaginol, desacetyl-cinobufagin, desacetylcinobufaginol, bufotalinin	RPS12	6206	STITCH
Resibufogenin, resibufagin, gamabufotalin (gamabufogenin), 1β-hydroxybufalin, bufotalin, 19-oxo-desacetyl-cinobufotalin, resibufogenol, cinobufaginol, desacetyl-cinobufagin, desacetylcinobufaginol, bufotalinin	TAF1	6872	STITCH
Resibufogenin, resibufagin, gamabufotalin (gamabufogenin), 1β-hydroxybufalin, bufotalin, 19-oxo-desacetyl-cinobufotalin, resibufogenol, cinobufaginol, desacetyl-cinobufagin, desacetylcinobufaginol, bufotalinin	ECEL1	9427	STITCH

Table S4 SBP's target proteins—cont'd

Compounds	Gene symbol	Entrez	Database
Resibufogenin, resibufagin, gamabufotalin (gamabufogenin), 1β-hydroxybufalin, bufotalin, 19-oxo-desacetyl-cinobufotalin, resibufogenol, cinobufaginol, desacetyl-cinobufagin, desacetylcinobufaginol, bufotalinin	GCN1L1	10985	STITCH
Resibufogenin, resibufagin, gamabufotalin (gamabufogenin), 1β-hydroxybufalin, bufotalin, 19-oxo-desacetyl-cinobufotalin, resibufogenol, cinobufaginol, desacetyl-cinobufagin, desacetylcinobufaginol, bufotalinin	RWDD1	51389	STITCH
Resibufogenin, resibufagin, gamabufotalin (gamabufogenin), 1β-hydroxybufalin, bufotalin, 19-oxo-desacetyl-cinobufotalin, resibufogenol, cinobufaginol, desacetyl-cinobufagin, desacetylcinobufaginol, bufotalinin	ZC3H15	55854	STITCH
Protocatechuic acid, transcinnamic acid	MGA	23269	HIT
Protocatechuic acid	PRKACA	5566	HIT
Protocatechuic acid	PRKCA	5578	HIT
Protocatechuic acid	PRKCG	5582	HIT
Protocatechuic acid	PRKCZ	5590	HIT
Procyanidin	CDK1	983	STITCH
Procyanidin	FOXO1	2308	STITCH
Pimaric acid?	FCER1G	2207	STITCH
Pimaric acid?	KCNMA1	3778	STITCH
Pimaric acid?	KCNMB1	3779	STITCH
Pimaric acid?	SART1	9092	STITCH
p-Cymene(thymol)	ELANE	1991	HIT
Panaxadiol, panaxatrio1, oleanolic acid, 3-epioleanolic acid, cinnzeylanine, cinncassiols A, cinncassiols B	NR3C1	2908	HIT,STITCH
Panaxadiol, panaxatrio1, ginsenoside Rg$_3$, bufalin, vanillin	MMP9	4318	HIT,STITCH
Palmitic acid	IL10	3586	HIT
Palmitic acid	PCYT1A	5130	HIT
Palmitic acid	PTEN	5728	HIT
Palmitic acid	SLC22A5	6584	HIT
Palmitic acid	TEP1	7011	HIT
Oleanonic acid, normuscone, 3-methylcyclotridecan-2-one, cyclotetradecanone, oleanolic acid, cholic acid, 3-epioleanolic acid	GPBAR1	151306	STITCH

Continued

Table S4 SBP's target proteins—cont'd

Compounds	Gene symbol	Entrez	Database
Oleanolic acid, ginsenoside Rf (dammarane,β-D-glucopyranoside deriv), ginsenoside Rg$_3$, ginsenoside Rh$_2$, deoxycholic acid, 3-epioleanolic acid, linalool, cinnamaldehyde	PTGS2	5743	STITCH, HIT,HIT
Oleanolic acid, ginsenoside Fc, ginsenoside Ra$_1$, ginsenoside Ra$_2$, ginsenoside Ra$_3$, ginsenoside Rb$_2$(20-[(6-O-alpha-L-arabinopyranosyl-beta-D-glucopyranosyl)oxy]-12beta-hydroxydammar-24-en-3beta-yl 2-O-beta-D-glucopyranosyl-beta-D-glucopyranoside), ginsenoside Rb$_3$ (dammarane,β-D-glucopyranoside deriv), ginsenoside Rs$_1$, ginsenoside Rs$_2$, notoginsenoside Fa, quinquenoside R1,3-epioleanolic acid, cinnamaldehyde, cinnamoside	NFE2L2	4780	STITCH,HIT
Oleanolic acid, 5-hydroxyindoleacetic acid (5-HIAA)(5-hydroxyindole-3-acetic acid), 3-epioleanolic acid	TOP1	7150	STITCH
Oleanolic acid, 3-epioleanolic acid, epoxycinnamyl cinnamate, cinnamtannin A2, cinnamtannin A3, (procyanidin B-2 6-C-β-D-glucopyranoside), cassioside	TOP2A	7153	STITCH
Oleanolic acid, 3-epioleanolic acid, dehydroabietic acid, linoleic acid	PPARA	5465	STITCH
Oleanolic acid, 3-epioleanolic acid	CASP8	841	STITCH
Oleanolic acid, 3-epioleanolic acid	MAPK14	1432	STITCH
Oleanolic acid, 3-epioleanolic acid	PTGIR	5739	STITCH
Oleanolic acid, 3-epioleanolic acid	PTGIS	5740	STITCH
Oleanolic acid, 3-epioleanolic acid	PTPN1	5770	STITCH
Oleanolic acid, 3-epioleanolic acid	AKR1B10	57016	STITCH
Notoginsenoside R1	SELE	6401	HIT
Normuscone, 3-methylcyclotridecan-3-one, cyclotetradecanone, testosterone	AR	367	STITCH
Normuscone, 3-methylcyclotridecan-1-one, cyclotetradecanone	HACL1	26061	STITCH
Nicotinamide, cinncassiols C3	PARP1	142	STITCH
Nicotinamide, adenine, uracil	PNP	4860	STITCH
Nicotinamide	PARP4	143	STITCH
Nicotinamide	ART3	419	STITCH
Nicotinamide	BST1	683	STITCH
Nicotinamide	CD38	952	STITCH
Nicotinamide	NNMT	4837	STITCH
Nicotinamide	PARP3	10039	STITCH
Nicotinamide	NAMPT	10135	STITCH

Table S4 SBP's target proteins—cont'd

Compounds	Gene symbol	Entrez	Database
Nicotinamide	SIRT5	23408	STITCH
Nicotinamide	SIRT1	23411	STITCH
Nicotinamide	SIRT6	51548	STITCH
Nicotinamide	NMNAT1	64802	STITCH
Nicotinamide	TNKS2	80351	STITCH
Nicotinamide	PARP9	83666	STITCH
Nicotinamide	NAPRT1	93100	STITCH
Nicotinamide	ART5	116969	STITCH
Nicotinamide	PARP15	165631	STITCH
Nicotinamide	NMNAT3	349565	STITCH
Myrcene	ATP6V1E1	529	STITCH
Myrcene	HOXA9	3205	STITCH
Myrcene	HOXD9	3235	STITCH
Myrcene	IPP	3652	STITCH
Myrcene	RPS3A	6189	STITCH
Myrcene	ZNF224	7767	STITCH
Myrcene	GGPS1	9453	STITCH
Myrcene	PDSS1	23590	STITCH
Myrcene	SAGE1	55511	STITCH
Myrcene	PDSS2	57107	STITCH
Myrcene	SDR16C5	195814	STITCH
Muscopyridine, hydroxymuscopyridine A, hydroxymuscopyridine B, beta-pinene	CNGA2	1260	STITCH
Muscopyridine, hydroxymuscopyridine A, hydroxymuscopyridine B, beta-pinene	CNGA3	1261	STITCH
Muscopyridine, hydroxymuscopyridine A, hydroxymuscopyridine B	OR8D1	283159	STITCH
Muscopyran, testosterone	CYP17A1	1586	STITCH
Muscopyran, cholic acid, benzoic acid	CES1	1066	STITCH
Muscol, estradiol, oleanolic acid, 3-epioleanolic acid	CYP1A2	1544	STITCH
Muscol, deoxycholic acid	VCAM1	7412	STITCH,HIT
Muscol, butanoic acid, 4-terpineol	BCHE	590	STITCH
Muscol	ACHE	43	STITCH
Muscol	CD63	967	STITCH
Muscol	CFTR	1080	STITCH
Muscol	CYP2B6	1555	STITCH
Muscol	CYP2C19	1557	STITCH
Muscol	CYP2E1	1571	STITCH
Methyl 4-hydroxycinnamate(methyl *p*-Couma)	AKR1B1	231	STITCH
Marinobufagenin, marinobufagin	ATP4B	496	STITCH
Marinobufagenin, marinobufagin	CTSS	1520	STITCH
Marinobufagenin, marinobufagin	DNAH8	1769	STITCH

Continued

Table S4 SBP's target proteins—cont'd

Compounds	Gene symbol	Entrez	Database
Marinobufagenin, marinobufagin	ERG	2078	STITCH
Marinobufagenin, marinobufagin	FGF10	2255	STITCH
Marinobufagenin, marinobufagin	FLI1	2313	STITCH
Marinobufagenin, marinobufagin	GNB3	2784	STITCH
Marinobufagenin, marinobufagin	REN	5972	STITCH
Marinobufagenin, marinobufagin	SRC	6714	STITCH
Marinobufagenin, marinobufagin	ATP11A	23250	STITCH
Lyoniresinol-3α-O-β-D-glucopyranoside	MAP2K1	5604	STITCH
Linoleic acid	ALOX15	246	STITCH
Linoleic acid	ALOX15B	247	STITCH
Linoleic acid	ACSL1	2180	STITCH
Linoleic acid	GPX2	2877	STITCH
Linoleic acid	FADS1	3992	STITCH
Linoleic acid	PLA2G1B	5319	STITCH
Linoleic acid	FADS2	9415	STITCH
Linoleic acid	ELOVL2	54898	STITCH
Linoleic acid	ELOVL5	60481	STITCH
Linoleic acid	ACSBG2	81616	STITCH
Linoleic acid	PLA2G12B	84647	STITCH
Linoleic acid	PLA2G4D	283748	STITCH
Linalool	ADORA2A	135	HIT
Linalool	KATNA1	11104	HIT
Limonene	BAD	572	HIT
Leucine	DROSHA	29102	STITCH
L-cis-Diltiazem HCl	CNGA1	1259	STITCH
1-Benzoyl-3-phenylpropyne	NUCB1	4924	STITCH
1,8-Cineole	IL5	3567	HIT
1,8-Cineole	PRODH	5625	HIT
Isopimaric acid	PTGER2	5732	STITCH
Isoborneol	SLC7A1	6541	STITCH
Isoborneol	SLC7A2	6542	STITCH
Isoborneol	SLC7A4	6545	STITCH
Isoborneol	DICER1	23405	STITCH
Isoborneol	SLC7A14	57709	STITCH
Isoborneol	SLC7A3	84889	STITCH
Hyodeoxycholic acid, bilirubin	UGT2B4	7363	STITCH
Hyodeoxycholic acid	GHDC	84514	STITCH
Glycocholic acid, cinncassiols D4	CLPS	1208	STITCH
Glycocholic acid	BAAT	570	STITCH
Glycocholic acid	CEL	1056	STITCH
Glycocholic acid	ODC1	4953	STITCH
Glycocholic acid	PNLIP	5406	STITCH
Glycocholic acid	SCP2	6342	STITCH

Table S4 SBP's target proteins—cont'd

Compounds	Gene symbol	Entrez	Database
Glycocholic acid	SLCO1A2	6579	STITCH
Glycocholic acid	ABCC3	8714	STITCH
Glycocholic acid	SLCO1B1	10599	STITCH
Glycocholic acid	SLCO1B3	28234	STITCH
Ginsenoside Ro	AKTIP	64400	STITCH
Ginsenoside Rh_2, cinnamaldehyde	NFKBIA	4792	HIT,HIT
Ginsenoside Rh_2	ADCYAP1	116	HIT
Ginsenoside Rh_2	CASP1	834	HIT
Ginsenoside Rh_2	MAP2K4	6416	HIT
Ginsenoside Rh_2	SLC2A4	6517	HIT
Ginsenoside Rh_2	PSMG1	8624	HIT
Ginsenoside Rh_1, ginsenoside Rh_2	BCL2A1	597	STITCH
Ginsenoside Rh_1, ginsenoside Rh_2	RHAG	6005	STITCH
Ginsenoside Rg_3, 5-hydroxyindoleacetic acid (5-HIAA)(5-hydroxyindole-3-acetic acid)	PPARG	5468	HIT,STITCH
Ginsenoside Rg_3	HTR3A	3359	HIT
Ginsenoside Rg_3	PRKAG2	51422	HIT
Ginsenoside Rg_2, notoginsenoside R_2	GSK3B	2932	STITCH
Ginsenoside Rg_2, notoginsenoside R_2	STK11	6794	STITCH
Ginsenoside Rg_2, notoginsenoside R_2	NR0B2	8431	STITCH
Ginsenoside Rg_1, protocatechuic acid	PRKCB	5579	HIT,HIT
Ginsenoside Rg_1, palmitic acid	COL1A1	1277	HIT,HIT
Ginsenoside Rg_1, butanoic acid, (−)-epicatechin	IL2	3558	HIT, STITCH, HIT
Ginsenoside Rg_1	ACTA2	59	HIT
Ginsenoside Rg_1	ADRB2	154	HIT
Ginsenoside Rg_1	CDH1	999	HIT
Ginsenoside Rg_1	FN1	2335	HIT
Ginsenoside Rg_1	SMAD2	4087	HIT
Ginsenoside Rg_1	TGFB1	7040	HIT
Ginsenoside Rg_1	THBS1	7057	HIT
Ginsenoside Rf (dammarane,β-D-glucopyranoside deriv), ginsenoside Rg_3, ginsenoside Rh_2, limonene	IFNG	3458	HIT,HIT
Ginsenoside Rf (dammarane,β-D-glucopyranoside deriv), ginsenoside Rg_3, ginsenoside Rh_2, 1,8-cineole, palmitic acid, (−)-epicatechin	TNF	7124	HIT,HIT
Ginsenoside Rf (dammarane,β-D-glucopyranoside deriv), ginsenoside Rg_3, ginsenoside Rh_2, 1,8-cineole	IL1B	3553	HIT,HIT
Ginsenoside Rf (dammarane,β-D-glucopyranoside deriv), ginsenoside Rg_1, ginsenoside Rg_3, limonene, 1,8-cineole	IL4	3565	HIT,HIT

Continued

Table S4 SBP's target proteins—cont'd

Compounds	Gene symbol	Entrez	Database
Ginsenoside Re, oleanolic acid, ginsenoside Rd, ginsenoside Rh$_2$, bufalin, butanoic acid, 3-epioleanolic acid, (−)-epicatechin, cinncassiols C3	CASP3	836	HIT, STITCH, HIT
Ginsenoside Re, ginsenoside Rg$_3$, ginsenoside Rh$_2$, linalool	NOS2	4843	HIT,HIT
Ginsenoside Re	NOS3	4846	HIT
Ginsenoside Rd, ginsenoside Re, ursodeoxycholic acid, limonene, palmitic acid	BCL2	596	HIT,HIT
Ginsenoside Rd, ginsenoside Re, ginsenoside Rh$_2$, bufalin, cinncassiols C3	BAX	581	HIT,STITCH
Ginsenoside Rd	PSMD3	5709	HIT
Ginsenoside Rc, ginsenoside Re	FOS	2353	HIT
Ginsenoside Rc	CYP2C9	1559	HIT
Ginsenoside Rb$_1$, ginsenoside Rg$_1$	AHR	196	HIT
Ethylcinnamate	PDCL2	132954	STITCH
Estradiol, ginsenoside Rg$_1$, bufoserotonins A, bufoserotonins B, benzyl cinnamate	CYP1A1	1543	STITCH,HIT
Estradiol, ginsenoside Rb$_1$	ESR2	2100	STITCH,HIT
Estradiol, bufoserotonins B, abietatriene-3β-ol,4-ethyphenol	ESR1	2099	STITCH
Estradiol, abietatriene-3β-ol	HSD17B1	3292	STITCH
Estradiol, 5-hydroxymethyl-2-furaldehyde	SULT1A1	6817	STITCH
Estradiol	GLUL	2752	STITCH
Estradiol	OXTR	5021	STITCH
Estradiol	ABCB1	5243	STITCH
Estradiol	SULT1E1	6783	STITCH
Estradiol	TFF1	7031	STITCH
Estradiol	NCOA3	8202	STITCH
Estradiol	HSD17B7	51478	STITCH
Dihydrocoumarone	PON1	5444	STITCH
Dihydrocoumarone	PON2	5445	STITCH
Dihydrocoumarone	PON3	5446	STITCH
Desacetylbufotalin	POLI	11201	STITCH
Deoxycholic acid, procyanidin, cinncassiols C3	TP53	7157	HIT,STITCH
Deoxycholic acid, limonene	HMGCR	3156	HIT,HIT
Deoxycholic acid	BIRC2	329	HIT
Deoxycholic acid	BAK1	578	HIT
Deoxycholic acid	EGFR	1956	HIT
Deoxycholic acid	GPT	2875	HIT
Deoxycholic acid	ICAM1	3383	HIT
Deoxycholic acid	L1CAM	3897	HIT
Deoxycholic acid	MCL1	4170	HIT
Deoxycholic acid	MUC2	4583	HIT

Table S4 SBP's target proteins—cont'd

Compounds	Gene symbol	Entrez	Database
Deoxycholic acid	PTPRG	5793	HIT
Deoxycholic acid	BAG3	9531	HIT
D–Borneol	OXT	5020	STITCH
D–Borneol	PPA1	5464	STITCH
D–Borneol	RB1	5925	STITCH
D–Borneol	ULK1	8408	STITCH
D–Borneol	CAMKK2	10645	STITCH
D–Borneol	CAMKK1	84254	STITCH
Coumarin	CYP2A13	1553	STITCH
Cinobufagin, muscone, muscol, testosterone, oleanolic acid, ginsenoside Rf (dammarane,β-D-glucopyranoside deriv), bufalin, ursodeoxycholic acid, hyodeoxycholic acid, 3-epioleanolic acid	CYP3A4	1576	STITCH,HIT
Cinobufagin 3-acetate, 1-hydroxy-cinobufagin, cinobufotalin, 19-oxo-cinobufotalin	GLRA1	2741	STITCH
Cinobufagin 3-acetate, 1-hydroxy-cinobufagin, cinobufotalin, 19-oxo-cinobufotalin	RRM2	6241	STITCH
Cinnzeylanine, cinncassiols D1	ACADL	33	STITCH
Cinnzeylanine, cinncassiols D1	TBL1X	6907	STITCH
Cinnzeylanine, cinncassiols D1	CDK5RAP1	51654	STITCH
Cinnzeylanine, cinncassiols D1	EXOSC4	54512	STITCH
Cinnzeylanine, cinncassiols D1	IFT80	57560	STITCH
Cinnzeylanine, cinncassiols D1	TBL1XR1	79718	STITCH
Cinnzeylanine, cinncassiols D1	TBL1Y	90665	STITCH
Cinnzeylanine, cinncassiols D1	WDR17	116966	STITCH
Cinnzeylanine, cinncassiols D1	EXOSC6	118460	STITCH
Cinnzeylanine, Cinncassiols A, Cinncassiols B	ADCY1	107	STITCH
Cinncassiols, cinncassiols D3	MT1X	4501	STITCH
Cinncassiols, cinncassiols D3	DOCK4	9732	STITCH
Cinncassiols D4	AGA	175	STITCH
Cinncassiols D4	CHIT1	1118	STITCH
Cinncassiols D4	HEXA	3073	STITCH
Cinncassiols D4	HEXB	3074	STITCH
Cinncassiols D4	RAB27A	5873	STITCH
Cinncassiols D4	SI	6476	STITCH
Cinncassiols D4	RPL23	9349	STITCH
Cinncassiols D4	SF3B4	10262	STITCH
Cinncassiols D4	CHIA	27159	STITCH
Cinncassiols D4	SIAE	54414	STITCH
Cinncassiols D4	TASP1	55617	STITCH
Cinncassiols D4	ASRGL1	80150	STITCH
Cinncassiols D4	OVCA2	124641	STITCH

Continued

Table S4 SBP's target proteins—cont'd

Compounds	Gene symbol	Entrez	Database
Cinncassiols D4	ASPG	374569	STITCH
Cinncassiols C3	CCND1	595	STITCH
Cinnamyl acetate, myrcene, cinnamyl acetate	TKT	7086	STITCH
Cinnamyl acetate, myrcene, cinnamyl acetate	TKTL1	8277	STITCH
Cinnamyl acetate, myrcene, cinnamyl acetate	TKTL2	84076	STITCH
Cinnamyl acetate, cinnamyl acetate	CPT1A	1374	STITCH
Cinnamyl acetate, cinnamyl acetate	CPT1B	1375	STITCH
Cinnamyl acetate, cinnamyl acetate	ARL5A	26225	STITCH
Cinnamyl acetate, cinnamyl acetate	CPT1C	126129	STITCH
Cinnamaldehyde	C5AR1	728	HIT
Cinnamaldehyde	IFNB1	3456	HIT
Cinnamaldehyde	IRF3	3661	HIT
Cinnamaldehyde	RELA	5970	HIT
Cinnamaldehyde	TLR4	7099	HIT
Cinnamaldehyde	TXNRD1	7296	HIT
Cinnamaldehyde	TRPV1	7442	HIT
Cinnamaldehyde	TRPV4	59341	HIT
Cholic acid, glycocholic acid	SLC10A1	6554	STITCH
Cholic acid, glycocholic acid	SLC10A2	6555	STITCH
Cholic acid, glycocholic acid	ABCB11	8647	STITCH
Cholic acid, glycocholic acid	SLC27A5	10998	STITCH
Cholic acid, chenodeoxycholic acid, glycocholic acid	NR1H4	9971	STITCH,HIT
Cholic acid	COX5B	1329	STITCH
Cholic acid	COX6A2	1339	STITCH
Cholic acid	COX6B1	1340	STITCH
Cholic acid	COX7A1	1346	STITCH
Cholic acid	COX7C	1350	STITCH
Cholic acid	ESRRG	2104	STITCH
Cholic acid	FECH	2235	STITCH
Cholic acid	COX5A	9377	STITCH
Cholesterol, notoginsenoside R_2	SREBF2	6721	STITCH
Cholesterol, glycocholic acid	ALB	213	STITCH
Cholesterol, deoxycholic acid	LDLR	3949	STITCH,HIT
Cholesterol	ABCA1	19	STITCH
Cholesterol	APOA1	335	STITCH
Cholesterol	APOB	338	STITCH
Cholesterol	APOE	348	STITCH
Cholesterol	CAV1	857	STITCH
Cholesterol	CETP	1071	STITCH
Cholesterol	CYP11A1	1583	STITCH
Cholesterol	CYP27A1	1593	STITCH
Cholesterol	LCAT	3931	STITCH

Table S4 SBP's target proteins—cont'd

Compounds	Gene symbol	Entrez	Database
Cholesterol	LPA	4018	STITCH
Cholesterol	LPL	4023	STITCH
Cholesterol	SOAT1	6646	STITCH
Cholesterol	SCAP	22937	STITCH
Cholesterol	ABCG8	64241	STITCH
Cholest-4-en-4-one, testosterone	AKR1D1	6718	STITCH
Cholest-4-en-3-one, cholesterol, cholic acid, deoxycholic acid	CYP7A1	1581	STITCH,HIT
Cassioside	FDFT1	2222	STITCH
Cassioside	LSS	4047	STITCH
Cassioside	RPE65	6121	STITCH
Cassioside	BCMO1	53630	STITCH
Cassioside	BCO2	83875	STITCH
Cassioside	ZNF644	84146	STITCH
Cassioside	ISPD	729920	STITCH
Camphene	CNR1	1268	STITCH
Calamenene	HTR1A	3350	STITCH
Butanoic acid	CCK	885	STITCH
Butanoic acid	GAST	2520	STITCH
Butanoic acid	GCG	2641	STITCH
Butanoic acid	GCGR	2642	STITCH
Butanoic acid	FFAR1	2864	STITCH
Butanoic acid	FFAR2	2867	STITCH
Butanoic acid	GSN	2934	STITCH
Butanoic acid	NTS	4922	STITCH
Butanoic acid	PTAFR	5724	STITCH
Butanoic acid	TAC1	6863	STITCH
Butanoic acid	TACR2	6865	STITCH
Butanoic acid	TACR1	6869	STITCH
Butanoic acid	TACR3	6870	STITCH
Butanoic acid	TRH	7200	STITCH
Butanoic acid	LPAR2	9170	STITCH
Butanoic acid	NPS	594857	STITCH
Bufoserotonins B,5-hydroxyindoleacetic acid (5-HIAA)(5-hydroxyindole-3-acetic acid)	SPR	6697	STITCH
Bufoserotonins A, bufoserotonins B, 5-hydroxyindoleacetic acid (5-HIAA) (5-hydroxyindole-3-acetic acid)	ASMT	438	STITCH
Bufoserotonins A, bufoserotonins B	AANAT	15	STITCH
Bufoserotonins A, bufoserotonins B	IDO1	3620	STITCH
Bufoserotonins A, bufoserotonins B	MTNR1A	4543	STITCH
Bufoserotonins A, bufoserotonins B	MTNR1B	4544	STITCH
Bufoserotonins A, bufoserotonins B	NQO2	4835	STITCH

Continued

Table S4 SBP's target proteins—cont'd

Compounds	Gene symbol	Entrez	Database
Bufoserotonins A	HTR1D	3352	STITCH
Bufoserotonins A	HTR2A	3356	STITCH
Bufalin, cinnamtannin A2, cinnamtannin A3, (procyanidin B-2 6-C-β-D-glucopyranoside)	CASP9	842	STITCH
Bufalin, cinnamtannin A2, Cinnamtannin A3, (procyanidin B-2 6-C-β-D-glucopyranoside)	MAPK1	5594	STITCH
Bufalin, cinnamtannin A2, cinnamtannin A3, (procyanidin B-2 6-C-β-D-glucopyranoside)	MAPK3	5595	STITCH
Bufalin	GNRH1	2796	STITCH
Bufalin	MAPK8	5599	STITCH
Bufalin	MAPK9	5601	STITCH
Bufalin	TF	7018	STITCH
Bufalin	EIF2AK3	9451	STITCH
Bufalin	ZNF263	10127	STITCH
Bilirubin, vanillin, vanillic acid, β-phenylpropionic acid	UGT1A10	54575	STITCH
Bilirubin, vanillin, vanillic acid, β-phenylpropionic acid	UGT1A8	54576	STITCH
Bilirubin, vanillin, vanillic acid, β-phenylpropionic acid	UGT1A7	54577	STITCH
Bilirubin, D-borneol	UGT1A5	54579	STITCH
Bilirubin, D-borneol	UGT1A9	54600	STITCH
Bilirubin, D-borneol	UGT1A4	54657	STITCH
Bilirubin, D-borneol	UGT1A3	54659	STITCH
Bilirubin, coumarin	UGT2B15	7366	STITCH
Bilirubin	ALPL	249	STITCH
Bilirubin	ALPP	250	STITCH
Bilirubin	ALPPL2	251	STITCH
Bilirubin	BLVRA	644	STITCH
Bilirubin	HMOX1	3162	STITCH
Bilirubin	HMOX2	3163	STITCH
Bilirubin	UGT2B7	7364	STITCH
Bilirubin	UGT2B10	7365	STITCH
Bilirubin	UGT2B11	10720	STITCH
Beta-pinene, myrcene	COLQ	8292	STITCH
Beta-pinene, myrcene	SPEN	23013	STITCH
Beta-pinene, myrcene	TPSD1	23430	STITCH
Beta-pinene	ALAS1	211	STITCH
Beta-pinene	ST3GAL3	6487	STITCH
Benzyl cinnamate	AKR1C2	1646	STITCH
Benzyl cinnamate	NQO1	1728	STITCH
Benzyl cinnamate	MT1A	4489	STITCH
Benzyl cinnamate	MT2A	4502	STITCH

Table S4 SBP's target proteins—cont'd

Compounds	Gene symbol	Entrez	Database
Benzyl cinnamate	TXN	7295	STITCH
Benzyl cinnamate	MAFF	23764	STITCH
Benzyl cinnamate	FAM60A	58516	STITCH
Benzoic acid	RAB9A	9367	STITCH
Benzoic acid	HRSP12	10247	STITCH
Benzoic acid	GLYAT	10249	STITCH
Benzoic acid	PRDX5	25824	STITCH
Benzoic acid	ACSM1	116285	STITCH
Benzoic acid	ACSM2B	348158	STITCH
Benzaldehyde	ALDH1A2	8854	STITCH
Benzaldehyde	ALDH8A1	64577	STITCH
α-Terpineol, (−)-epicatechin	IL6	3569	HIT
Arenobufagin, bufarenogin, Ψ-bufarenogin (psi-bufarenogin), telocinobufagin, bufotalidin (hellebrigenin)	SDF4	51150	STITCH
Alpha-pinene	LHFPL5	222662	STITCH
Adenine, uracil	SLC29A2	3177	STITCH
Adenine, cassioside	SLC29A3	55315	STITCH
Adenine	ACACB	32	STITCH
Adenine	ACP1	52	STITCH
Adenine	ACVR2B	93	STITCH
Adenine	ADA	100	STITCH
Adenine	APRT	353	STITCH
Adenine	HSP90AA1	3320	STITCH
Adenine	MTAP	4507	STITCH
Adenine	PNMT	5409	STITCH
Adenine	PYGM	5837	STITCH
Adenine	SRPK2	6733	STITCH
Adenine	STK24	8428	STITCH
Adenine	SF3B1	23451	STITCH
Adenine	SF3B14	51639	STITCH
Adenine	CHFR	55743	STITCH
Adenine	PECR	55825	STITCH
Adenine	MRI1	84245	STITCH
Adenine	ADAT3	113179	STITCH
Abietatriene-3β-ol	STS	412	STITCH
Abietatriene-3β-ol	RXRA	6256	STITCH
5-Hydroxyindoleacetic acid (5-HIAA) (5-hydroxyindole-3-acetic acid), calamenene	TH	7054	STITCH
5-Hydroxyindoleacetic acid (5-HIAA) (5-hydroxyindole-3-acetic acid)	ALDH2	217	STITCH
5-Hydroxyindoleacetic acid (5-HIAA) (5-hydroxyindole-3-acetic acid)	ALDH1B1	219	STITCH
5-Hydroxyindoleacetic acid (5-HIAA) (5-hydroxyindole-3-acetic acid)	ALDH9A1	223	STITCH

Continued

Table S4 SBP's target proteins—cont'd

Compounds	Gene symbol	Entrez	Database
5-Hydroxyindoleacetic acid (5-HIAA) (5-hydroxyindole-3-acetic acid)	ALDH3A2	224	STITCH
5-Hydroxyindoleacetic acid (5-HIAA) (5-hydroxyindole-3-acetic acid)	AOX1	316	STITCH
5-Hydroxyindoleacetic acid (5-HIAA) (5-hydroxyindole-3-acetic acid)	CBR1	873	STITCH
5-Hydroxyindoleacetic acid (5-HIAA) (5-hydroxyindole-3-acetic acid)	DDC	1644	STITCH
5-Hydroxyindoleacetic acid (5-HIAA) (5-hydroxyindole-3-acetic acid)	GCH1	2643	STITCH
5-Hydroxyindoleacetic acid (5-HIAA) (5-hydroxyindole-3-acetic acid)	MAOA	4128	STITCH
5-Hydroxyindoleacetic acid (5-HIAA) (5-hydroxyindole-3-acetic acid)	MAOB	4129	STITCH
5-Hydroxyindoleacetic acid (5-HIAA) (5-hydroxyindole-3-acetic acid)	SLC6A4	6532	STITCH
5-Hydroxyindoleacetic acid (5-HIAA) (5-hydroxyindole-3-acetic acid)	TPH1	7166	STITCH
4-Ethyphenol	GPATCH1	55094	STITCH
3-Ethyphenol, β-phenylpropionic acid	TYR	7299	STITCH
3′-O-Methyl-(−)-epicatechin, 5,3′-di-O-methylate-(−)-epicatechin, 5,7,3′-tri-O-methylate-(−)-epicatechin, (4′-O-methyl-(+)-catechin), (7,4′-di-O-methylate-(+)-catechin), (5,7,4′-tri-O-methylate-(+)-catechin), 5,7-dimethyl-3′,4′-di-O-methylene-(±)-epicatechin	CA3	761	STITCH
3′-O-Methyl-(−)-epicatechin, 5,3′-Di-O-methylate-(−)-epicatechin, 5,7,3′-tri-O-methylate-(−)-epicatechin, (4′-O-methyl-(+)-catechin), (7,4′-di-O-methylate-(+)-catechin), (5,7,4′-tri-O-methylate-(+)-catechin), 5,7-dimethyl-3′,4′-di-O-methylene-(±)-epicatechin	CA4	762	STITCH
3′-O-methyl-(−)-epicatechin, 5,3′-di-O-methylate-(−)-epicatechin, 5,7,3′-tri-O-methylate-(−)-epicatechin, (4′-O-methyl-(+)-catechin), (7,4′-di-O-methylate-(+)-catechin), (5,7,4′-tri-O-methylate-(+)-catechin), 5,7-dimethyl-3′,4′-di-O-methylene-(±)-epicatechin	CA5A	763	STITCH

Table S4 SBP's target proteins—cont'd

Compounds	Gene symbol	Entrez	Database
3′-O-Methyl-(−)-epicatechin, 5,3′-di-O-methylate-(−)-epicatechin, 5,7,3′-tri-O-methylate-(−)-epicatechin, (4′-O-methyl-(+)-catechin), (7,4′-di-O-methylate-(+)-catechin), (5,7,4′-tri-O-methylate-(+)-catechin), 5,7-dimethyl-3′,4′-di-O-methylene-(±)-epicatechin	CA6	765	STITCH
3′-O-Methyl-(−)-epicatechin, 5,3′-di-O-methylate-(−)-epicatechin, 5,7,3′-tri-O-methylate-(−)-epicatechin, (4′-O-methyl-(+)-catechin), (7,4′-di-O-methylate-(+)-catechin), (5,7,4′-tri-O-methylate-(+)-catechin), 5,7-dimethyl-3′,4′-di-O-methylene-(±)-epicatechin	CA7	766	STITCH
3′-O-Methyl-(−)-epicatechin, 5,3′-di-O-methylate-(−)-epicatechin, 5,7,3′-tri-O-methylate-(−)-epicatechin, (4′-O-methyl-(+)-catechin), (7,4′-di-O-methylate-(+)-catechin), (5,7,4′-tri-O-methylate-(+)-catechin), 5,7-dimethyl-3′,4′-di-O-methylene-(±)-epicatechin	CA9	768	STITCH
3′-O-Methyl-(−)-epicatechin, 5,3′-di-O-methylate-(−)-epicatechin, 5,7,3′-tri-O-methylate-(−)-epicatechin, (4′-O-methyl-(+)-catechin), (7,4′-di-O-methylate-(+)-catechin), (5,7,4′-tri-O-methylate-(+)-catechin), 5,7-dimethyl-3′,4′-di-O-methylene-(±)-epicatechin	CA12	771	STITCH
3′-O-Methyl-(−)-epicatechin, 5,3′-di-O-methylate-(−)-epicatechin, 5,7,3′-tri-O-methylate-(−)-epicatechin, (4′-O-methyl-(+)-catechin), (7,4′-di-O-methylate-(+)-catechin), (5,7,4′-tri-O-methylate-(+)-catechin), 5,7-dimethyl-3′,4′-di-O-methylene-(±)-epicatechin	CA5B	11238	STITCH
3,4,5-Trimethoxyphenol-β-D-apiofuranosyl (1→6)-β-D-glucopyranoside	AMY2A	279	STITCH
3,4,5-Trimethoxyphenol-β-D-apiofuranosyl (1→6)-β-D-glucopyranoside	GANC	2595	STITCH
3,4,5-trimethoxyphenol-β-D-apiofuranosyl (1→6)-β-D-glucopyranoside	TGM4	7047	STITCH
3,4,5-Trimethoxyphenol-β-D-apiofuranosyl (1→6)-β-D-glucopyranoside	GANAB	23193	STITCH
2-Piperidinecarboxylic acid, benzoic acid	DAO	1610	STITCH
2-Piperidinecarboxylic acid, 5-hydroxyindoleacetic acid (5-HIAA) (5-hydroxyindole-3-acetic acid)	ALDH7A1	501	STITCH

Continued

Table S4 SBP's target proteins—cont'd

Compounds	Gene symbol	Entrez	Database
2-Piperidinecarboxylic acid	ATP5A1	498	STITCH
2-Piperidinecarboxylic acid	ATP5B	506	STITCH
2-Piperidinecarboxylic acid	ATP5C1	509	STITCH
2-Piperidinecarboxylic acid	CAT	847	STITCH
2-Piperidinecarboxylic acid	F2	2147	STITCH
2-Piperidinecarboxylic acid	PEX1	5189	STITCH
2-Piperidinecarboxylic acid	PHYH	5264	STITCH
2-Piperidinecarboxylic acid	PIN1	5300	STITCH
2-Piperidinecarboxylic acid	PREP	5550	STITCH
2-Piperidinecarboxylic acid	CLPP	8192	STITCH
2-Piperidinecarboxylic acid	GNPAT	8443	STITCH
2-Piperidinecarboxylic acid	PREPL	9581	STITCH
2-Piperidinecarboxylic acid	AASS	10157	STITCH
2-Piperidinecarboxylic acid	PIPOX	51268	STITCH
2-Piperidinecarboxylic acid	PEX26	55670	STITCH
2-Ethyphenol	FTL	2512	STITCH
?Benzyl benzoate (Ascabin), benzyl benzoate	LIPE	3991	STITCH
?5-Hydroxymethyl-2-furaldehyde	DCX	1641	STITCH
?5-Hydroxymethyl-2-furaldehyde	HBA2	3040	STITCH
?5-Hydroxymethyl-2-furaldehyde	HBB	3043	STITCH
?5-Hydroxymethyl-2-furaldehyde	SULT1A2	6799	STITCH
(?(−)-Epicatechin 3-O-β-D-glucopyranoside)	RPL8	6132	STITCH
(?(−)-epicatechin 3-O-β-D-glucopyranoside)	SLC5A1	6523	STITCH
(?(−)-Epicatechin 3-O-β-D-glucopyranoside)	TBP	6908	STITCH
(?(−)-Epicatechin 3-O-β-D-glucopyranoside)	TBPL1	9519	STITCH
(?(−)-Epicatechin 3-O-β-D-glucopyranoside)	MRPL2	51069	STITCH
(?(−)-Epicatechin 3-O-β-D-glucopyranoside)	TBPL2	387332	STITCH
(−)-Epicatechin	COMT	1312	HIT
(−)-Epicatechin	CREB1	1385	HIT
(−)-Epicatechin	ACE	1636	HIT
(−)-Epicatechin	GCLC	2729	HIT
(−)-Epicatechin	GRIA2	2891	HIT
(−)-Epicatechin	GRIN1	2902	HIT
(−)-Epicatechin	GSS	2937	HIT
(−)-Epicatechin	HAS2	3037	HIT
(−)-Epicatechin	IL1A	3552	HIT
(−)-Epicatechin	PLAT	5327	HIT
(−)-Epicatechin	PLAU	5328	HIT
(−)-Epicatechin	POR	5447	HIT
(−)-Epicatechin	CCL2	6347	HIT
(−)-Epicatechin	DUOX2	50506	HIT
(−)-Epicatechin	CRTC2	200186	HIT
((−)-Epicatechin 8-C-β-D-glucopyranoside)	MANBA	4126	STITCH
((−)-Epicatechin 6-C-β-D-glucopyranoside)	SLC5A2	6524	STITCH

Table S5 SBP's plasma absorbed compounds and their targets

Component	Medicinal materials	Target	Database
Muscone	Moschus	CYP3A4	STITCH
Ginsenoside Rb$_1$	Total ginsenoside ginseng root	AHR	HIT
		BHLHE76	
		ESR2	
		ESTRB	
		NR3A2	
Ginsenoside Rb$_2$(20-[(6-O-alpha-L-arabinopyranosyl-beta-D-glucopyranosyl)oxy]-12beta-hydroxydammar-24-en-3beta-yl 2-O-Beta-D-glucopyranosyl-beta-D-glucopyranoside)	Total ginsenoside ginseng root	NFE2L2	STITCH
		AKT1	
Ginsenoside Rb$_3$ (dammarane,β-D-glucopyranoside deriv)	Total ginsenoside ginseng root	NFE2L2	STITCH
		AKT1	
Ginsenoside Rd	Total ginsenoside ginseng root	CASP3	HIT
		CPP32	
		PSMD3	
		BCL2	
		BCL2L4	
		BAX	
Ginsenoside Rc	Total ginsenoside ginseng root	FOS	HIT
		G0S7	
		CYP2C9	
		CYP2C10	
Ginsenoside Re	Total ginsenoside ginseng root	NOS3	HIT
		BAX	
		BCL2L4	
		NOS2	
		NOS2A	
		CASP3	
		CPP32	
		BCL2	
		FOS	
		G0S7	
Ginsenoside Rg$_1$	Total ginsenoside ginseng root	AHR	HIT
		BHLHE76	
		CYP1A1	
		ACTA2	
		ACTSA	
		ACTVS	
		GIG46	
		TGFB1	
		TGFB	

Continued

Table S5 SBP's plasma absorbed compounds and their targets—cont'd

Component	Medicinal materials	Target	Database
		SMAD2	
		MADH2	
		MADR2	
		THBS1	
		TSP	
		TSP1	
		CDH1	
		CDHE	
		UVO	
		COL1A1	
		FN1	
		FN	
		PRKCB	
		PKCB	
		PRKCB1	
		IL2	
		IL4	
Resibufogenin	Bufonis Venenum	PHKA1	STITCH
		ECEL1	
		TAF1	
		ZC3H15	
		DRG1	
		SERPINA6	
		RPS12	
		PGK1	
		RWDD1	
		GCN1L1	
Gamabufotalin (gamabufogenin)	Bufonis Venenum	PHKA1	STITCH
		ECEL1	
		TAF1	
		ZC3H15	
		DRG1	
		SERPINA6	
		RPS12	
		PGK1	
		RWDD1	
		GCN1L1	
Arenobufagin	Bufonis Venenum	SDF4	STITCH

Table S5 SBP's plasma absorbed compounds and their targets—cont'd

Component	Medicinal materials	Target	Database
Bufalin	Bufonis Venenum	CYP3A4	STITCH
		CASP3	
		BAX	
		CASP9	
		EIF2AK3	
		GNRH1	
		TF	
		ZNF263	
		MMP9	
		MAPK8	
		MAPK9	
		MAPK3	
		MAPK1	
1β–Hydroxybufalin	Bufonis Venenum	PHKA1	STITCH
		ECEL1	
		TAF1	
		ZC3H15	
		DRG1	
		SERPINA6	
		RPS12	
		PGK1	
		RWDD1	
		GCN1L1	
Bufotalin	Bufonis Venenum	PHKA1	STITCH
		ECEL1	
		TAF1	
		ZC3H15	
		DRG1	
		SERPINA6	
		RPS12	
		PGK1	
		RWDD1	
		GCN1L1	
Telocinobufagin	Bufonis Venenum	SDF4	STITCH
Cinobufotalin	Bufonis Venenum	RRM2	STITCH
		GLRA1	
Ursodeoxycholic acid	Bovis Calculus Artifactus	CYP3A4	HIT
		CYP3A3	
		FABP6	HIT
		ILBP	
		ILLBP	
		NCOA1	HIT
		BHLHE74	

Continued

Table S5 SBP's plasma absorbed compounds and their targets—cont'd

Component	Medicinal materials	Target	Database
		SRC1	
		BCL2	HIT
		E2F1	HIT
		RBBP3	
Cholic acid	Bovis Calculus Artifactus	ABCB11	STITCH
		FABP6	
		CES1	
		FECH	
		NR1H4	
		ESRRG	
		MT-CO2	
		COX5A	
		COX7A1	
		COX6A2	
		MT-CO3	
		MT-CO1	
		GPBAR1	
		COX5B	
		COX6B1	
		CYP7A1	
		SLC10A2	
		COX7C	
		SLC10A1	
		SLC27A5	
Deoxycholic acid	Bovis Calculus Artifactus	BAG3	HIT
		BIS	
		BIRC2	
		API1	
		IAP2	
		MIHB	
		RNF48	
		MCL1	
		BCL2L3	
		BAK1	
		BAK	
		BCL2L7	
		CDN1	
		TP53	
		P53	
		MUC2	
		SMUC	
		ICAM1	
		VCAM1	
		L1CAM	

Table S5 SBP's plasma absorbed compounds and their targets—cont'd

Component	Medicinal materials	Target	Database
		PTGS2	
		COX2	
		PTPRG	
		PTPG	
		EGFR	
		ERBB1	
		CYP7A1	
		CYP7	
		LDLR	
		GPT	
		AAT1	
		GPT1	
		HMGCR	
Chenodeoxycholic acid	Bovis Calculus Artifactus	NR1H4	HIT
		BAR	
		FXR	
		HRR1	
		RIP14	
Hyodeoxycholic acid	Bovis Calculus Artifactus	UGT2B4	STITCH
		CYP3A4	
		GHDC	
Cinnamaldehyde	Styrax	C5AR1	HIT
		C5AR	
		C5R1	
		TRPV1	
		VR1	
		TRPV4	
		VRL2	
		VROAC	
		NFKBIA	
		IKBA	
		MAD3	
		NFKBI	
		NFE2L2	
		NRF2	
		TXNRD1	
		GRIM12	
		KDRF	
		RELA	
		NFKB3	
		IRF3	
		TLR4	
		PTGS2	
		COX2	
		IFNB1	

Continued

Table S5 SBP's plasma absorbed compounds and their targets—cont'd

Component	Medicinal materials	Target	Database
cis–cinnamic acid	Styrax	IFB IFNB CA1 CA2	STITCH
Benzyl benzoate	Styrax	LIPE	STITCH
D–Borneol	Borneolum Syntheticum	RB1 UGT1A5 UGT1A4 CAMKK2 CAMKK1 UGT1A3 UGT1A9 PPA1 UGT1A1 ULK1 OXT	STITCH
Isoborneol	Borneolum Syntheticum	SLC7A2 SLC7A4 SLC7A1 ENSG00000188666 SLC7A3 SLC7A14 DICER1 RNASEN	STITCH

Table S6 Significant expressed genes and corresponding fold change values

Gene_symbol	Entrez_gene	Fold change
TRAF3IP3	80342	0.049808
GAD2	2572	18.57932
CYLC1	1538	18.10809
SYNGR1	9145	0.061548
NLGN4Y	22829	0.063076
MME	4311	15.64419
TACC1	6867	15.50599
TOX3	27324	15.42795
PRKDC	5591	0.065013
LCN2	3934	14.43118
ZKSCAN8	7745	0.069429

Table S6 Significant expressed genes and corresponding fold change values—cont'd

Gene_symbol	Entrez_gene	Fold change
C3orf18	51161	0.06987
LAMA4	3910	0.073016
HEXA-AS1	80072	0.074715
LOXL2	4017	13.0397
RBMXL2	27288	13.02746
TNIP3	79931	0.078097
ELTD1	64123	12.73362
KRT83	3889	0.079213
TNFSF14	8740	0.079748
EPS15L1	58513	12.24958
PRX	57716	0.082222
ZC2HC1C	79696	0.084623
TEX13A	56157	11.79943
MBL2	4153	0.086092
ANXA13	312	11.44103
Igk	243469	0.088902
PELO	53918	0.088978
BAI3	577	0.089595
CFI	3426	0.093251
IGFBP7	3490	0.093929
CDH20	28316	0.094785
ECM2	1842	10.5127
SPAM1	6677	0.095205
EFCAB1	79645	0.095469
DIAPH3	81624	10.46563
SLC7A8	23428	10.42589
SAP30	8819	10.38012
PTPRT	11122	10.37189
DPEP3	64180	10.33414
CDH15	1013	10.28328
ATXN3	4287	0.097484
MUSK	4593	0.099133
XYLB	9942	0.10109
LAMP3	27074	0.101299
BHMT	635	9.857221
MCM3AP	8888	9.822597
ZNF135	7694	0.10245
MMP1	4312	9.705378
ISG20L2	81875	9.703212
OPRL1	4987	0.104977
DOCK5	80005	0.105559
CAMK1D	57118	0.106208

Continued

Table S6 Significant expressed genes and corresponding fold change values—cont'd

Gene_symbol	Entrez_gene	Fold change
ANGPTL2	23452	0.106298
TTLL7	79739	0.106309
PTK2B	2185	0.107349
SEMA3D	223117	9.211773
GABRA5	2558	0.109001
ELF5	2001	9.153281
EPM2A	7957	0.109313
TLL1	7092	0.109628
ERV9-1	1.01E+08	9.060175
PPP1R3A	5506	0.110831
PARVB	29780	0.110934
TTC22	55001	0.111884
RASL12	51285	0.112133
ELL2	22936	8.895335
FGF20	26281	0.112481
C14orf105	55195	0.112763
DSC2	1824	8.817805
CIB2	10518	8.79141
MIR1257///TAF4	6874///100302168	8.785914
PRKG1	5592	0.113837
ENTPD3	956	8.776766
CASR	846	8.762664
TTTY2///TTTY2B	60439///100101117	8.760013
ADAM22	53616	0.114552
PCCA	5095	0.115014
TRPC6	7225	8.684741
UGT2B4	7363	8.669116
LZTS1	11178	0.115721
CD4	920	0.116837
AQP4	361	0.116923
CRHR1	1394	0.11697
FGB	2244	8.526688
PDLIM4	8572	0.11729
NFATC4	4776	0.117306
GABRG2	2566	0.117487
MSR1	4481	0.117944
CCIN	881	8.473448
FAM65B	9750	0.11856
CALD1	800	0.118984
GCM2	9247	8.381394
SPOCK3	50859	0.119771
SOCS1	8651	0.120055

Table S6 Significant expressed genes and corresponding fold change values—cont'd

Gene_symbol	Entrez_gene	Fold change
CDKN1C	1028	8.310353
SIRPB1	10326	0.12066
IGH///IGHA1///IGHG1///IGHG2///IGHG3///IGHM	3492///3493///3500///3501///3502///3507	8.282598
ADH1B	125	0.120986
ARPP21	10777	0.122065
CAMP	820	0.12253
RECK	8434	8.156001
PLA2R1	22925	0.123234
SCG3	29106	0.123401
SPON1	10418	0.12396
HAL	3034	0.124515
CCDC134	79879	0.125059
SELPLG	6404	7.97903
LINC00965	349196	0.125383
PDPN	10630	0.127127
DYRK3	8444	0.127329
CCDC102B	79839	0.127625
IL5RA	3568	0.128061
TIAM2	26230	7.80199
TEK	7010	0.129225
PAK3	5063	0.129631
MST1L	11223	0.129675
LOC101060620///MAPK8IP1	9479///101060620	7.70517
PDLIM5	10611	0.130006
HGF	3082	7.691901
TNKS	8658	7.673146
TAZ	6901	0.130691
PCLO	27445	0.130696
CD69	969	7.629999
VSNL1	7447	7.629885
PTN	5764	7.629177
CWH43	80157	7.613785
PSMB9	5698	0.131491
ABCB11	8647	7.597977
DCX	1641	7.581249
TCF21	6943	7.553765
PTRF	284119	0.132907
ECRP	643332	7.508783
CDH6	1004	7.48641
CGA	1081	0.133665
CALY	50632	7.472534

Continued

Table S6 Significant expressed genes and corresponding fold change values—cont'd

Gene_symbol	Entrez_gene	Fold change
C16orf70	80262	0.133868
ASTN1	460	7.46684
SMARCA4	6597	7.460428
IGHD	3495	7.406807
SMG7-AS1	284649	0.135044
DCHS2	54798	0.13511
CYP1B1	1545	7.394989
LOC100507388	1.01E+08	0.135247
LOC100996400///NOL4	8715///100996400	0.135313
EDA	1896	0.13577
PTPN20A///PTPN20B	26095///653129	0.137094
MAGI2	9863	0.137344
CASP1	834	7.280741
CCL23	6368	7.246165
SCGB1D1	10648	7.220643
CYP1A1	1543	7.197823
GPR98	84059	0.139598
DAB2	1601	0.139781
PTCD2	79810	0.139878
ADAM28	10863	0.139939
CCDC85B	11007	7.123477
ALB	213	0.140735
MYF5	4617	0.142132
ENG	2022	0.142194
IGF2BP3	10643	6.975194
PTGS2	5743	0.144067
CDKN2A	1029	0.144933
HBA1///HBA2	3039///3040	0.144972
DUSP1	1843	6.875058
PER2	8864	6.858962
CDKL5	6792	0.146056
IGHA1///IGHG1///IGHM///IGHV3-23///IGHV4-31	3493///3500///3507///28396///28442	0.146131
EMX2	2018	0.146491
MORN1	79906	0.146525
GIMAP1-GIMAP5///GIMAP5	55340///100527949	6.815763
GPLD1	2822	6.783258
PCSK5	5125	6.767327
APOB	338	0.148074
BAIAP3	8938	0.148099
ANKRD2	26287	6.744425
SLC23A2	9962	0.148304

Table S6 Significant expressed genes and corresponding fold change values—cont'd

Gene_symbol	Entrez_gene	Fold change
RTDR1	27156	0.148858
MAP2K2	5605	0.148968
SLC16A4	9122	6.709282
AURKC	6795	0.149083
BGN	633	0.149102
CMKLR1	1240	0.14968
LHCGR	3973	0.149763
GRIP1	23426	6.671348
APOBEC3F///APOBEC3G	60489///200316	0.150016
GYPA	2993	6.663177
CYP4F12	66002	6.642306
MAGEB4	4115	6.626046
EDNRA	1909	6.608504
BIN1	274	6.601771
KAT6A	7994	6.595417
LINC00939	400084	0.151836
SLC4A7	9497	6.584317
LOC100130331	1E+08	6.582577
SV2B	9899	0.151986
PPFIA2	8499	0.152439
NEFL	4747	6.548001
TMEM257	9142	0.152855
CXCL14	9547	0.153303
SYNE1	23345	6.508186
NBLA00301	79804	0.153963
LOC441666	441666	6.490143
SOSTDC1	25928	6.488516
KRT33B	3884	6.470345
FUT7	2529	6.454396
SRPX2	27286	6.446732
SEMA3G	56920	0.156687
CCL5	6352	0.156795
GHSR	2693	0.157019
SCN7A	6332	6.367043
UTS2	10911	0.157085
SLCO2B1	11309	6.36024
PNPLA3	80339	6.345309
BRDT	676	6.342818
P2RX1	5023	0.157827
ABCA6	23460	6.322789
GNA15	2769	0.158296
PICK1	9463	6.311152

Continued

Table S6 Significant expressed genes and corresponding fold change values—cont'd

Gene_symbol	Entrez_gene	Fold change
CFHR5	81494	6.305242
CD44	960	6.300612
IGF1	3479	0.158977
KCNJ4	3761	0.159144
PARVB	29780	6.283343
PLN	5350	0.15949
CCR9	10803	6.262108
TCF4	6925	0.159695
ICAM2	3384	6.212491
TM6SF2	53345	0.162673
PTGES	9536	0.162882
SLC39A9	55334	6.133942
MRC1	4360	0.16316
GFI1	2672	0.164101
SEC14L4	284904	0.164126
GFAP	2670	0.164137
CACNG2	10369	0.164205
MAF	4094	0.164989
ZNF132	7691	6.059267
CDK5R1	8851	0.165179
MLXIP	22877	6.039835
CSAG2///CSAG3	389903///728461	5.990051
HCP5	10866	0.167732
HSD17B2	3294	5.949833
C4BPB	725	5.945282
LRRN3	54674	0.168342
EPHB1	2047	0.168436
KIAA1045	23349	0.168494
GMFG	9535	5.918256
CHM	1121	0.169363
EFNA5	1946	0.169618
CHI3L1	1116	0.16966
FGF2	2247	0.170339
SMPX	23676	5.85365
GPR17	2840	0.171199
MEG3	55384	5.825222
FGF2	2247	0.171904
RHCE	6006	0.172181
KNG1	3827	0.172281
SPATA31C2	645961	0.172453
LALBA	3906	5.784084
ACTL6B	51412	0.173061

Table S6 Significant expressed genes and corresponding fold change values—cont'd

Gene_symbol	Entrez_gene	Fold change
C9orf38	29044	5.759905
RAG1	5896	5.756218
CMKLR1	1240	0.173813
POPDC3	64208	0.173852
FKRP	79147	5.747948
MTSS1	9788	5.745005
VCAN	1462	5.739205
6-Sep	23157	0.174491
FABP7	2173	0.174907
ELK1	2002	0.174992
LGALS7///LGALS7B	3963///653499	5.706515
SNAP91	9892	5.696224
LOC100506403///RUNX1	861///100506403	5.69353
LEF1	51176	5.689237
ESR1	2099	5.678731
CIITA	4261	5.671998
GTPBP10	85865	0.176417
HPR	3250	5.653687
FBXO17	115290	5.649747
GPX1	2876	0.177258
SCN3A	6328	0.177369
DDC	1644	5.629318
HLF	3131	0.177756
B3GALT2	8707	0.177996
F13B	2165	0.178002
PRDM10	56980	0.178138
VCAN	1462	0.178211
PRPF31	26121	5.603477
FSHR	2492	5.597511
CDA	978	0.178766
F2RL3	9002	5.582876
RECQL5	9400	0.179167
TAT	6898	5.571299
MGC4294	79160	5.565525
PECAM1	5175	0.179789
TRIM31	11074	0.179794
NPL	80896	0.179887
CES1///LOC100653057	1066///100653057	0.180399
IL7	3574	0.180538
CYP4F2	8529	5.532467
CEACAM21	90273	5.530934
TLL2	7093	0.180842

Continued

Table S6 Significant expressed genes and corresponding fold change values—cont'd

Gene_symbol	Entrez_gene	Fold change
PRKAA2	5563	0.181181
SMOX	54498	0.181637
FAM5B	57795	0.181702
AVPR2	554	0.182131
U2AF2	11338	0.182384
FAM5C	339479	5.482328
B3GALT1	8708	0.182514
KIAA1661	85375	0.182538
PDCD1LG2	80380	0.182757
KCNB2	9312	0.182843
CEACAM1	634	5.46452
KMT2A	4297	5.464303
NEUROD2	4761	0.183135
COPE	11316	0.18324
POLDIP3	84271	0.183289
BGN	633	5.452267
UGT1A1///UGT1A10///UGT1A3///UGT1A4///UGT1A5///UGT1A6///UGT1A7///UGT1A8///UGT1A9	54575///54576///54577///54578///54579///54600///54657///54658///54659	5.444446
JAK3	3718	0.184047
PPFIA4	8497	5.424242
GPR3	2827	5.391927
ZAP70	7535	5.377475
CADM4	199731	5.371842
CACNA1I	8911	0.186231
CXCL11	6373	5.368142
ACTL7B	10880	0.186855
PTGER1	5731	5.345205
ADCYAP1	116	5.335639
HDAC9	9734	5.333859
KIAA1967	57805	5.332472
AP4E1	23431	5.318138
CLUL1	27098	5.315793
CDKN1C	1028	5.312103
PLCB2	5330	5.302396
RAB40A	142684	5.299368
KCNG1	3755	0.188731
MLLT4	4301	5.294704
DAGLA	747	0.188877
LAPTM5	7805	5.291987
IGLC1	3537	5.288474

Table S6 Significant expressed genes and corresponding fold change values—cont'd

Gene_symbol	Entrez_gene	Fold change
CLCN7	1186	5.285575
PCDHGA10///PCDHGA11///PCDHGA12///PCDHGA3///PCDHGA5///PCDHGA6///PCDHGC3	5098///26025///56105///56106///56109///56110///56112	5.281698
PSG5	5673	5.277557
C14orf1	11161	5.253942
BCL11A	53335	0.190902
TRPC3	7222	0.191277
ANGPT2	285	5.227882
PLXNC1	10154	0.191511
BTN2A2	10385	0.191971
DNASE1	1773	5.195785
ATP2A3	489	0.19254
STAB2	55576	0.192576
HOXA7	3204	0.192689
GRIP2	80852	5.174947
DNAJB5	25822	0.193616
CRYBA1	1411	5.153648
MC2R	4158	5.150732
FAM182B///FAM27A///FAM27B///FAM27C	548321///728882///100132948///100133121	0.194155
SPRR1A	6698	0.194298
MYH4	4622	5.137494
MUC4	4585	0.194662
FOLH1	2346	5.133513
MPPE1	65258	0.194899
LAMA4	3910	0.195065
GRM8	2918	5.126296
NOTCH3	4854	5.126225
SLC6A6	6533	5.123775
NR2F6	2063	0.195601
BUB1	699	0.195997
MFAP3L	9848	0.196999
PSG2	5670	5.065988
TRIM15	89870	5.064375
CCL20	6364	0.198221
GPA33	10223	5.039552
C1orf186///LOC100505650	440712///100505650	0.198569
TNMD	64102	0.198714
CBLN1	869	0.198716
LOC101060181///ZNF44	51710///101060181	5.031502

Continued

Table S6 Significant expressed genes and corresponding fold change values—cont'd

Gene_symbol	Entrez_gene	Fold change
KIR3DL2///LOC727787	3812///727787	0.199451
ADAM3A	1587	5.011363
SCGB1D2	10647	0.199663
SLC26A3	1811	5.007883
LTC4S	4056	0.199985
VGLL1	51442	0.200052
LRRC32	2615	0.200356
N4BP2L1	90634	0.200382
IFNB1	3456	0.200548
LOC100506124///TTC21B	79809///100506124	0.200596
FCER2	2208	4.984489
NCKIPSD	51517	0.200682
TACR1	6869	0.200781
CRTAM	56253	0.20086
IGHV5-78	28387	0.200963
CSN3	1448	4.949852
ZNF154	7710	0.202151
FLT1	2321	0.202276
PDPN	10630	4.940035
FUT3	2525	4.931013
LOC100507472///PCSK6	5046///100507472	0.203107
CPM	1368	4.922866
GPR132	29933	4.922575
PCDHGB6	56100	4.913877
XCL1	6375	0.203546
HIC2	23119	4.90501
MYCN	4613	0.203975
PKD2L2	27039	4.901526
MOGAT2	80168	0.204024
GALR2	8811	4.897788
CEACAM3	1084	0.204564
ID2B	84099	0.205304
SLC24A1	9187	0.205461
CDH6	1004	0.20581
HBE1	3046	4.844616
HCRP1	387535	4.842431
LIPE	3991	0.206557
SLC15A1	6564	0.206567
GPR85	54329	0.206874
SLC7A8	23428	0.207573
TNIK	23043	4.814631
KLK7	5650	0.207762

Table S6 Significant expressed genes and corresponding fold change values—cont'd

Gene_symbol	Entrez_gene	Fold change
MASP1	5648	4.812777
WNT5B	81029	0.208045
ERC2-IT1	711	0.208058
KCNAB1	7881	0.2081
CDY1	9085	0.208255
AJAP1	55966	0.208435
C6orf15	29113	0.208688
MTNR1B	4544	0.208781
ESRRG	2104	4.777049
HOXA11	3207	4.77543
CDC42EP3	10602	4.774433
GATA4	2626	4.774418
KCNH1	3756	4.765713
DPT	1805	4.764085
C20orf195	79025	0.210178
DPYSL4	10570	4.747357
DNMT3L	29947	0.210937
MUC7	4589	0.211101
FOXO3///FOXO3B	2309///2310	4.736416
PDE4A	5141	0.211139
TIE1	7075	4.73281
ZNF204P	7754	0.211383
KIR2DL3	3804	0.211516
GULP1	51454	0.211794
BTN3A2	11118	0.211922
CEL	1056	0.211981
F10	2159	4.717063
FEZF2	55079	0.212006
HS3ST1	9957	4.712031
KANSL3	55683	0.212244
CXCR2	3579	0.212573
WNT7B	7477	4.703215
NRXN1	9378	4.698906
CACNA1H	8912	0.212866
NFE2	4778	0.212897
HLA-DRA	3122	4.695531
YME1L1	10730	0.21345
MAP4K2	5871	0.213893
MAGEA10-MAGEA5///MAGEA5	4104///100533997	0.214282
TSHZ2	128553	0.214409
IGH///IGHA2///IGHD///IGHG1	3492///3494///3495///3500	0.21443
OR3A1	4994	4.661118

Continued

Table S6 Significant expressed genes and corresponding fold change values—cont'd

Gene_symbol	Entrez_gene	Fold change
TRIM46	80128	4.656649
SLC7A8	23428	0.214914
GAGE1	2543	0.215561
CD1D	912	4.623247
GRIN1	2902	0.216345
SLC34A2	10568	0.216387
GNRHR	2798	4.61118
ADD3-AS1	1.01E+08	0.217093
MS4A1	931	4.600435
STAT2	6773	0.217624
TRIM3	10612	4.59444
ENTPD1	953	4.591823
CELF2	10659	4.587314
KLHL35	283212	0.218049
INPP5D	3635	4.582542
COL4A4	1286	0.218448
IPW///LOC100506948///SNORD107///SNORD115-13///SNORD115-26///SNORD115-7///SNORD116-28///SNRPN	3653///6638///91380///100033444///100033450///100033802///100033820///100506948	4.575452
MCHR1	2847	4.573281
PARVB	29780	4.570383
PHYHIP	9796	0.21885
INSL6	11172	4.56706
RFPL1	5988	0.219027
CCL13	6357	0.219075
NR0B2	8431	4.563859
CST1	1469	0.220249
IGFBP3	3486	0.220257
NRG2	9542	4.53621
PDYN	5173	4.534907
CYP4F8	11283	4.531935
GPR12	2835	0.220786
ITGA8	8516	0.220864
VCX2	51480	0.221083
SUGP1	57794	0.221275
ATP8A1	10396	0.22131
KLK14	43847	0.221328
CLCA2	9635	4.514545
CXCR3	2833	4.512124
FBLN1	2192	4.502183
FOXE1	2304	4.492598

Table S6 Significant expressed genes and corresponding fold change values—cont'd

Gene_symbol	Entrez_gene	Fold change
OPN1SW	611	4.487854
RPL35A	6165	4.486049
DCHS1	8642	0.223215
GALR1	2587	4.476715
MNDA	4332	0.223473
ICAM1	3383	4.473712
PPP1R3A	5506	0.22368
LTF	4057	0.223887
SAFB2	9667	4.466275
FGFR2	2263	4.455691
ACAA2	10449	0.22453
CHP2	63928	4.451845
KCNJ13	3769	4.448025
CCDC28B	79140	4.447669
MDFIC	29969	4.438573
CLCA1	1179	0.225814
SLC52A1	55065	0.226566
HMGCS2	3158	0.226632
LOC100129973	1E+08	4.406954
G6PC	2538	0.227037
ZNF862	643641	0.22724
PNMA2	10687	0.227415
FCAR	2204	0.227796
JAM2	58494	4.379757
CALD1	800	4.376271
TRIM29	23650	0.228748
SNPH	9751	4.360747
TCF7L2	6934	4.359842
DSCR4	10281	4.354692
TPSAB1	7177	0.229838
CDHR5	53841	0.230038
HFE	3077	0.230202
GFRA2	2675	4.34122
LINC00652	29075	4.333482
GPM6B	2824	4.324861
LZTS1	11178	4.323023
CD5L	922	0.231402
PDE4A	5141	4.318118
CYTIP	9595	0.231725
CLCN4	1183	0.232038
CD84	8832	0.23233
PON3	5446	0.232415

Continued

Table S6 Significant expressed genes and corresponding fold change values—cont'd

Gene_symbol	Entrez_gene	Fold change
NEK9	91754	0.23262
SNX29	92017	0.232661
IGHA1///IGHA2///IGHG1///IGHG4///IGHM///IGHV4-31	3493///3494///3500///3503///3507///28396	4.297695
CDC42EP4	23580	0.232809
APOL3	80833	0.232852
CDHR5	53841	4.29162
PAX3	5077	0.233321
GART	2618	4.282222
TRIO	7204	4.27639
MYH6	4624	4.272645
MS4A5	64232	0.234066
AHSG	197	4.268815
METTL10	399818	4.26673
LAMB4	22798	0.234445
DOC2B	8447	4.254913
ADRBK1	156	0.235038
CASR	846	0.235447
TAS2R8	50836	0.235545
OR2B6	26212	0.235546
OR12D3///OR5V1	81696///81797	0.235565
ALDOB	229	0.23574
OSM	5008	0.235816
ADAMTS8	11095	0.235901
SNN	8303	0.235994
MAPK8IP3	23162	4.231425
EFCAB6	64800	0.236646
HMOX1	3162	4.208924
SLC6A6	6533	4.208891
ANXA10	11199	4.208301
KLF8	11279	0.237918
BANK1	55024	0.237967
KLRF1	51348	0.238122
HAO1	54363	0.238156
EIF2S2	8894	0.238174
PRMT2	3275	4.197706
HP///HPR	3240///3250	0.238402
LPAR1	1902	0.238816
HRH1	3269	0.238876
FBN1	2200	4.183925
PLIN1	5346	0.239106
CXCL2	2920	0.23943

Table S6 Significant expressed genes and corresponding fold change values—cont'd

Gene_symbol	Entrez_gene	Fold change
LCMT2	9836	0.239463
ADAM29	11086	0.239472
AFF3	3899	4.172102
SMARCA1	6594	4.169445
POU2F3	25833	0.239999
OR6A2	8590	0.240191
KMT2A	4297	4.162907
ASIC1	41	0.240353
KRT4	3851	4.158364
TGM2	7052	0.240736
PZP	5858	4.153531
MYH13	8735	0.241222
CYLD	1540	0.241303
C22orf43	51233	4.139056
TGFA	7039	0.241808
SCN2B	6327	4.133081
HGD	3081	4.127912
C1S	716	0.242311
WISP1	8840	4.126851
ERGIC3	51614	0.242881
SLAMF7	57823	4.112216
BAALC	79870	4.11185
HGD	3081	0.243276
TONSL	4796	4.109574
CELA3A	10136	0.243468
COL13A1	1305	0.243818
SOX18	54345	0.244025
ZNF221	7638	0.244298
NID2	22795	0.244729
ALDH1A1	216	0.245012
NCDN	23154	4.073453
NRP2	8828	0.245619
RND1	27289	0.245666
CACNA1E	777	0.245667
CRYAB	1410	4.070503
ALDH3B1	221	0.245739
COL4A1	1282	0.246131
IGLJ3	28831	0.246152
TRMT1	55621	0.246197
IL2RA	3559	4.060918
OSBPL10	114884	0.246424
IL5RA	3568	0.246707

Continued

Table S6 Significant expressed genes and corresponding fold change values—cont'd

Gene_symbol	Entrez_gene	Fold change
BPY2	9083	4.053234
TRAC///TRAJ17///TRAV20	28663///28738///28755	0.246803
HUWE1	10075	4.048871
PYGO1	26108	0.24699
PPARGC1A	10891	0.247075
GTPBP1	9567	4.039788
GPR15	2838	4.032832
CXorf57	55086	0.248201
TOX3	27324	4.016068
NCLN	56926	0.249145
SLC12A3	6559	4.010562
PIK3R4	30849	0.249425
MMP11	4320	0.249503
ACACB	32	0.249538
IL37	27178	4.006777
RNASE3	6037	4.005261
OGDHL	55753	0.249677
NPTX2	4885	4.003965
CALD1	800	4.001629

Table S7 The 63 experimentally validated CVD pathways regulated by both SBPac and SBPc

Pathway ID	Pathway name	Pathway URL
636	PID_LYMPHANGIOGENESIS_PATHWAY	http://www.broadinstitute.org/gsea/msigdb/cards/ PID_LYMPHANGIOGENESIS_PATHWAY
630	PID_S1P_S1P2_PATHWAY	http://www.broadinstitute.org/gsea/msigdb/cards/ PID_S1P_S1P2_PATHWAY
613	PID_SYNDECAN_2_PATHWAY	http://www.broadinstitute.org/gsea/msigdb/cards/ PID_SYNDECAN_2_PATHWAY
601	PID_VEGFR1_PATHWAY	http://www.broadinstitute.org/gsea/msigdb/cards/ PID_VEGFR1_PATHWAY
595	PID_AR_NONGENOMIC_PATHWAY	http://www.broadinstitute.org/gsea/msigdb/cards/ PID_AR_NONGENOMIC_PATHWAY
574	PID_ECADHERIN_KERATINOCYTE_PATHWAY	http://www.broadinstitute.org/gsea/msigdb/cards/ PID_ECADHERIN_KERATINOCYTE_ PATHWAY
567	PID_ERBB2ERBB3PATHWAY	http://www.broadinstitute.org/gsea/msigdb/cards/ PID_ERBB2ERBB3PATHWAY
548	PID_IL2_PI3KPATHWAY	http://www.broadinstitute.org/gsea/msigdb/cards/ PID_IL2_PI3KPATHWAY
536	PID_ERBB1_RECEPTOR_PROXIMAL_PATHWAY	http://www.broadinstitute.org/gsea/msigdb/cards/ PID_ERBB1_RECEPTOR_PROXIMAL_ PATHWAY
533	PID_IL2_1PATHWAY	http://www.broadinstitute.org/gsea/msigdb/cards/ PID_IL2_1PATHWAY
521	PID_S1P_S1P1_PATHWAY	http://www.broadinstitute.org/gsea/msigdb/cards/ PID_S1P_S1P1_PATHWAY
515	PID_ANGIOPOIETINRECEPTOR_PATHWAY	http://www.broadinstitute.org/gsea/msigdb/cards/ PID_ANGIOPOIETINRECEPTOR_ PATHWAY
493	PID_AVB3_OPN_PATHWAY	http://www.broadinstitute.org/gsea/msigdb/cards/ PID_AVB3_OPN_PATHWAY

Continued

Table S7 The 63 experimentally validated CVD pathways regulated by both SBPac and SBPpc—cont'd

Pathway ID	Pathway name	Pathway URL
409	SA_B_CELL_RECEPTOR_COMPLEXES	http://www.broadinstitute.org/gsea/msigdb/cards/ SA_B_CELL_RECEPTOR_COMPLEXES
4030	TCGA_GLIOBLASTOMA_MUTATED	http://www.broadinstitute.org/gsea/msigdb/cards/ TCGA_GLIOBLASTOMA_MUTATED
4028	DING_LUNG_CANCER_MUTATED_RECURRENTLY	http://www.broadinstitute.org/gsea/msigdb/cards/ DING_LUNG_CANCER_MUTATED_ RECURRENTLY
398	BIOCARTA_ARF_PATHWAY	http://www.broadinstitute.org/gsea/msigdb/cards/ BIOCARTA_ARF_PATHWAY
397	BIOCARTA_TRKA_PATHWAY	http://www.broadinstitute.org/gsea/msigdb/cards/ BIOCARTA_TRKA_PATHWAY
396	BIOCARTA_TFF_PATHWAY	http://www.broadinstitute.org/gsea/msigdb/cards/ BIOCARTA_TFF_PATHWAY
394	BIOCARTA_CREB_PATHWAY	http://www.broadinstitute.org/gsea/msigdb/cards/ BIOCARTA_CREB_PATHWAY
393	BIOCARTA_TPO_PATHWAY	http://www.broadinstitute.org/gsea/msigdb/cards/ BIOCARTA_TPO_PATHWAY
381	BIOCARTA_TGFB_PATHWAY	http://www.broadinstitute.org/gsea/msigdb/cards/ BIOCARTA_TGFB_PATHWAY
366	BIOCARTA_MET_PATHWAY	http://www.broadinstitute.org/gsea/msigdb/cards/ BIOCARTA_MET_PATHWAY
353	BIOCARTA_ERK5_PATHWAY	http://www.broadinstitute.org/gsea/msigdb/cards/ BIOCARTA_ERK5_PATHWAY
3521	BIERIE_INFLAMMATORY_RESPONSE_TGFB1	http://www.broadinstitute.org/gsea/msigdb/cards/ BIERIE_INFLAMMATORY_RESPONSE_ TGFB1
352	BIOCARTA_HER2_PATHWAY	http://www.broadinstitute.org/gsea/msigdb/cards/ BIOCARTA_HER2_PATHWAY
351	BIOCARTA_CARDIACEGF_PATHWAY	http://www.broadinstitute.org/gsea/msigdb/cards/ BIOCARTA_CARDIACEGF_PATHWAY
331	BIOCARTA_PTEN_PATHWAY	http://www.broadinstitute.org/gsea/msigdb/cards/ BIOCARTA_PTEN_PATHWAY

321	BIOCARTA_CCR5_PATHWAY	http://www.broadinstitute.org/gsea/msigdb/cards/BIOCARTA_CCR5_PATHWAY
3118	WU_HBX_TARGETS_3_DN	http://www.broadinstitute.org/gsea/msigdb/cards/WU_HBX_TARGETS_3_DN
311	BIOCARTA_NTHI_PATHWAY	http://www.broadinstitute.org/gsea/msigdb/cards/BIOCARTA_NTHI_PATHWAY
308	BIOCARTA_NGF_PATHWAY	http://www.broadinstitute.org/gsea/msigdb/cards/BIOCARTA_NGF_PATHWAY
299	BIOCARTA_EGFR_SMRTE_PATHWAY	http://www.broadinstitute.org/gsea/msigdb/cards/BIOCARTA_EGFR_SMRTE_PATHWAY
298	BIOCARTA_PYK2_PATHWAY	http://www.broadinstitute.org/gsea/msigdb/cards/BIOCARTA_PYK2_PATHWAY
292	BIOCARTA_INSULIN_PATHWAY	http://www.broadinstitute.org/gsea/msigdb/cards/BIOCARTA_INSULIN_PATHWAY
291	BIOCARTA_GLEEVEC_PATHWAY	http://www.broadinstitute.org/gsea/msigdb/cards/BIOCARTA_GLEEVEC_PATHWAY
290	BIOCARTA_RACCYCD_PATHWAY	http://www.broadinstitute.org/gsea/msigdb/cards/BIOCARTA_RACCYCD_PATHWAY
282	BIOCARTA_IL6_PATHWAY	http://www.broadinstitute.org/gsea/msigdb/cards/BIOCARTA_IL6_PATHWAY
280	BIOCARTA_IL4_PATHWAY	http://www.broadinstitute.org/gsea/msigdb/cards/BIOCARTA_IL4_PATHWAY
276	BIOCARTA_IGF1_PATHWAY	http://www.broadinstitute.org/gsea/msigdb/cards/BIOCARTA_IGF1_PATHWAY
275	BIOCARTA_HIF_PATHWAY	http://www.broadinstitute.org/gsea/msigdb/cards/BIOCARTA_HIF_PATHWAY
273	BIOCARTA_HCMV_PATHWAY	http://www.broadinstitute.org/gsea/msigdb/cards/BIOCARTA_HCMV_PATHWAY
250	BIOCARTA_EPO_PATHWAY	http://www.broadinstitute.org/gsea/msigdb/cards/BIOCARTA_EPO_PATHWAY
246	BIOCARTA_EGF_PATHWAY	http://www.broadinstitute.org/gsea/msigdb/cards/BIOCARTA_EGF_PATHWAY
2288	GALIE_TUMOR_ANGIOGENESIS	http://www.broadinstitute.org/gsea/msigdb/cards/GALIE_TUMOR_ANGIOGENESIS

Continued

Table S7 The 63 experimentally validated CVD pathways regulated by both SBPac and SBPpc—cont'd

Pathway ID	Pathway name	Pathway URL
214	BIOCARTA_CDMAC_PATHWAY	http://www.broadinstitute.org/gsea/msigdb/cards/BIOCARTA_CDMAC_PATHWAY
2083	AGARWAL_AKT_PATHWAY_TARGETS	http://www.broadinstitute.org/gsea/msigdb/cards/AGARWAL_AKT_PATHWAY_TARGETS
207	BIOCARTA_BCELLSURVIVAL_PATHWAY	http://www.broadinstitute.org/gsea/msigdb/cards/BIOCARTA_BCELLSURVIVAL_PATHWAY
204	BIOCARTA_SPPA_PATHWAY	http://www.broadinstitute.org/gsea/msigdb/cards/BIOCARTA_SPPA_PATHWAY
199	BIOCARTA_AT1R_PATHWAY	http://www.broadinstitute.org/gsea/msigdb/cards/BIOCARTA_AT1R_PATHWAY
1956	DEBOSSCHER_NFKB_TARGETS_REPRESSED_BY_GLUCOCORTICOIDS	http://www.broadinstitute.org/gsea/msigdb/cards/DEBOSSCHER_NFKB_TARGETS_REPRESSED_BY_GLUCOCORTICOIDS
1954	SCHEIDEREIT_IKK_TARGETS	http://www.broadinstitute.org/gsea/msigdb/cards/SCHEIDEREIT_IKK_TARGETS
1942	BAKER_HEMATOPOIESIS_STAT3_TARGETS	http://www.broadinstitute.org/gsea/msigdb/cards/BAKER_HEMATOPOIESIS_STAT3_TARGETS
1941	BAKER_HEMATOPOIESIS_STAT1_TARGETS	http://www.broadinstitute.org/gsea/msigdb/cards/BAKER_HEMATOPOIESIS_STAT1_TARGETS
1932	TURJANSKI_MAPK14_TARGETS	http://www.broadinstitute.org/gsea/msigdb/cards/TURJANSKI_MAPK14_TARGETS
1930	TURJANSKI_MAPK7_TARGETS	http://www.broadinstitute.org/gsea/msigdb/cards/TURJANSKI_MAPK7_TARGETS
1929	TURJANSKI_MAPK8_AND_MAPK9_TARGETS	http://www.broadinstitute.org/gsea/msigdb/cards/TURJANSKI_MAPK8_AND_MAPK9_TARGETS
1928	TURJANSKI_MAPK1_AND_MAPK2_TARGETS	http://www.broadinstitute.org/gsea/msigdb/cards/TURJANSKI_MAPK1_AND_MAPK2_TARGETS

1891	MARKS_HDAC_TARGETS_DN	http://www.broadinstitute.org/gsea/msigdb/cards/ MARKS_HDAC_TARGETS_DN
1851	BUSA_SAM68_TARGETS_DN	http://www.broadinstitute.org/gsea/msigdb/cards/ BUSA_SAM68_TARGETS_DN
172	KEGG_BLADDER_CANCER	http://www.broadinstitute.org/gsea/msigdb/cards/ KEGG_BLADDER_CANCER
165	KEGG_PANCREATIC_CANCER	http://www.broadinstitute.org/gsea/msigdb/cards/ KEGG_PANCREATIC_CANCER
1088	REACTOME_ACTIVATION_OF_THE_AP1_ FAMILY_OF_TRANSCRIPTION_FACTORS	http://www.broadinstitute.org/gsea/msigdb/cards/ REACTOME_ACTIVATION_OF_THE_AP1_ FAMILY_OF_TRANSCRIPTION_FACTORS

REFERENCES

1. http://www.who.int/mediacentre/factsheets/fs317/en/index.htL.
2. http://www.healthknowledge.org.uk/public-health-textbook/disease-causation-diagnostic/2b-epidemiology-diseases-phs/chronic-diseases/coronary-heart-disease.
3. Falk E. Pathogenesis of atherosclerosis. *J Am Coll Cardiol* 2006;**47**:C7–12.
4. Bui QT, Prempeh M, Wilensky RL. Atherosclerotic plaque development. *Int J Biochem Cell Biol* 2009;**41**:2109–13.
5. Li AC, Glass CK. The macrophage foam cell as a target for therapeutic intervention. *Nat Med* 2002;**8**:1235–42.
6. Robertson AK, Hansson GK. T cells in atherogenesis: for better or for worse? *Arterioscler Thromb Vasc Biol* 2006;**26**:2421–32.
7. Bachelet I, Levi-Schaffer F. Mast cells as effector cells: a co-stimulating question. *Trends Immunol* 2007;**28**:360–5.
8. Niessner A, Weyand CM. Dendritic cells in atherosclerotic disease. *Clin Immunol* 2010;**134**:25–32.
9. Huo YQ, Ley KF. Role of platelets in the development of atherosclerosis. *Trends Cardiovasc Med* 2004;**14**:18–22.
10. Taddei S, Vanhoutte PM. Role of endothelium in endothelin-evoked contractions in the rat aorta. *Hypertension* 1993;**21**:9–15.
11. Ross R, Glomset JA. Atherosclerosis and the arterial smooth muscle cell: proliferation of smooth muscle is a key event in the genesis of the lesions of atherosclerosis. *Science* 1973;**180**:1332–9.
12. Förstermann U, Münzel T. Endothelial nitric oxide synthase in vascular disease: from marvel to menace. *Circulation* 2006;**113**:1708–14.
13. Mallat Z, Tedgui A. Current perspective on the role of apoptosis in atherothrombotic disease. *Circ Res* 2001;**88**:998–1003.
14. Mohamad N, Judith AB, Andrew DW, et al. The Yin and Yang of oxidation in the development of the fatty streak. A review based on the 1994 George Lyman Duff Memorial Lecture. *Arterioscler Thromb Vasc Biol* 1996;**16**:831–42.
15. Hansson GK. Inflammation, atherosclerosis, and coronary artery disease. *New Engl J Med* 2005;**352**:1685–95.
16. Willerson JT, Kereiakes DJ. Clinical research and future improvement in clinical care: the Health Insurance Portability and Accountability Act (HI PAA) and future difficulties but optimism for the way forward. *Circulation* 2003;**108**:919–20.
17. Ruiz-Ortega M, Lorenzo O, Ruperez M, et al. Role of the renin-angiotensin system in vascular diseases: expanding the field. *Hypertension* 2001;**38**:1382–7.
18. Brunner F, Brás-Silva C, Cerdeira AS, et al. Cardiovascular endothelins: essential regulators of cardiovascular homeostasis. *Pharmacol Ther* 2006;**111**:508–31.
19. Kingsley K, Huff JL, Rust WL, et al. ERK1/2 mediates PDGF-BB stimulated vascular smooth muscle cell proliferation and migration on laminin-5. *Biochem Biophys Res Commun* 2002;**293**:1000–6.
20. Nguyen LL, D'Amore PA. Cellular interactions in vascular growth and differentiation. *Int Rev Cytol* 2001;**204**:1–48.
21. Raines EW, Koyama H, Carragher NO, et al. The extracellular matrix dynamically regulates smooth muscle cell responsiveness to PDGF. *Ann N Y Acad Sci* 2000;**902**:39–51.
22. Gilbert RE, Douglas SA, Krum H. Urotensin-II as a novel therapeutic target in the clinical management of cardiorenal disease. *Curr Opin Investig Drugs* 2004;**5**:276–82.
23. Qi YF, Xia CF, Chen YH, et al. Effects of adrenomedullin on proliferation of vascular smooth muscle cells induced by urotensin II. *Chin J Pathophysiol* 2002;**18**:230–2.
24. Manuel M, Xu QB. Smooth muscle cell apoptosis in arteriosclerosis. *Exp Gerontol* 2001;**36**:969–87.
25. Kockx MM, Knaapen WM. The role of apoptosis in vascular disease. *J Pathol* 2000;**190**:267–80.
26. Bennett MR, Boyle JJ. Apoptosis of vascular smooth muscle cells in atherosclerosis. *Atherosclerosis* 1998;**138**:3–9.
27. Harrington JR. The role of MCP-1 in atherosclerosis. *Stem Cells* 2000;**18**:65–6.

28. Qiao JH, Tripathi J, Mishra NK, et al. Role of macrophage colony-stimulating factor in atherosclerosis: studies of osteopetrotic mice. *Am J Pathol* 1997;**150**:1687–99.

29. Esther L, Dirk L, Linda B, et al. CD40 and its ligand in atherosclerosis. *Trends Cardiovasc Med* 2007;**17**:118–23.

30. Bradley MN, Tontonoz P. LXR: a nuclear receptor target for cardiovascular disease? *Drug Discov Today* 2005;**2**:97–103.

31. GD1 B, Evans RM. PPARs and LXRs: atherosclerosis goes nuclear. *Trends Endocrinol Metab* 2004;**15**:158–65.

32. Schiller NK, Boisvert WA, Curtiss LK. Inflammation in atherosclerosis. *Nature* 2002;**420**:868–74.

33. Mach F, Schönbeck U, Libby P. CD40 signaling in vascular cells: a key role in atherosclerosis? *Atherosclerosis* 1998;**137**(Suppl):S89–95.

34. Schönbeck U, Mach F, Sukhova GK, et al. Regulation of matrix metalloproteinase expression in human vascular smooth muscle cells by T Lymphocytes a role for cd40 signaling in plaque rupture? *Circ Res* 1997;**81**:448–54.

35. Stemme S, Faber B, Holm J, et al. T lymphocytes from human atherosclerotic plaques recognize oxidized low density lipoprotein. *PNAS* 1995;**92**:3893–7.

36. Wick G, Romen M, Amberger A, et al. Atherosclerosis, autoimmunity, and vascular-associated lymphoid tissue. *FASEB J* 1997;**11**:1199–207.

37. Taleb S, Tedgui A, Mallat Z. Regulatory T-cell immunity and its relevance to atherosclerosis. *J Intern Med* 2008;**263**:489–99.

38. Mekori YA, Metcalfe DD. Mast cell–T cell interactions. *J Allergy Clin Immunol* 1999;**104**(3 Pt 1):517–23.

39. Mor A, Mekori YA. Mast cells and atherosclerosis. *Isr Med Assoc J* 2001;**3**:216–21.

40. Kelley JL, Chi DS, Abou-Auda W, et al. The molecular role of mast cells in atherosclerotic cardiovascular disease. *Mol Med Today* 2000;**6**(8):304.

41. Kovanen PT, Lee M, Leskinen MJ, et al. The mast cell, a rich source of neutral proteases in atherosclerotic plaques. *Int Congr Ser* 2004;**1262**:494–7.

42. Lee M, Lindstedt LK, Kovanen PT. Mast cell-mediated inhibition of reverse cholesterol transport. *Arterioscler Thromb* 1992;**12**:1329–35.

43. Di-Girolamo N, Wakefield D. In vitro and in vivo expression of interstitial collagenase/MMP-1 by human mast cells. *Dev Immunol* 2000;**7**:131–42.

44. Kanbe N, Tanaka A, Kanbe M, et al. Human mast cells produce matrix metalloproteinase 9. *Eur J Immunol* 1999;**29**:2645–9.

45. Maija K, Allard CW, Chris ML, et al. Mast cell infiltration in acute coronary syndromes: implications for plaque rupture. *J Am Coll Cardiol* 1998;**32**:606–12.

46. Sun J, Sukhova GK, Wolters PJ, et al. Mast cells promote atherosclerosis by releasing proinflammatory cytokines. *Nat Med* 2007;**13**:719–24.

47. Leskinen MJ, Heikkila HM, Speer MY, et al. Mast cell chymase induces smooth muscle cell apoptosis by disrupting NF-kappaB-mediated survival signaling. *Exp Cell Res* 2006;**312**:1289–98.

48. Lord RS, Bobryshev YV. Clustering of dendritic cells in athero-prone areas of the aorta. *Atherosclerosis* 1999;**146**:197–8.

49. Bobryshev YV, Lord RS, Rainer SP, et al. VCAM-1 expression and network of VCAM-1 positive vascular dendritic cells in advanced atherosclerotic lesions of carotid arteries and aortas. *Acta Histochem* 1996;**98**:185–94.

50. Alvarez D, Vollmann EH, von Andrian UH. Mechanisms and consequences of dendritic cell migration. *Immunity* 2008;**29**:325–42.

51. Shortman K, Naik SH. Steady-state and inflammatory dendritic-cell development. *Nat Rev Immunol* 2007;**7**:19–30.

52. Alderman CJ, Bunyard PR, Chain BM, et al. Effects of oxidised low density lipoprotein on dendritic cells: a possible immunoregulatory component of the atherogenic micro-environment? *Cardiovasc Res* 2002;**55**:806–19.

53. Zhang X, Niessner A, Nakajima T, et al. Interleukin 12 induces T-cell recruitment into the atherosclerotic plaque. *Circ Res* 2006;**98**:524–31.

54. Ruggeri ZM. Platelets in atherothrombosis. *Nat Med* 2002;**8**:1227–34.

55. Gawaz M. Platelets in the onset of atherosclerosis. *Blood Cells Mol Dis* 2006;**36**:206–10.

56. Massberg S, Gawaz M, Grüner S, et al. A crucial role of glycoprotein VI for platelet recruitment to the injured arterial wall in vivo. *J Exp Med* 2003;**197**:41–9.

57. Arya M, López JA, Romo GM, et al. Glycoprotein Ib–IX-mediated activation of integrin αIIbβ3: effects of receptor clustering and von Willebrand factor adhesion. *J Thromb Haemost* 2003;**1**:1150–7.

58. Kahn ML. Platelet-collagen responses: molecular basis and therapeutic promise. *Semin Thromb Hemost* 2004;**30**:419–25.

59. Coughlin SR. Thrombin signalling and protease-activated receptors. *Nature* 2000;**407**:258–64.

60. Covic L, Gresser AL, Kuliopulos A. Biphasic kinetics of activation and signaling for PAR1 and PAR4 thrombin receptors in platelets. *Biochemistry* 2000;**39**:5458–67.

61. Gachet C. Platelet activation by ADP: the role of ADP antagonists. *Ann Med* 2000;**32**(Suppl. 1):15–20.

62. Savage B, Cattaneo M, Ruggeri ZM. Mechanisms of platelet aggregation. *Curr Opin Hematol* 2001;**8**:270–6.

63. Henn V, Slupsky JR, Grafe M, et al. CD40 ligand on activated platelets triggers an inflammatory reaction of endothelial cells. *Nature* 1998;**391**:591–4.

64. Whitmer JT, Idell-Wenger JA, Rovetto MJ, et al. Control of fatty acid metabolism in ischemic and hypoxic hearts. *J Biol Chem* 1978;**253**:4305–9.

65. Ussher JR, Lopaschuk GD. Targeting malonyl CoA inhibition of mitochondrial fatty acid uptake as an approach to treat cardiac ischemia/reperfusion. *Basic Res Cardiol* 2009;**104**:203–10.

66. Grover GJ, Marone PA, Koetzner L, et al. Energetic signalling in the control of mitochondrial F1F0 ATP synthase activity in health and disease. *Int J Biochem Cell Biol* 2008;**40**:2698–701.

67. Fillingame RH, Jiang W, Dmitriev OY, Coupling H. (+) Transport to rotary catalysis in F-type ATP synthases: structure and organization of the transmembrane rotary motor. *J Exp Biol* 2000;**203**(Pt 1):9–17.

68. Duchen MR. Mitochondria in health and disease: perspectives on a new mitochondrial biology. *Mol Asp Med* 2004;**25**:365–451.

69. To KK, Huang LE. Suppression of hypoxia-inducible factor 1α (HIF-1α) transcriptional activity by the HIF prolyl hydroxylase EGLN1. *J Biol Chem* 2005;**280**:38102–7.

70. Zolk O, Solbach TF, Eschenhagen T, et al. Activation of negative regulators of the hypoxia-inducible factor (HIF) pathway in human end-stage heart failure. *Biochem Biophys Res Commun* 2008;**376**:315–20.

71. Dulhunty AF, Beard NA, Pouliquin P, et al. Agonists and antagonists of the cardiac ryanodine receptor: potential therapeutic agents. *Pharmacol Ther* 2007;**113**:247–63.

72. Benjamin IJ, Schneider MD. Learning from failure: congestive heart failure in the postgenomic age. *J Clin Invest* 2005;**115**:495–9.

73. Shimizu Y, Minatoguchi S, Hashimoto K, et al. The role of serotonin in ischemic cellular damage and the infarct size-reducing effect of sarpogrelate, a 5-hydroxytryptamine-2 receptor blocker, in rabbit hearts. *J Am Coll Cardiol* 2002;**40**:1347–55.

74. Maurel A, Hernandez C, Kunduzova O, et al. Age-dependent increase in hydrogen peroxide production by cardiac monoamine oxidase A in rats. *Am J Physiol Heart Circ Physiol* 2003;**284**:H1460–7.

75. Chen M, Zsengeller Z, Xiao CY, et al. Mitochondrial-to-nuclear translocation of apoptosis-inducing factor in cardiac myocytes during oxidant stress: potential role of poly(ADP-ribose) polymerase-1. *Cardiovasc Res* 2004;**63**:682–8.

76. Szabó C. Cardioprotective effects of poly(ADP-ribose) polymerase inhibition. *Pharmacol Res* 2005;**52**:34–43.

77. Sommerschild HT, Kirkeboen KA. Adenosine and cardioprotection during ischaemia and reperfusion – an overview. *Acta Anaesthesiol Scand* 2000;**44**:1038–55.

78. Headrick JP, Hack B, Ashton KJ. Acute adenosinergic cardioprotection in ischemic-reperfused hearts. *Am J Physiol Heart Circ Physiol* 2003;**285**:H1797–818.

79. Wang L, Luo X, Wang Y. Evaluation on tolerability and safety of long-term administration with Shexiang Baoxin Pill in patients with coronary heart disease of stable angina pectoris. *Chin J Integr Med* 2008;**28**(5):399–401.

80. Li TQ, Li Y, Fan WH. Effects of She Xiang Bao Xin Pill and simvastatin on stability of atherosclerotic plaque in rabbit femoral artery. *Chin J Geriatr Heart Brain Vessel Dis* 2006;**5**:002.

81. Shen W, Fan W, Shi H. Effects of Shexiang Baoxin Pill on angiogenesis in atherosclerosis plaque and ischemic myocardium. *Chin J Integr Med* 2010;**30**(12):1284–7.

82. Wu D, Hong H, Jiang Q. Effect of Shexiang Baoxin Pill in alleviating myocardial fibrosis in spontaneous hypertensive rats. *Chin J Integr Med* 2005;**25**(4):350–3.

83. Kario K, Pickering TG, Umeda Y, Hoshide S, Hoshide Y, Morinari M, et al. Morning surge in blood pressure as a predictor of silent and clinical cerebrovascular disease in elderly hypertensives a prospective study. *Circulation* 2003;**107**(10):1401–6.

84. Ouriel K. Peripheral arterial disease. *Lancet* 2001;**358**(9289):1257–64.

85. Mendis S, Puska P, Norrving B. *Global atlas on cardiovascular disease prevention and control.* Geneva: World Health Organization; 2011.

86. Collaborators MCOD. Global, regional, and national age-sex specific all-cause and cause-specific mortality for 240 causes of death, 1990-2013: a systematic analysis for the Global Burden of Disease Study 2013. *Lancet* 2015;**41**(9963):119.

87. Zhao J, Jiang P, Zhang W. Molecular networks for the study of TCM pharmacology. *Brief Bioinform* 2010;**11**(4):417–30.

88. Jiang P, Dai W, Yan S, Chen Z, Xu R, Ding J, et al. Potential biomarkers in the urine of myocardial infarction rats: a metabolomic method and its application. *Mol BioSyst* 2011;**7**(7):824–31.

89. Xiang L, Jiang P, Zhan C, Chen Z, Liu X, Huang X, et al. The serum metabolomic study of intervention effects of the traditional Chinese medicine Shexiang Baoxin Pill and a multi-component medicine polypill in the treatment of myocardial infarction in rats. *Mol BioSyst* 2012;**8**(9):2434–42.

90. Jiang P, Dai W, Yan S, Chen Z, Xu R, Ding J, et al. Biomarkers in the early period of acute myocardial infarction in rat serum and protective effects of Shexiang Baoxin Pill using a metabolomic method. *J Ethnopharmacol* 2011;**138**(2):530–6.

91. Xiang L, Jiang P, Wang S, Hu Y, Liu X, Yue R, et al. Metabolomic strategy for studying the intervention and the synergistic effects of the Shexiang Baoxin Pill for treating myocardial infarction in rats. *Evid Based Complement Alternat Med* 2013;**2013**(1):823121.

92. Jiang P, Liu R, Dou S, Liu L, Zhang W, Chen Z, et al. Analysis of the constituents in rat plasma after oral administration of Shexiang Baoxin Pill by HPLC-ESI-MS/MS. *Biomed Chromatogr* 2009;**23**(12):1333–43.

93. Quan Y, Zhang YM. Efect of Shexiang Baoxin Wan on blood vessel endothelial function in patients with atrial fibrillation complicated with hypertension. *Cent South Pharm* 2011;**10**:010.

94. Xuezhong W, Ping Z, Yuesong W. The expression of MMP-2 and the effect of Shexiangbaoxin Pill on it in DHR heart. *J Emerg Tradit Chin Med* 2006;**8**:060.

95. Shao L, Zhang B. Traditional Chinese medicine network pharmacology: theory, methodology and application. *Chin J Nat Med* 2013;**11**(2):110–20.

96. Zhang Y, Bai M, Zhang B, Liu C, Guo Q, Sun Y, et al. Uncovering pharmacological mechanisms of Wu-tou decoction acting on rheumatoid arthritis through systems approaches: drug-target prediction, network analysis and experimental validation. *Sci Rep* 2015;**5**:srep09463.

97. Wang X, Sun H, Zhang A, Jiao G, Sun W, Yuan Y. Pharmacokinetics screening for multi-components absorbed in the rat plasma after oral administration traditional Chinese medicine formula Yin-Chen-Hao-Tang by ultra performance liquid chromatography-electrospray ionization/quadrupole-time-of-flight mass spectrometry combined with pattern recognition methods. *Analyst* 2011;**136**(23):5068–76.

98. Yan Z, Chen Y, Li T, Zhang J, Yang X. Identification of metabolites of Si-Ni-San, a traditional Chinese medicine formula, in rat plasma and urine using liquid chromatography/diode array detection/triple–quadrupole spectrometry. *J Chromatogr B* 2012;**885**:73–82.

99. Fang H, Wang Y, Yang T, Ga Y, Zhang Y, Liu R, et al. Bioinformatics analysis for the antirheumatic effects of huang-lian-jie-du-tang from a network perspective. *Evid Based Complement Alternat Med* 2013;**2013**:245357.

100. Piñero J, Queralt-Rosinach N, Bravo À, Deu-Pons J, Bauer-Mehren A, Baron M, et al. DisGeNET: a discovery platform for the dynamical exploration of human diseases and their genes. *Database* 2015;**2015**:bav028.

101. Ren T, Liu X, Gao J. Introduction of basic database system of traditional Chinese medicine. *J Tradit Chin Med* 2001;**8**(11):90–1.

102. Ye H, Ye L, Kang H, Zhang D, Tao L, Tang K, et al. HIT: linking herbal active ingredients to targets. *Nucleic Acids Res* 2011;**39**(Suppl. 1):D1055–9.

103. Chen YC. TCM Database@Taiwan. The world's largest traditional Chinese medicine database for drug screening in silico. *PLoS One* 2011;**6**(1):e15939.

104. Xue R, Fang Z, Zhang M, Yi Z, Wen C, Shi T. TCMID: traditional Chinese medicine integrative database for herb molecular mechanism analysis. *Nucleic Acids Res* 2013;**41**(d1):D1089–95.

105. Qiao X, Hou T, Zhang W, Guo SL, Xu X. ChemInform Abstract: a 3D structure database of components from chinese traditional medicinal herbs. *ChemInform* 2002;**33**(33):481–9.

106. Kuhn M, von Mering C, Campillos M, Jensen LJ, Bork P. STITCH: interaction networks of chemicals and proteins. *Nucleic Acids Res* 2008;**36**(Suppl. 1):D684–8.

107. Liana G, Shupingb W, Xiang L, Pengb J, Zhang W-D, Liu RH. Identification of volatility components of Shexiang Baoxin Pill in rat plasma by GC-MS. *J Pharm Pract* 2012;**3**:014.

108. Mering CV, Huynen M, Jaeggi D, Schmidt S, Bork P, Snel B. STRING: a database of predicted functional associations between proteins. *Nucleic Acids Res* 2003;**31**(1):258–61.

109. Liberzon A, Subramanian A, Pinchback R, Thorvaldsdóttir H, Tamayo P, Mesirov JP. Molecular signatures database (MSigDB) 3.0. *Bioinformatics* 2011;**27**(12):1739–40.

110. Lamb J. The connectivity map: a new tool for biomedical research. *Nat Rev Cancer* 2007;**7**(1):54–60.

111. XA Q, Rajpal DK. Applications of connectivity map in drug discovery and development. *Drug DiscovToday* 2012;**17**(23–24):1289–98.

112. Lamb J, Crawford ED, Peck D, Modell JW, Blat IC, Wrobel MJ, et al. The connectivity map: using gene-expression signatures to connect small molecules, genes, and disease. *Science* 2006;**313**(5795):1929–35.

113. Wen ZN, Wang ZJ, Wang S, Ravula R, Yang L, Xu J, et al. Discovery of molecular mechanisms of traditional chinese medicinal formula si-wu-tang using gene expression microarray and connectivity map. *PLoS One* 2011;**6**(3):1118–36.

114. Tong H, Faloutsos C, Pan J-Y. Random walk with restart: fast solutions and applications. *Knowl Inf Syst* 2008;**14**(3):327–46.

115. Macropol K, Can T, Singh AK. RRW: repeated random walks on genome-scale protein networks for local cluster discovery. *BMC Bioinf* 2009;**10**(1):1.

116. Köhler S, Bauer S, Horn D, Robinson PN. Walking the interactome for prioritization of candidate disease genes. *Am J Hum Genet* 2008;**82**(4):949–58.

117. Erten MS. *Network based prioritization of disease genes* [Master's thesis]. Case Western Reserve University; 2009.

118. Zhao J, Yang P, Li F, Tao L, Ding H, Rui Y, et al. Therapeutic effects of astragaloside iv on myocardial injuries: multi-target identification and network analysis. *PLoS One* 2012;**7**(9):e44938.

119. Colinge J, Rix U, Superti-furga G. In: *Novel global network scores to analyze kinase inhibitor profiles. The fourth international conference on computational systems biology, Suzhou, China*; 2010. p. 305–13.

120. Peng J, Dou SS, Liu L, Zhang WD, Chen ZL, RL X, et al. Identification of multiple constituents in the TCM-formula Shexiang Baoxin Pill by LC coupled with DAD-ESI-MS-MS. *Chromatographia* 2009;**70**(1):133–42.

121. Yıldırım MA, Goh K-I, Cusick ME, Barabási A-L, Vidal M. Drug-target network. *Nat Biotechnol* 2007;**25**(10):1119–26.

122. Elia L, Condorelli G. RNA (Epi) genetics in cardiovascular diseases. *J Mol Cell Cardiol* 2015;**89**:11–6.

123. Karaźniewicz-Łada M, Danielak D, Burchardt P, Kruszyna Ł, Komosa A, Lesiak M, et al. Clinical pharmacokinetics of clopidogrel and its metabolites in patients with cardiovascular diseases. *Clin Pharmacokinet* 2014;**53**(2):155–64.

124. Rexrode KM, Ridker PM, Hegener HH, Buring JE, Manson JE, Zee RY. Polymorphisms and haplotypes of the estrogen receptor-β gene (ESR2) and cardiovascular disease in men and women. *Clin Chem* 2007;**53**(10):1749–56.

125. Demerath E, Towne B, Blangero J, Siervogel R. The relationship of soluble ICAM-1, VCAM-1, P-selectin and E-selectin to cardiovascular disease risk factors in healthy men and women. *Ann Hum Biol* 2001;**28**(6):664–78.

126. Van Gaal LF, Mertens IL, Christophe E. Mechanisms linking obesity with cardiovascular disease. *Nature* 2006;**444**(7121):875–80.

127. Chen K-C, Wang Y-S, C-Y H, Chang W-C, Liao Y-C, Dai C-Y, et al. OxLDL up-regulates microRNA-29b, leading to epigenetic modifications of MMP-2/MMP-9 genes: a novel mechanism for cardiovascular diseases. *FASEB J* 2011;**25**(5):1718–28.

128. Álvarez R, González P, Batalla A, Reguero JR, Iglesias-Cubero G, Hevia S, et al. Association between the NOS3 (−786 T/C) and the ACE (I/D) DNA genotypes and early coronary artery disease. *Nitric Oxide* 2001;**5**(4):343–8.

129. Skarke C, Schuss P, Kirchhof A, Doehring A, Geisslinger G, Lötsch J. Pyrosequencing of polymorphisms in the COX-2 gene (PTGS2) with reported clinical relevance. *Pharmacogenomics* 2007;**8**(12):1643–60.

130. Azhar M, Schultz JEJ, Grupp I, Dorn GW, Meneton P, Molin DG, et al. Transforming growth factor beta in cardiovascular development and function. *Cytokine Growth Factor Rev* 2003;**14**(5):391–407.

131. Stoll LL, Denning GM, Weintraub NL. Endotoxin, TLR4 signaling and vascular inflammation: potential therapeutic targets in cardiovascular disease. *Curr Pharm Des* 2006;**12**(32):4229–45.

132. Hwang S-J, Ballantyne CM, Sharrett AR, Smith LC, Davis CE, Gotto AM, et al. Circulating adhesion molecules VCAM-1, ICAM-1, and E-selectin in carotid atherosclerosis and incident coronary heart disease cases the Atherosclerosis Risk In Communities (ARIC) study. *Circulation* 1997;**96**(12):4219–25.

133. Zhao Y, Chen X, Cai L, Yang Y, Sui G, Fu S. Angiotensin II/angiotensin II type I receptor (AT1R) signaling promotes MCF-7 breast cancer cells survival via PI3-kinase/Akt pathway. *J Cell Physiol* 2010;**225**(1):168–73.

134. Sasaki A, Yasukawa H, Shouda T, Kitamura T, Dikic I, Yoshimura A. CIS3/SOCS-3 suppresses erythropoietin (EPO) signaling by binding the EPO receptor and JAK2. *J Biol Chem* 2000;**275**(38):29338–47.

135. Ziello JE, Jovin IS, Huang Y. Hypoxia-Inducible Factor (HIF)-1 regulatory pathway and its potential for therapeutic intervention in malignancy and ischemia. *Yale J Biol Med* 2007;**80**(2):51–60.

136. Khaled WT, Read EK, Nicholson SE, Baxter FO, Brennan AJ, Came PJ, et al. The IL-4/IL-13/Stat6 signalling pathway promotes luminal mammary epithelial cell development. *Development* 2007;**134**(15):2739–50.

137. Grivennikov S, Karin M. Autocrine IL-6 signaling: a key event in tumorigenesis? *Cancer Cell* 2008;**13**(1):7–9.

138. Zhao L, Yang G, Zhao X. Rho-associated protein kinases play an important role in the differentiation of rat adipose-derived stromal cells into cardiomyocytes in vitro. *PLoS One* 2014;**9**(12):e115191.

139. Chanprasert S, Geddis AE, Barroga C, Fox NE, Kaushansky K. Thrombopoietin (TPO) induces c-myc expression through a PI3K-and MAPK-dependent pathway that is not mediated by Akt, PKC ζ or mTOR in TPO-dependent cell lines and primary megakaryocytes. *Cell Signal* 2006;**18**(8):1212–8.

140. Fukuhara S, Sako K, Noda K, Zhang J, Minami M, Mochizuki N. Angiopoietin-1/Tie2 receptor signaling in vascular quiescence and angiogenesis. *Histol Histopathol* 2010;**25**(3):387–96.

141. Rosen H, Goetzl EJ. Sphingosine 1-phosphate and its receptors: an autocrine and paracrine network. *Nat Rev Immunol* 2005;**5**(7):560–70.

142. Roberts DM, Kearney JB, Johnson JH, Rosenberg MP, Kumar R, Bautch VL. The vascular endothelial growth factor (VEGF) receptor Flt-1 (VEGFR-1) modulates Flk-1 (VEGFR-2) signaling during blood vessel formation. *Am J Pathol* 2004;**164**(5):1531–5.

143. Wissmann C, Detmar M. Pathways targeting tumor lymphangiogenesis. *Clin Cancer Res* 2006;**12**(23):6865–8.

144. Kortylewski M, Kujawski M, Wang T, Wei S, Zhang S, Pilon-Thomas S, et al. Inhibiting Stat3 signaling in the hematopoietic system elicits multicomponent antitumor immunity. *Nat Med* 2005;**11**(12):1314–21.

INDEX

Note: Page numbers followed by *f* indicate figures, and *t* indicate tables.